BMA LIBRARY

British Medical Association
BMA House
Tavistock Square
London
WC1H 9JP

Tel: 020 7383 6625
Email: bma-library@bma.org.uk
Web: www.bma.org.uk/library

Location: QV 735

WITHDRAWN FROM LIBRARY

BMA

D1145401

Pocket
Prescriber
Emergency Medicine

Anthony FT Brown MB ChB FRCP FRCSEd FACEM FCEM
Professor of Emergency Medicine, Discipline of Anaesthesiology
and Critical Care, School of Medicine, University of Queensland,
Brisbane, Australia
Senior Staff Specialist, Department of Emergency Medicine, Royal
Brisbane and Women's Hospital, Brisbane, Australia

**Timothy RJ Nicholson MBBS BSc MSc PhD MRCP
MRCPsych**
Academic Clinical Lecturer, Section of Cognitive Neuropsychiatry,
Institute of Psychiatry, London, UK

Donald RJ Singer BMedBiol MD FRCP
Professor of Clinical Pharmacology and Therapeutics, Clinical
Sciences Research, Warwick Medical School, University of Warwick
and University Hospitals Coventry and Warwickshire, Coventry, UK

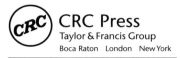

CRC Press
Taylor & Francis Group
Boca Raton   London   New York

CRC Press is an imprint of the
Taylor & Francis Group, an **informa** business

CRC Press
Taylor & Francis Group
6000 Broken Sound Parkway NW, Suite 300
Boca Raton, FL 33487-2742

© 2014 by Anthony Brown, Timothy Nicholson and Donald Singer
CRC Press is an imprint of Taylor & Francis Group, an Informa business

No claim to original U.S. Government works

Printed on acid-free paper
Version Date: 20130607

International Standard Book Number-13: 978-1-4441-7664-3 (Paperback)

This book contains information obtained from authentic and highly regarded sources. While all reasonable efforts have been made to publish reliable data and information, neither the author[s] nor the publisher can accept any legal responsibility or liability for any errors or omissions that may be made. The publishers wish to make clear that any views or opinions expressed in this book by individual editors, authors or contributors are personal to them and do not necessarily reflect the views/opinions of the publishers. The information or guidance contained in this book is intended for use by medical, scientific or health-care professionals and is provided strictly as a supplement to the medical or other professional's own judgement, their knowledge of the patient's medical history, relevant manufacturer's instructions and the appropriate best practice guidelines. Because of the rapid advances in medical science, any information or advice on dosages, procedures or diagnoses should be independently verified. The reader is strongly urged to consult the drug companies' printed instructions, and their websites, before administering any of the drugs recommended in this book. This book does not indicate whether a particular treatment is appropriate or suitable for a particular individual. Ultimately it is the sole responsibility of the medical professional to make his or her own professional judgements, so as to advise and treat patients appropriately. The authors and publishers have also attempted to trace the copyright holders of all material reproduced in this publication and apologize to copyright holders if permission to publish in this form has not been obtained. If any copyright material has not been acknowledged please write and let us know so we may rectify it in any future reprint.

Except as permitted under U.S. Copyright Law, no part of this book may be reprinted, reproduced, transmitted, or utilized in any form by any electronic, mechanical, or other means, now known or hereafter invented, including photocopying, microfilming, and recording, or in any information storage or retrieval system, without written permission from the publishers.

For permission to photocopy or use material electronically from this work, please access www.copyright.com (http://www.copyright.com/) or contact the Copyright Clearance Center, Inc. (CCC), 222 Rosewood Drive, Danvers, MA 01923, 978-750-8400. CCC is a not-for-profit organization that provides licenses and registration for a variety of users. For organizations that have been granted a photocopy license by the CCC, a separate system of payment has been arranged.

Trademark Notice: Product or corporate names may be trademarks or registered trademarks, and are used only for identification and explanation without intent to infringe.

Library of Congress Cataloging-in-Publication Data

Pocket prescriber emergency medicine / edited by Anthony F.T. Brown, Timothy R.J. Nicholson, and Donald R.J. Singer.
    p. ; cm. -- (Pocket prescriber)
    Emergency medicine
    Includes bibliographical references and index.
    ISBN 978-1-4441-7664-3 (paperback : alk. paper)
    I. Brown, Anthony F. T., editor. II. Nicholson, Timothy R. J., editor. III. Singer, Donald R. J., editor. IV. Title:
Emergency medicine. V. Series: Pocket prescriber.
    [DNLM: 1. Drug Prescriptions--Handbooks. 2. Emergency Medicine--methods--Handbooks. 3. Emergency
Treatment--methods--Handbooks. 4. Pharmaceutical Preparations--administration & dosage--Handbooks. QV 735]

RS57
615.1′4--dc23
                                                                              2013018418

Visit the Taylor & Francis Web site at
http://www.taylorandfrancis.com

and the CRC Press Web site at
http://www.crcpress.com

DEDICATION

To my Mum and Dad for their inspiration and zest for life, and to my sister Alison for being so supportive and kind.

Tony Brown
July 2013

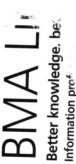

www.bma

BMA LI

Better knowledge, be
Information prof

By borro

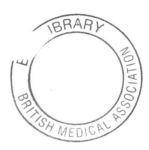

LIBRARY
BRITISH MEDICAL ASSOCIATION

CONTENTS

Contributors   ix
Foreword   xi
Preface   xiii
Acknowledgements   xiv
How to use this book   xv
List of abbreviations   xvii
How to prescribe safely in the ED   xxvii

Common/useful drugs   1

Drug selection   177
Analgesia in the ED   178
Antiemetics in the ED   179
Local anaesthesia   181
Procedural sedation and analgesia   182
Rapid sequence induction   184
Drug infusion guideline   186

How to prescribe   195
Intravenous fluids   196
Insulin   204
Anticoagulants   209
Steroids   217
Sedation in the ED   219
Controlled drugs   221

Medical emergencies   223
Cardiopulmonary resuscitation (CPR)   225
Anaphylaxis   225
Acute coronary syndrome (ACS)   226
Acute LVF   234
Hypertension and accelerated hypertension   235
Atrial fibrillation   240
Acute severe asthma   242

Pneumonia 244
COPD exacerbation 247
Pulmonary embolism 248
Acute upper GI haemorrhage 249
Hypoglycaemia 251
DKA 252
HHS (HONK) 255
Addisonian crisis 256
Myxoedema coma/crisis 257
Thyrotoxic crisis/thyroid storm 257
Meningitis 258
Seizures 260
TIA and stroke 261
Severe sepsis or septic shock 264
Febrile neutropenia 265
Urinary tract infections 265
GI infections 266
TB pneumonia 267
Malaria 267
Electrolyte disturbances 269
Alcohol withdrawal 271
Acute poisoning 274

Surgical emergencies **285**
Acute abdomen 286
Orthopaedic infections 287
ENT infections 288
Eye infections 288

Reference information **291**
Glasgow coma scale 292
Mental state examination 293
Acid-base nomogram 294
Useful formulae 295
Common laboratory reference values 297

Index 301

CONTRIBUTORS

Adam MC Archibald BSc(Hons) MBChB
FY2 Simpson Centre for Reproductive Health, Royal Infirmary of Edinburgh

Peter J Barnes DM DSc FRCP FMedSci FRS
Professor and Consultant in Respiratory Medicine, National Heart and Lung Institute, Imperial College London

Alison Bedlow BSc MBBS FRCP
Consultant Dermatologist, South Warwickshire NHS Foundation Trust

Aodhan Breathnach MD FRCPath
Consultant Medical Microbiologist, Department of Medical Microbiology St George's Hospital, London

Emma C Derrett-Smith BSc MBBS MRCP
Clinical Research Fellow, Centre for Rheumatology and Connective Tissue Diseases, UCL Medical School, London

Timothy WR Doulton BSc MBBS MRCP MD
Consultant Nephrologist, Kent Kidney Care Centre, East Kent Hospitals University NHS Foundation Trust

Thomas M Galliford MBBS BSc(Hons) MRCP
SpR Department of Diabetes and Endocrinology, Imperial College NHS Healthcare Trust, London

Beth D Harrison MA BM BCh DM FRCP FRCPath
Consultant Haematologist, University Hospital Coventry and Warwickshire NHS Trust

Steven Harsum MBBS BSc PhD FRCOphth
Consultant Ophthalmologist, Sutton Eye Unit, Epsom and St Helier NHS Trust

Robin DC Kumar MBBS BSc FRCA
Clinical Fellow in Neuroanaesthesia, National Hospital for Neurology and Neurosurgery, Queen Square, London

Simon J Little BA(Cantab) MBBS MRCP
SpR St Georges Hospital, London; and Wellcome Trust Research
Fellow, Functional Neurosurgery and Experimental Neurology,
Oxford University

Ramsay Singer MA(Oxon) MBBS MRCP
Registrar in General Medicine and Paediatrics, Kivunge
Hospital, Zanzibar.

Allison C Morton BMedSci MBChB MRCP PhD
Consultant Cardiologist, Sheffield Teaching Hospitals NHS Foundation
Trust; and Clinical Research Manager, NIHR Cardiovascular
Biomedical Research Unit, Northern General Hospital, Sheffield

Victor Pace FRCP
Consultant in Palliative Medicine, St Christopher's Hospice,
Sydenham, London

Stephen D Quinn MB BS BSc MRCOG
Clinical Research Fellow, Imperial College London; and Honorary
Specialist Registrar, Imperial College Healthcare NHS Trust, London

Ricardo Sainz-Fuertes LMS MSc MRCPsych
MRC Clinical Research Training Fellow, Institute of Psychiatry,
King's College London and Honorary Specialist Registrar in
Psychiatry, South London and Maudsley NHS Foundation Trust

Biba Stanton BMedSci MBBS MRCP PhD
Specialist Registrar, National Hospital for Neurology and
Neurosurgery, Queen Square, London

Rudolf Uher MD PhD MRCPsych
Clinical Lecturer, Social, Genetic and Developmental Psychiatry
Centre, Institute of Psychiatry, King's College London

Esther Unitt BMedSci MBBS MRCP DM
Consultant Gastroenterologist and Hepatologist at the University
Hospital, Coventry and Warwickshire Hospitals NHS Trust

W Stephen Waring PhD FRCP(Edin)
Consultant in Acute Medicine and Toxicology, Acute Medical Unit,
York Teaching Hospital NHS Foundation Trust

FOREWORD

Busy clinicians in every specialty must, in an age when all are overwhelmed by instant data at the touch of a button, be able to access straightforward didactic information that is reliable, consistent and useful at the bedside. Sometimes a small, *vade mecum* style pocket book fulfils the task perfectly and can be easier and quicker to use than any digital equivalent.

Arguably the most important part of clinical practice demanding this type of book is clinical pharmacology and drug prescribing. Drug errors continue to be a major barrier to the delivery of safe health care. Systematic attempts to reduce unnecessary patient morbidity and mortality are underway; any practical and simple aid that will help is welcomed.

This book does its job admirably. It is the first member of a new suite of books with the generic title *Pocket Prescriber*, but each is targeted at a specific audience, in this case emergency medicine care. The main section on over 500 **common/useful drugs** remains identical in each volume, with other sections adapted to the needs of the target group.

The structure of this new book is easy to follow and logical; all relevant information for a specific drug can be readily absorbed and digested, making the translation to safer prescribing smooth and more consistent. This volume includes important content on drugs, fluids and algorithms used in the emergency department, vastly expanded sections on medical and surgical emergencies, as well as a wealth of practical information around the use and delivery of medications.

This excellent book will prove itself an invaluable prescribing guide for all front line clinical staff who work in an emergency department, whether they are permanent or in-training members of the team.

Geoff Hughes, Associate Professor
MBBS FRCP FCEM FACEM DRCOG
Editor-in-Chief, *Emergency Medicine Journal*, BMJ Group UK
Executive Director, Critical Care Services
Central Adelaide Local Health Network,
South Australia

PREFACE

This specialty edition of the hugely popular *Pocket Prescriber* series retains the same distinct format with the **Common/Useful Drugs** section essentially unchanged and content from the other sections rearranged and reformatted to best align with emergency department practice.

New content has been added including CPR, anaphylaxis, procedural sedation, local anaesthesia and rapid sequence induction, as well as vastly expanded medical and surgical emergencies sections. Finally all content has been updated to include the latest evidence-based guidelines to bring you the essence of emergency medicine prescribing in one compact source.

Tony Brown
July 2013

ACKNOWLEDGEMENTS

Particular thanks to Caroline Makepeace, head of Postgraduate and Professional Publishing, Health Sciences, and Stephen Clausard, senior project editor of Hodder Education, for their efficiency, enthusiasm and advice – both are an absolute delight to work with.

Also to Tim and Donald for so generously sharing their intellectual property to expand their concept into new specialty areas – again a pure pleasure to work with.

The information in this book has been collated from many sources, including manufacturer's information sheets ('SPCs' – Summary of Product Characteristics sheets), the *British National Formulary* (BNF), national and international guidelines, as well as numerous pharmacology and general medical books, journals and papers. Where information is not consistent between these sources, that from the SPCs has generally been taken as definitive.

Tony Brown
July 2013

STANDARD LAYOUT OF DRUGS

DRUG/TRADE NAME

Class/action: More information is given for generic forms, especially for the original and most commonly used drug(s) of each class.

Use: use^x (correlating to dose as below).

CI: contraindications; **L** (liver failure), **R** (renal failure), **H** (heart failure), **P** (pregnancy), **B** (breastfeeding). *Allergy to active drug, or any excipients (other substances in the preparation) assumed too obvious to mention.*

Caution: **L** (liver failure), **R** (renal failure), **H** (heart failure), **P** (pregnancy), **B** (breastfeeding), **E** (elderly patients). If a contraindication is given for a drug it is assumed too obvious to mention that a caution is also inherently implied.

SE: side effects; listed in order of frequency encountered. Common/important side effects set in **bold**.

Warn: information to give to patients before starting drug.

Monitor: parameters that need to be monitored during treatment.

Interactions: included only if very common or potentially serious; ↑/↓**P450** (induces/inhibits cytochrome P450 metabolism), **W+** (increases effect of warfarin), **W–** (decreases effect of warfarin).

Dose: dose^x (for Use^x as above). *NB Doses are for adults only.*

Important points highlighted at end of drug entry.

Use/dose^{NICE}: National Institute of Health and Clinical Excellence guidelines exist for the drug (basics often in BNF – see www.nice.org.uk for full details).

Dose$^{BNF/SPC}$: dose regimen complicated; please refer to BNF and/or SPC (Summary of Product Characteristics sheet; the manufacturer's information sheet enclosed with drug packaging – can also be viewed at or downloaded from www.emc.medicines.org.uk).

Asterisks (*) and **daggers (†)** denote links between information within local text.

> **Only relevant sections are included** for each drug. **Trade names** (in OUTLINE font) are given only if found regularly on drug charts or if non-proprietary (generic, non-trade-name) drug does not exist yet.

KEY

☠ Potential dangers highlighted with skull and crossbones

▼ New drug or new indication under intense surveillance by Committee on Safety of Medicines (CSM): *important to report all suspected drug reactions via Yellow Card scheme* (accurate as going to press: from June 2013 CSM list)

☺ *Good for:* reasons to give a certain drug when choice exists

☹ *Bad for:* reasons to not give a certain drug when choice exists

⇒ Causes/goes to

∴ Therefore

Δ Change/disturbance

Ψ Psychiatric

↑ Increase/high

↓ Decrease/low

 ↑/↓ electrolytes refers to serum levels, unless stated otherwise.

DOSES

od	once daily	nocte	at night
bd	twice daily	mane	in the morning
tds	three times daily	prn	as required
qds	four times daily	stat	at once

ROUTES

im	intramuscular	po	oral
inh	inhaled	pr	rectal
iv	intravenous	sc	subcutaneous
ivi	intravenous infusion	top	topical
neb	via nebuliser	sl	sublingual

 Routes are presumed po, unless stated otherwise.

LIST OF ABBREVIATIONS

5-ASA	5-aminosalicylic acid
5HT	5-hydroxytryptamine (= serotonin)
AAA	abdominal aortic aneurysm
AAC	antibiotic-associated colitis
Ab	antibody
ABPM	ambulatory blood pressure monitoring
ACC	American College of Cardiology
ACCP	American College of Chest Physicians
ACE-i	ACE inhibitor
ACh	acetylcholine
ACS	acute coronary syndrome
ADP	adenosine diphosphate
AF	atrial fibrillation
Ag	antigen
AHA	American Heart Association
AKI	acute kidney injury
ALL	acute lymphoblastic leukaemia
ALP	alkaline phosphatase
ALS	advanced life support (algorithm of European Resuscitation Council)
ALT	alanine(-amino) transferase
AMI	acute myocardial infarction
AMTS	abbreviated mental test score (same as MTS)
ANA	anti-nuclear antigens
APTT	activate partial thromboplastin time
ARB(s)	angiotensin receptor blocker(s)
ARDS	adult respiratory distress syndrome
AS	aortic stenosis
ASAP	as soon as possible
assoc	associated
AST	aspartate transaminase
AV	arteriovenous
AVM	arteriovenous malformation
AVN	atrioventricular node

AZT	zidovudine
BBB	bundle branch block
BCSH	British Committee for Standards in Haematology
BCT	broad complex tachycardia
BF	blood flow
BG	serum blood glucose in mmol/l; *see also* CBG
BHS	British Hypertension Society
BIH	benign intracranial hypertension
BIPAP	bilevel/biphasic positive airway pressure
BLS	basic life support (algorithm of European Resuscitation Council)
BM	bone marrow (NB: BM is often used, confusingly, to signify finger-prick glucose; CBG - capillary blood glucose - is used instead in this book)
BMI	body mass index
BNF	British National Formulary
BP	blood pressure
BPH	benign prostatic hypertrophy
BTS	British Thoracic Society
Bx	biopsy
C	constipation
CA^{2+}	calcium
Ca	cancer (NB: note calcium is written as CA^{2+})
CAH	congenital adrenal hyperplasia
cAMP	cyclic adenosine monophosphate
CAP	community-acquired pneumonia
CBF	cerebral blood flow
CBG	capillary blood glucose in mmol/l on finger-prick testing. (NB: BM is often used to denote this, but is confusing and less accurate, thus not used in this book)
CCF	congestive cardiac failure
cf	compared with
CI	contraindicated
CK	creatine kinase
CKD	chronic kidney disease
CLL	chronic lymphocytic leukaemia

CML	chronic myelogenous leukaemia
CMV	cytomegalovirus
CNS	central nervous system
CO	cardiac output
CO_2	carbon dioxide
COPD	chronic obstructive pulmonary disease
COX	cyclo-oxygenase
CPR	cardiopulmonary resuscitation
CRF	chronic renal failure
CRP	C reactive protein
CSF	cerebrospinal fluid
CSM	Committee on Safety of Medicines
CT	computerised tomography
CVA	cerebrovascular accident
CVP	central venous pressure
CXR	chest X-ray
CYP	cytochrome P450
D	diarrhoea
D&V	diarrhoea and vomiting
$D_{1/2/3 \, ...}$	dopamine receptor subtype 1/2/3...
DA	dopamine
DCT	distal convoluted tubule
dfx	defects
DI	diabetes insipidus
DIC	disseminated intravascular coagulation
DIGAMI	glucose, insulin and potassium intravenous infusion used in acute myocardial infarction
DKA	diabetic ketoacidosis
DM	diabetes mellitus
DMARD	disease-modifying anti-rheumatoid arthritis drug
dt	due to
DWI	diffusion weighted imaging (specialist MRI mostly used for stroke/TIA)
Dx	diagnosis
EØ	eosinophils
e'lyte	electrolyte

EBV	Epstein-Barr virus
ECG	electrocardiogram
ECT	electroconvulsive therapy
ED	emergency department
EF	ejection fraction
ENT	ear, nose and throat
EPSE	extrapyramidal side effects
ERC	European Resuscitation Council
ESC	European Society of Cardiology
esp	especially
ESR	erythrocyte sedimentation rate
EST	exercise stress test
ETT	endotracheal tube
exac	exacerbates
FBC	full blood count
Fe	iron
FFP	fresh frozen plasma
FHx	family history
FiO_2	inspired O_2 concentration
FMF	familial Mediterranean fever
fx	effects
G6PD	glucose-6-phosphate dehydrogenase
GABA	gamma aminobutyric acid
GBS	Guillain-Barré syndrome
GCS	Glasgow Coma Scale
GFR	glomerular filtration rate
GI	gastrointestinal
GIFTASUP	Guidelines on Intravenous Fluid Therapy for Adult Surgical Patients
GIK	glucose, insulin and K^+ infusion
GMC	General Medical Council (of UK)
GTN	glyceryl trinitrate
GU	genitourinary
h	hour(s)
H(O)CM	hypertrophic (obstructive) cardiomyopathy
Hb	haemoglobin

HB	heart block
HBPM	home blood pressure monitoring
HCM	hypertrophic cardiomyopathy (formerly known as HOCM)
Hct	haematocrit
HDL	high density lipoprotein
HF	heart failure
HHS	hyperosmolar, hyperlycaemic state (formerly known as HONK)
Hib	*H. influenzae*, type b
HIV	human immunodeficiency virus
HLA	human leucocyte antigen
HMG-CoA	3-hydroxy-3-methyl-glutaryl coenzyme A
HONK	hyperosmolar non-ketotic state (see HHS above)
hrly	hourly
HSV	herpes simplex virus
HTN	hypertension
HUS	haemolytic uraemic syndrome
Hx	history
IBD	inflammatory bowel disease
IBS	irritable bowel syndrome
IBW	ideal body weight
ICH	intracranial haemorrhage
ICP	intracranial pressure
ICU	intensive care unit
IHD	ischaemic heart disease
IL-2	interleukin 2
im	intramuscular
inc	including
inh	inhaled
INR	international normalised ratio (prothrombin ratio)
IOP	intraocular pressure
ITP	immune/idiopathic thrombocytopenic purpura
ITU	intensive therapy unit
iv	intravenous
IVDU	intravenous drug user

ivi	intravenous infusion
Ix	investigation
K^+	potassium (serum levels unless stated otherwise)
LØ	lymphocytes
LA	long-acting
LBBB	left bundle branch block
LDL	low density lipoprotein
LF	liver failure
LFTs	liver function tests
LMWH	low-molecular-weight heparin
LP	lumbar puncture
LVF	left ventricular failure
MØ	macrophages
mane	in the morning
MAOI	monoamine oxidase inhibitor
MAP	mean arterial pressure
MCA	middle cerebral artery
MCV	mean corpuscular volume
metab	metabolised
Mg^{2+}	magnesium
MG	myasthenia gravis
MHRA	Medicines and Healthcare Products Regulatory Authority (UK)
MI	myocardial infarction
MMF	mycophenolate mofetil
MMSE	Mini-Mental State Examination (scored out of 30*)
MR	modified-release (drug preparation)†
MRI	magnetic resonance imaging
MRSA	methicillin-resistant *Staphylococcus aureus*
MS	multiple sclerosis
MSU	mid-stream urine
MTS	(abbreviated) Mental Test Score (scored out of 10*)
MUST	malnutrition universal screening tool
Mx	management
N	nausea
N&V	nausea and vomiting

NØ	neutrophils
NA	noradrenaline (norepinephrine)
Na^+	sodium (serum levels unless stated otherwise)
NBM	nil by mouth
NCT	narrow complex tachycardia
NDRI	noradrenaline and dopamine reuptake inhibitor
neb	via nebuliser
NGT	nasogastric tube
NH	non-Hodgkin's (lymphoma)
NIHSS	National (US) Institute of Health Stroke Scale
NIV	non-invasive ventilation
NMJ	neuromuscular junction
NMS	neuroleptic malignant syndrome
NPIS	National Poisons Information Service
NSAID	nonsteroidal anti-inflammatory drug
NSTEMI	non-ST elevation myocardial infarction
NYHA	New York Heart Association
OCD	obsessive compulsive disorder
OCP	oral contraceptive pill
OD	overdose (NB: *od* = once daily!)
OGD	oesophagogastroduodenoscopy
p'way(s)	pathway(s)
PAN	polyarteritis nodosa
PBC	primary biliary cirrhosis
PCI	percutaneous coronary intervention (preferred term for percutaneous transluminal coronary angioplasty (PTCA), which is a type of PCI)
PCOS	polycystic ovary syndrome
PCP	*Pneumocystis carinii* pneumonia
PCR	polymerase chain reaction
PCV	packed cell volume
PDA	patent ductus arteriosus
PE	pulmonary embolism
PEA	pulseless electrical activity
PEG	percutaneous endoscopic gastrostomy
PG(x)	prostaglandin (receptor subtype *x*)

phaeo	phaeochromocytoma
PHx	past history (of)
PID	pelvic inflammatory disease
PML	progressive multifocal leukoencephalopathy
PMR	polymyalgia rheumatica
po	by mouth
PO_4	phosphate (serum levels, unless stated otherwise)
PPI	proton pump inhibitor
pr	rectal
PR	per rectal (digital examination)
prep(s)	preparation(s)
prn	as required
PSA	prostate specific antigen
Pt	platelet(s)
PT	prothrombin time
PTH	parathyroid hormone
PTSD	post-traumatic stress disorder
PU	peptic ulcer
PUO	pyrexia of unknown origin
PVD	peripheral vascular disease
Px	prophylaxis
QT(c)	QT interval (corrected for rate)
RA	rheumatoid arthritis
RAD	right axis deviation
RAS	renal artery stenosis
RBBB	right bundle branch block
RBF	renal blood flow
RF	renal failure
RLS	restless legs syndrome
ROSIER	Recognition Of Stroke In Emergency Room scale for diagnosis of stroke/TIA
RR	respiratory rate
RRT	renal replacement therapy
RSI	rapid sequence induction
RSV	respiratory syncytial virus
RTI	respiratory tract infection

RV	right ventricle
RVF	right ventricular failure
Rx	treatment
SAH	subarachnoid haemorrhage
SAN	sinoatrial node
SBE	subacute bacterial endocarditis
sc	subcutaneous
SE(s)	side effect(s)
sec	second(s)
SIADH	syndrome of inappropriate antidiuretic hormone
SIGN	Scottish Intercollegiate Guidelines Network
SJS	Stevens-Johnson syndrome
sl	sublingual
SLE	systemic lupus erythematosus
SOA	swelling of ankles
SOB (OE)	shortness of breath (on exertion)
SPC	Summary of Product Characteristics drug sheet
spp	species
SR	slow/sustained release (drug preparation)
SSRI	selective serotonin reuptake inhibitor
SSS	sick sinus syndrome
STEMI	ST elevation myocardial infarction
supp	suppository
SVT	supraventricular tachycardia
$t_{1/2}$	half-life
T_3	triiodothyronine/liothyronine
T_4	thyroxine ($\uparrow/\downarrow T_4$ = hyper/hypothyroid)
TBG	thyroid binding globulin
TCA	tricyclic antidepressant
TE	thromboembolism
TEDS	thromboembolism deterrent stockings
TEN	toxic epidermal necrolysis
TFTs	thyroid function tests
TG	triglyceride
TIBC	total iron binding capacity

TIMI score	risk score for UA/NSTEMI named after TIMI (thrombolysis in MI) trial
TNF	tumour necrosis factor
top	topical
TPMT	thiopurine methyltransferase
TPR	total peripheral resistance
TTA(s)	(drugs) to take away, i.e. prescriptions for inpatients on discharge/leave (aka TTO)
TTO(s)	see TTA
TTP	thrombotic thrombocytopenic purpura
U&Es	urea and electrolytes
UA(P)	unstable angina (pectoris)
UC	ulcerative colitis
URTI	upper respiratory tract infection
USS	ultrasound scan
UTI	urinary tract infection
UV	ultraviolet
V	vomiting
VBG	venous blood gas
VE(s)	ventricular ectopic(s)
VF	ventricular fibrillation
vit	vitamin
VLDL	very low density lipoprotein
VT	ventricular tachycardia
VTE	venous thromboembolism
VZV	varicella zoster virus (chickenpox/shingles)
w	with
w/in	within
w/o	without
WCC	white cell count
WE	Wernicke's encephalopathy
wk	week
WPW	Wolff–Parkinson–White syndrome
Wt	weight
xs	excess
ZE	Zollinger–Ellison syndrome

HOW TO PRESCRIBE SAFELY IN THE ED

Take time/care to ↓risk to patients (and to protect yourself).

Always check the following are correct for *all* prescriptions:

Patient, indication and drug, **legible** format (generic name, clarity, handwriting, **identifiable signature**, your contact number), dosage, frequency, time(s) of day, date, duration of treatment, route of administration.

Know where to find information, if you are uncertain:

Look up the drug dose, contraindication, caution, side effect or interaction, whenever you are unsure. Whether in a book (this one!), online, smart phone, app or even by asking a colleague, get into the habit of checking, then rechecking.

DO

- Make a clear, accurate record in the notes of all medicines prescribed, written at the time of prescription
- Complete allergy box and alert labels, where relevant
- Include on all drug charts and TTAs the patient's surname and given name, date of birth, date of admission and consultant (if possible use a printed label for patient details)
- **PRINT** (i.e. use upper case) all drugs as approved (generic) names, e.g. 'IBUPROFEN' *not* 'nurofen'
- State dose, route and frequency, giving strength of solutions/creams
- Write the word microgram in full; avoid abbreviations such as mcg or μ
- Shorten the word gram to 'g' (rather than 'gm' which is easily confused with mg)
- Write the word 'units' in full, preceded by a space; abbreviating to 'U' can be misread as zero (a 10-fold error)
- Document weight where dosing is weight-dependent
- Write quantities <1 g in mg (e.g. 400 mg *not* 0.4 g)
- Write quantities <1 mg in micrograms (e.g. 200 micrograms *not* 0.2 mg)

- Not use trailing zeroes (10 mg *not* 10.0 mg)
- Precede decimal points with another figure (e.g 0.8 ml *not* .8 ml) and only use decimals where unavoidable
- Check and recheck calculations
- Provide clear additional instructions, e.g. for monitoring, review of antibiotic route and duration, maximum daily/24 h dose for PRN drugs
- Specify solution to be used and duration of any iv infusions/injections
- Avoid using abbreviated/non-standard drug names
- Avoid writing 'T' (tablet sign) for non-tablet formulations, e.g. sprays
- Amend a prescribed drug by drawing a line through it, date and initial this, then rewrite as new prescription
- Check and count number of drugs when rewriting a drug chart

IMPORTANT FURTHER ADVICE

1   Make sure choice of drug and dose is right for the patient, their condition and significant comorbidity, with particular attention to age*, gender, ethnicity, renal or liver dysfunction, risk of drug–drug and drug–disease interactions, and risks in pregnancy (and those of child-bearing age who may become pregnant) and during breastfeeding. Anticipate possible effects of over-the-counter and herbal medicines and lifestyle (e.g. dietary salt and alcohol intake).

   *Although arbitrary, age of >65 yrs denotes 'elderly', but the fx of age can occur earlier/later and are continuous across age spectrum.

2   Common settings where drug problems occur are often predictable if you understand relevant pathology, routes of drug metabolism (liver, P450, renal, etc) and drug mechanisms of action. Take particular care with:
    - Renal or liver disease
    - Pregnancy/breastfeeding: use safest options (in the UK consider consulting the National Teratology Information Service; tel: 0191 232 1525)

- NSAIDs/bisphosphonates and peptic ulcer disease
- Asthma and β-blockers
- Conditions worsened by antimuscarinic drugs (see p. 276): urinary retention/BPH, glaucoma, paralytic ileus
- Rare conditions where drugs commonly pose risk, e.g. porphyria, myasthenia, G6PD deficiency, phaeo

3 Always obtain informed consent; agree proposed prescriptions with the patient (or carer if patient has authorised their involvement in their care or has lost capacity), explaining proposed benefits, nature and duration of treatment, clarifying concerns, warning of possible, especially severe, adverse effects, highlighting recommended monitoring and review arrangements and stating what the patient should do in the event of a suspected adverse reaction.

- Only in extreme emergencies is it justified to not do this. For drugs with common potentially fatal/severe side effects document that these risks have been explained to, and accepted by the patient, such as with thrombolysis (see p. 230).

4 Check that appropriate previous medicines are continued and over-the-counter and herbal medicine use is recorded.

5 Make sure that you are being objective. Prescribing should be for the benefit of the patient not the prescriber.

6 Keep up to date about medicines you are prescribing and the related conditions you are treating.

7 Follow CSM guidance on reporting suspected adverse reactions to medicines (see top right link at www.mhra.gov.uk for links to details of the Yellow Card reporting scheme and downloads of reported adverse drug reactions for specific medicines).

8 Ensure continuity of care by keeping the patient's GP (or other preferred medical adviser) informed about prescribing, monitoring and follow-up arrangements and responsibilities. Write a letter/summary.

9 Assume a letter given to the patient will be opened and read, so email, fax or post any discharge letter that may contain sensitive information.

10 See legal advice on eligibility to prescribe and use of unlicensed medicines on the GMC website (www.gmc-uk.org).

Common/useful drugs

ABCIXIMAB/REOPRO

Antiplatelet agent – monoclonal Ab against platelet glycoprotein IIb/IIIa receptor (involved in Pt aggregation).

Use: Px of ischaemic complications of PCI and Px of MI in unstable angina unresponsive to conventional Rx awaiting PCI[NICE] (see p. 233).

CI: active internal bleeding, CVA w/in 2 years, intracranial neoplasm, aneurysm or AVM. Major surgery, intracranial/intraspinal surgery or trauma w/in 2 months. Hypertensive retinopathy, vasculitis, ↓Pt, haemorrhagic diathesis, severe ↑BP. **L** (if severe)/**R** (if requiring haemodialysis)/**B**.

Caution: drugs that ↑bleeding risk, **L/R/P/E**.

SE: bleeding* /↓Pt*, N&V, ↓BP, ↓HR, pain (chest, back or pleuritic), headache, fever, oedema. Rarely, hypersensitivity, tamponade, ARDS.

Monitor: FBC* (baseline plus 2–4 h, 12 h and 24 h after giving) and clotting (baseline at least).

Dose: 250 microgram/kg iv over 1 min, then 0.125 microgram/kg/min (max 10 microgram/min) ivi; see BNF/product literature for dose timing. *NB: use iv non-pyrogenic, low protein binding filter. Needs concurrent heparin.* Specialist use only: get senior advice or contact on-call cardiology.

ACAMPROSATE/CAMPRAL EC

Modifies GABA transmission ⇒ ↓pleasurable fx of alcohol ∴ ↓s craving and relapse rate.

Use: maintaining alcohol abstinence supported by counselling.

CI: L (only if severe), **R/P/B**.

SE: GI upset, pruritus, rash, Δ libido.

Dose: 666 mg tds po if age 18–65 years (avoid outside this age range) and >60 kg (if <60 kg give 666 mg mane then 333 mg noon and nocte). *Start ASAP after alcohol stopped. Usually give for 1 year.*

ACARBOSE

Oral hypoglycaemic: intestinal α-glucosidase inhibitor. Delays digestion and ↓s absorption of starch and sucrose.

Use: IDDM not controlled by other oral hypoglycaemics and/or diet.

CI: IBD, hernia, Hx of abdominal surgery or obstruction **R** (if severe)
L/P/B.
SE: flatulence, GI upset, rarely hepatitis and ileus.
Monitor: LFTs.
Interactions: may ↑hypoglycaemic fx of sulphonylureas and insulin.
Dose: initially 50 mg od po, ↑up to 200 mg tds po.

ACIDEX

Alginate raft-forming oral suspension for acid reflux.
Dose: 10–20 ml after meals and at bedtime (NB: 3 mmol Na^+/5 ml)

ACETAZOLAMIDE/DIAMOX

Carbonic anhydrase inhibitor (sulphonamide-like).
Use: glaucoma (acute-angle closure, primary open-angle
unresponsive to maximal topical Rx, or secondary), ↑ICP. Rarely
epilepsy or diuresis.
CI: ↓K^+, ↓Na^+, ↑Cl^- acidosis, sulphonamide allergy, adrenocortical
insufficiency. **L/R**
Caution: acidosis, pulmonary obstruction **R/P/E**.
SE: nausea/GI upset, paraesthesia, drowsiness, mood Δ, headache,
Δ LFTs. If prolonged use acidosis (metabolic) and e'lyte Δs. Rarely
blood disorders and skin reactions (inc SJS/TENS).
Monitor: FBC, U&E if prolonged use.
Interactions: Many e.g.: ↑s levels of carbamazepine and phenytoin.
Can ↑cardiac toxicity (via ↓K^+) of disopyramide, flecainide, lidocaine
and cardiac glycosides. ↓s fx of methenamine and ↑ fx of quinidine.
Dose: 0.25–1 g/day po or iv^{SPC} (divided doses above 250 mg).
Also available as 250 mg MR preparation (as Diamox SR; max 2
capsules/day). Epilepsy: see BNF.

☠ Extravasation at injection site can ⇒ necrosis ☠.

ACETYLCYSTEINE/PARVOLEX

Precursor of glutathione, which detoxifies metabolites of paracetamol.
Use: paracetamol OD.
Caution: asthma* and atopy.

SE: allergy: rash, bronchospasm*, anaphylactoid reactions (esp if ivi too quick**).

Dose: initially 150 mg/kg in 200 ml 5% glucose as ivi over 60 min, then 50 mg/kg in 500 ml over 4 h, then 100 mg/kg in 1 litre over 16 h. NB: use max weight of 110 kg for dose calculation, even if patient weighs more. Ensure not given too quickly**. See p. 279 for Mx of paracetamol OD and treatment line graph.

ACICLOVIR (previously ACYCLOVIR)

Antiviral. Inhibits DNA polymerase *only in infected cells*: needs activation by viral thymidine kinase (produced by herpes spp).

Use: *iv:* severe HSV or VZV infections, e.g. meningitis, encephalitis and in immunocompromised patients (esp HIV – also used for Px); *po/top:* mucous membrane, genital, eye infections.

Caution: dehydration*, R/P/B.

SE: at ↑doses: **AKI, encephalopathy** (esp if dehydrated*). Also **hypersensitivity**, seizures, GI upset, blood disorders, skin reactions (including photosensitivity), headache, many non-specific neurological symptoms, ↓Pt, ↓WBC. Rarely Ψ reactions and hepatotoxicity.

Interactions: levels ↑d by probenecid and cimetidine.

Dose: 5 mg/kg tds ivi over 1 h (10 mg/kg if HSV encephalitis or VZV in immunocompromised patients); po/top^SPC/BNF.

☠ ivi leaks ⇒ severe local inflammation/ulceration ☠.

ACTIVATED CHARCOAL see Charcoal.

ACTRAPID Short-acting soluble insulin; see p. 204 for use.

ADENOSINE

Purine nucleoside. Slows AVN conduction time, dilates coronary arteries; acts on its own specific receptors.

Use: Rx of paroxysmal SVT (esp if accessory p'ways e.g. WPW) and Dx of SVT (NCT or BCT; ↓s rate to reveal underlying rhythm).

CI: ☠ asthma*, COPD (consider verapamil). ☠ **H**, ↓BP, ↑QTc, 2nd-/3rd-degree AV block or sick sinus syndrome (unless pacemaker fitted).

Caution: heart transplant (↓dose), AF/atrial flutter (↑s accessory pathway conduction).

SE: bronchospasm*, ↓BP. Rarely ↓HR/asystole/arrhythmias (mostly transient), angina (discontinue if occurs), flushing, respiratory failure.

Warn: can ⇒ transient unpleasant feelings: facial flushing, dyspnoea, choking feeling, nausea, chest pain and light-headedness.

Interactions: fx ↑by **dipyridamole**: ↓initial adenosine dose to 0.5–1 mg and watch for ↑bleeding (*anti-Pt fx of dipyridamole ↑d by adenosine*). fx ↓d by **theophyllines** and caffeine. Use with digoxin may ↑risk of VF.

Dose: 6 mg iv over 2 sec; if needed 12mg after 1-2 min, repeated after 1-2 min; stop if significant AV block (max 12 mg/dose); ↓quarter usual dose if dipyridamole essential. *NB: attach cardiac monitor and give via central (or large peripheral) vein, then flush.* $t_{1/2}$ <10 sec: often needs readministration (esp if given for Rx cf Dx).

ADRENALINE (im/iv)

Sympathomimetic: powerful stimulation of α (vasoconstriction), $β_1$(↑HR, ↑contractility) and $β_2$ (vasodilation, bronchodilation, uterine relaxation). Also ↓s immediate mast cell cytokine release.

Use: CPR and anaphylaxis (see algorithms on inside and outside front cover, respectively). Rarely for other causes of bronchospasm or shock (e.g. 2° to spinal/epidural anaesthesia).

Caution: cerebrovascular* and heart disease (esp arrhythmias and HTN), DM, ↑T_4, glaucoma (angle closure), labour (esp 2nd stage), phaeo. **H/E/R**.

SE: ↑HR, ↑BP, anxiety, sweats, tremor, headache, peripheral vasoconstriction, arrhythmias, pulmonary oedema (at ↑doses), N&V, weakness, dizziness, Ψ disturbance, hyperglycaemia, urinary retention (esp if ↑prostate), local reactions. Rarely CVA* (2° to HTN: monitor BP).

Interactions: fx ↑d by dopexamine, TCAs, ergotamine and oxytocin. Risk of: 1. ↑↑BP and ↓HR with non-cardioselective β-blockers (can also ⇒ ↓HR), TCAs, MAOIs and moclobemide. 2. arrhythmias with digoxin, quinidine and volatile liquid anaesthetics (e.g. halothane) and TCAs. Avoid use with tolazine or rasagiline.

Dose: CPR: 1 mg iv =10 ml of 1 in 10 000 (100 microgram/ml) then flush with ≥ 20 ml saline. If no or delayed iv access, try intraosseous route. Repeat as per ALS algorithm (see front cover). **Anaphylaxis:** 0.5 mg **im** (or sc) =0.5 ml of 1 in 1000 (1 mg/ml); repeat after 5 min if no response. (If cardiac arrest seems imminent or concerns over im absorption, give 0.5 mg **iv** slowly = 5 ml of 1 in 10 000 (100 microgram/ml) at 1 ml/min until response – get senior help first if possible as iv route ⇒ ↑risk of arrhythmias.)

☠ Don't confuse 1 in 1000 (im) with 1:10 000 (iv) solutions ☠.

ADVIL see Ibuprofen.

AGGRASTAT see Tirofiban; IIb/IIIa inhibitor (anti-Pt drug) for IHD.

AGOMELATINE/VALDOXAN

Antidepressant: synthetic melatonin analogue; melatonin receptor (MT1/MT2) agonist (also $5HT_{2C/B}$ antagonist); no effect on monoamine reuptake; resynchronises circadian rhythms and ↑s NA/DA in frontal cortex via $5HT_{2C}$ antagonism.

Use: depression; esp if inconsistent use (low risk of withdrawal syndrome on discontinuation) or if prominent insomnia/sleep reversal.

CI: dementia and see interactions below **L/B**.

Caution: elderly, history of mania (bipolar). **R/P/E.**

SE: nausea, diarrhoea, constipation, abdo pain, ΔLFTs (↑ transaminases in 5%; usually transient), drowsiness, headache, sweating, anxiety, suicidal behaviour.

Monitor: LFTs before and 3, 6, 12 and 24 wks after starting.

Interactions: levels ↑↑ by strong CYP1A2 inhibitors (e.g. fluvoxamine, ciprofloxacin – avoid) and ↑ by moderate inhibitors (e.g. propranolol, enoxacin, oestrogens, smoking). ↑ risk of convulsions with atomoxetine. Avoid with artemether/lumefantrine.

Dose: 25 mg nocte (can ↑ to 50 mg nocte after 2 wks).

ALENDRONATE (ALENDRONIC ACID)/FOSAMAX

Bisphosphonate: ↓s osteoclastic bone resorption.

Use: osteoporosis Rx and Px (esp if on corticosteroids).

CI: delayed GI emptying (esp achalasia and oesophageal stricture/
other abnormalities), ↓Ca^{2+}, unable to sit/stand upright ≥30 min, **R**
(if severe)/**P/B**.

Caution: upper GI disorders (inc gastritis/PU) **R**.

SE: oesophageal reactions*, GI upset/distension, ↓Ca^{2+}, ↓PO_4^{2-}
(transient), PU, hypersensitivity (esp skin reactions), myalgia. Rarely
osteonecrosis and femoral stress fractures (discontinue drug and
should receive no further bisphosphonates).

Warn: take upright with full glass of water on an empty stomach; stay
upright ≥30 min until breakfast* or other oral medicine. Stop tablets
and seek medical attention if symptoms of oesophageal irritation.

Dose: 10 mg mane[SPC/BNF] (10 mg od dosing can be given as once-
wkly 70-mg tablet *if for post-menopausal osteoporosis*).

ALFACALCIDOL

1-α-hydroxycholecalciferol: partially activated vitamin D (1α
hydroxy group normally added by kidney), but still requires hepatic
(25)-hydroxylation for full activation.

Use: severe vitamin D deficiency 2° to CRF.

CI/SE: ↑Ca^{2+}

Caution: nephrolithiasis, breast-feeding **E**.

Monitor: Ca^{2+}: monitor levels wkly, watch for symptoms (esp
N&V), rash, nephrocalcinosis.

Interactions: fx ↓d by barbiturates, anticonvulsants; ↑d by thiazides.

Dose: initially 1 microgram (=1000 nanograms) od po; maintenance
250–1000 nanograms od po. **NB:** ↓dose in elderly (initial dose 500
nanograms).

▼ ALISKIREN

Direct renin inhibitor (↓s angiotensinogen ⇒ angiotensin I).

Use: essential HTN (*for advice on stepped HTN Mx see p. 235*).

CI: potent P-glycoprotein inhibitors (*ciclosporin, itraconazole, verapamil, quinidine) **P/B**.

Caution: not recommended with ACE-i, ARBs, dehydration (risk of ↓BP), RAS, diuretics, ↓Na$^+$ diet, **↑K$^+$, moderate potent P-glycoprotein inhibitors (*ketaconazole, clari-/teli-/ery-thromycin, verapamil, amiodarone), DM***, **R**(if GFR <30 ml/min)/**H/P/B/E**.

SE: diarrhoea, dizziness, ↓BP, ↑K$^+$, ↓GFR. Rarely rash, angioedema, ↓Hb.

Monitor: U&Es esp **↑K$^+$ if taking ACE-i, ARBs, K$^+$ sparing diuretics, K$^+$ salts (inc dietary salt substitutes) or heparin. Check BG/HbA$_{1C}$ regularly***.

Interactions: metab by↓/↓/↑**P450** ∴ many; ↓s furosemide levels. Levels ↓ by irbesartan; levels ↑ by keto-/itra-conazole. fx ↓ by ↓Na$^+$ diet and NSAIDs. fx ↑ by P-glycoprotein inhibitors (see *CI/Caution).

Dose: initially 150 mg od, ↑ing to 300 mg od if required.

ALLOPURINOL

Xanthine oxidase inhibitor: ↓s uric acid synthesis.

Use: Px of **gout**, renal stones (urate or Ca^{2+} oxalate) and other ↑urate states (esp 2° to chemotherapy).

CI: acute gout: can worsen – don't start drug during attack (but don't stop drug if acute attack occurs during Rx).

Caution: **R** (↓dose), **L** (↓dose and monitor LFTs), **P/B**.

SE: GI upset, ☠ **severe skin reactions** ☠ (*stop drug if rash develops and allopurinol is implicated* – can reintroduce cautiously if mild reaction and no recurrence). Rarely, neuropathy (and many non-specific neurological symptoms), blood disorders, RF, hepatotoxicity, gynaecomastia, vasculitis.

Warn: report rashes, maintain good hydration.

Interactions: Include ↑s fx/toxicity of **azathioprine** (and possibly other cytotoxics, esp ciclosporin), chlorpropamide and theophyllines. Level ↓d by salicylates and probenecid. ↑rash with ampicillin and amoxicillin. **W+**.

Dose: initially 100 mg od po (↑if required to max of 900 mg/day in divided doses of up to 300 mg) after food. Usual dose 300 mg/day.

NB: ↓dose if ↑ fx other drugs or LF or RF.
Initial Rx can ↑gout: give colchicine or NSAID (e.g. indometacin or diclofenac – *not aspirin*) Px until ⩾1 month after urate normalised.

ALPHAGAN see Brimonidine; α-agonist eye drops for glaucoma.

ALTEPLASE ((recombinant) tissue-type plasminogen activator, rt-PA, TPA). Recombinant fibrinolytic.
Use: acute **MI**, acute massive **PE** (with haemodynamic instability). Acute ischaemic CVA w/in 4.5 h of onset (specialist use only).
CI/Caution/SE: See p. 230 for use in MI (for use in PE/CVA, see SPC). L (avoid if severe).
Dose: MI: total dose of 100 mg – regimen depends on time since onset of pain: *0–6 h*: 15 mg iv bolus, then 50 mg ivi over 30 min, then 35 mg ivi over 60 min; *6–12 h*: 10 mg iv bolus, then 50 mg ivi over 60 min, then four further 10 mg ivis, each over 30 min.
PE: 10 mg iv over 1–2 min then 90 mg ivi over 2 h.

> ☠ ↓doses if patient <65 kg; see SPC ☠. If MI concurrent unfractionated iv heparin needed for ⩾24 h; see p. 232. Heparin also needed if giving for PE; see SPC.

ALUMINIUM HYDROXIDE
Antacid, PO_4-binding agent (↓s GI absorption).
Use: dyspepsia, ↑PO_4 (which can ↑risk of bone disease; esp good if secondary to RF, when ↑Ca^{2+} can occur dt ↑PTH, as other PO_4 binders often contain Ca^{2+}).
CI: ↓PO_4, porphyria.
SE: constipation*. Aluminium can accumulate in RF (esp on dialysis) ⇒ ↑risk of encephalopathy, dementia, osteomalacia.
Interactions: can ↓absorption of oral antibiotics (e.g. tetracyclines).
Dose: 1–2 (500-mg) tablets or 5–10 ml of 4% suspension prn (qds often sufficient). ↑doses to individual requirements, esp if for ↑PO_4. Also available as 475 mg capsules as Alucaps (contains ↓Na^+). Most effective taken with meals and at bedtime. Consider laxative Px*.

AMANTADINE

Weak DA agonist; ↑s release and ↓s reuptake of DA. Also antiviral properties; ↓s release of viral nucleic acid.

Use: Parkinson's disease and dyskinesias. Also used for Px of influenza A (if immunocompromised, vaccine CI or in exposed health workers).

CI: gastric ulcer (inc Hx of), epilepsy, **R** (if creatinine clearance <15 ml/min), **P/B**.

Caution: confused or hallucinatory states **L/H/E**.

SE: confusion, hallucinations, leg oedema.

Warn: Can ↓skilled task performance (esp driving). Stop drug slowly*.

Interactions: memantine ↑risk of CNS toxicity, anticholinergics.

Dose: 100–400 mg daily[SPC/BNF]. NB: ↓dose in RF, E. ≥ 65 yrs
NB: stop slowly*: risk of withdrawal syndrome.

AMFEBUTAMONE see Bupropion; aid to smoking cessation.

AMILORIDE

K^+-sparing diuretic (weak): inhibits DCT Na^+ reabsorption and K^+ excretion.

Use: oedema (2° to HF, cirrhosis or ↑aldosterone), HTN (esp in conjunction with ↑K^+-wasting diuretics as combination preparations; see Co-amilofruse and Co-amilozide). *For advice on stepped HTN Mx see p. 235.*

CI: ↑K^+, Addison's, anuria **R**.

Caution: DM (as risk of RF; monitor U&E), ↑risk of acidosis, ↓Na^+, drugs causing low Na^+, high K^+ **P/B/E**.

SE: ↑K^+, GI upset, headache, dry mouth, ↓BP (esp postural), ↓Na^+, rash, confusion. Rarely encephalopathy, hepatic/renal dysfunction.

Interactions: ↑s lithium levels. Can ↑nephrotoxicity of NSAIDs.

Dose: 2.5–20 mg od (or divide into bd doses).

> ☠ Beware if on other drugs that ↑K^+, e.g. spironolactone, triamterene, ACE-i, ARBs and ciclosporin. Don't give oral K^+ supplements inc dietary salt-substitute tablets. ☠

AMINOPHYLLINE

Methylxanthine bronchodilator: as theophylline but ↑H_2O solubility (is mixed w ethylenediamine) and ↓hypersensitivity.

Use/CI/Caution/SE/Interactions: see Theophylline; also available iv for use in acute severe bronchospasm; see p. 243. ☠ NB: has many important interactions (dose adjustment may be needed) and can ⇒ arrhythmias (use cardiac monitor if giving iv). ☠

Monitor: serum levels at 6, 18 and 24 h after starting ivi. Also do levels initially if taking po.

Dose: po: MR preparation (**Phyllocontin continus**) ⇒ ↓SEs, has different doses at 225–450 mg bd (or 350–700 mg bd if Forte tablets – for smokers and others with short $t_{1/2}$). *If on a particular brand, ensure this is prescribed as they have different pharmacokinetics.* **iv:** load* with 5 mg/kg (usually = 250–500 mg) over ≥20 min, then 0.5 mg/kg ivi, then adjusted to keep plasma levels at 10–20 mg/l (= 55–110 micromol/l). If possible, contact pharmacy for dosing advice to consider interactions, obesity and liver/heart function.

☠ If already taking maintenance po aminophylline/theophylline, omit loading dose* and check levels ASAP to guide dosing ☠.

AMIODARONE

Class III antiarrhythmic: ↑s refractory period of conducting system; useful as has ↓negative inotropic fx than other drugs and can give when others ineffective/CI.

Use: tachyarrhythmias: esp paroxysmal SVT, AF, atrial flutter, nodal tachycardias, VT and VF. Also in CPR/periarrest arrhythmias.

CI: ↓HR (sinus), sinoatrial HB, SAN disease or severe conduction disturbance w/o pacemaker, Hx of thyroid disease/iodine sensitivity, **P/B**.

Caution: porphyria, ↓K^+ (↑risk of torsades), **L/R/H/E**.

SE: *Acute:* **N&V** (dose-dependent), ↓**HR/BP**. *Chronic:* rarely but seriously ↑**or** ↓**T4, interstitial lung disease** (e.g. fibrosis, *but reversible if caught early*), **hepatotoxicity, conduction disturbances**

(esp ↓HR). *Common:* **malaise**, **fatigue**, photosensitive skin (rarely 'grey-slate'), corneal deposits ± 'night glare' (reversible), tremor, sleep disorders. *Less commonly:* optic neuritis (rare but can ↓vision), peripheral neuropathy, blood disorders, hypersensitivity.

Monitor: TFTs and LFTs (baseline then 6-monthly). Also baseline K⁺ and CXR (watch for ↑SOB/alveolitis).

Warn: avoid sunlight/use sunscreen (inc several months after stopping).

Interactions: ↑s fx of phenytoin and digoxin. Other class III and many class Ia antiarrhythmics, antipsychotics, TCAs, lithium, erythromycin, co-trimoxazole, antimalarials, nelfinavir, ritonavir ⇒ ↑risk of ventricular arrhythmias. Verapamil, diltiazem and β-blockers ⇒ ↑risk of ↓HR and HB; CYP 3A4 dpt statins ↑myopathy **W +**.

Dose: **po:** load 200 mg tds in 1st wk, 200 mg bd in 2nd wk, then (usually od) maintenance dose according to response (long $t_{1/2}$: months before steady plasma concentration) *NB: initiate in hospital or specialist outpatient service;* **iv:** (extreme emergencies only) 150–300 mg in 10–20 ml 5% glucose over ⩾3 min (don't repeat for at least 15 min); **ivi:** 5 mg/kg over 20–120 min (max 1.2 g/day). For use in cardiac arrest/periarrest arrhythmias see ALS and tachycardia algorithms in the front and back cover flaps of this book respectively.

☠ iv doses: give via central line (if no time for insertion, give via largest cannula possible) with ECG monitoring. Avoid giving if severe respiratory failure or ↓BP (unless caused by arrhythmia) as can worsen. Avoid iv boluses if CCF/cardiomyopathy ☠.

AMITRIPTYLINE

Tricyclic antidepressant (TCA): blocks reuptake of NA (and 5HT).

Use: depression[1] (esp if insomnia, ↓appetite, psychomotor slowing or agitation prominent. NB: ↑danger in OD cf other antidepressants), neuropathic pain[2], migraine prophylaxis.

CI: recent MI (w/in 3 months), arrhythmias (esp HB), mania, **L** (if severe).

Caution: cardiac/thyroid disease, epilepsy*, glaucoma (angle closure), ↑prostate, phaeo, porphyria, anaesthesia. Also Hx of mania, psychosis or urinary retention, **L/H/P/B/E**.

SE: antimuscarinic fx (see p. 276), **cardiac fx** (arrhythmias, HB, HR, postural ↓BP, dizziness, syncope: **dangerous in OD**), ↑Wt, **sedation**** (often ⇒ 'hangover'), seizures*. Rarely mania, fever, blood disorders, hypersensitivity, ΔLFTs, ↓Na$^+$ (esp in elderly), neuroleptic malignant syndrome.

Warn: may impair driving**.

Interactions: 💀 MAOIs ⇒ HTN and CNS excitation. *Never give with, or <2 wks after, MAOI* 💀. Levels ↑d by SSRIs, phenothiazines and cimetidine. ↑Risk of arrhythmias with **amiodarone, pimozide** (is CI), thioridazine and some class I antiarrhythmics. ↑risk of paralytic ileus with antimuscarinics. ↑s sedative fx of alcohol. ↑CNS toxicity with **sibutramine** (is CI).

Dose: initially 75 mg (30–75 mg in elderly) nocte or in divided doses (↑if required to max 200 mg/day)[1]; initially 10 mg nocte ↑ing if required to 75 mg nocte[2].

AMLODIPINE/ISTIN

Ca^{2+} channel blocker (dihydropyridine): as nifedipine, but ⇒ no ↓contractility or ↑HF.

Use: HTN (*for advice on stepped HTN Mx see p. 229*), angina (esp 'Prinzmetal's' = coronary vasospasm).

CI: ACS, cardiogenic shock, significant aortic stenosis, **P/B**.

Caution: BPH (poly-/nocturia), acute porphyria, **L**.

SE: as nifedipine but ↑ankle swelling and possibly ↓vasodilator fx (headache, flushing and dizziness).

Interactions: may ↑fx of theophyllines; care with inducers of cytochrome 3A4; ↓simvastatin dose max. 20 mg od.

Dose: initially 5 mg od po (↑if required to 10 mg). **NB: consider ↓dose in LF.**

AMOXICILLIN

Broad-spectrum penicillin; good GI absorption (can give po and iv).

Use: mild pneumonias[1] (esp community-acquired), UTI, *Listeria* meningitis, endocarditis Px and many ENT/dental/other infections. *Often used with clavulanic acid as co-amoxiclav.*

CI/Caution/SE/Interactions: see Ampicillin.

Dose: 500–1000 mg tds po/iv[1]; for other severe infections see SPC/BNF (mild/moderate infections usually 250–500 mg tds po). **NB: ↓dose in RF.**

AMPICILLIN
Broad-spectrum penicillin for iv use: has ↓GI absorption cf amoxicillin, which is preferred po.
Use: Meningitis (esp *Listeria*; see p. 258)[1], Px pre-operative or for endocarditis during invasive procedures if valve lesions/prostheses, respiratory tract/ENT infections (esp community-acquired pneumonia dt *Haemophilus influenzae* or *Streptococcus pneumoniae*), UTIs (not for blind Rx, as *Escherichia coli* often resistant).
CI: penicillin hypersensitivity (NB: cross-reactivity with cephalosporins).
Caution: EBV/CMV infections, ALL, CLL (all ↑risk of rash), **R**.
SE: rash (erythematous, maculopapular: often does not reflect true allergy) commoner in RF or crystal nephropathy **N&V&D** (rarely AAC), **hypersensitivity**, CNS/blood disorders.
Interactions: levels ↑by probenecid. ↑effects of warfarin. ↑risk of rash with allopurinol. Can ↓fx of OCP (warn patient); ↑levels of methotrexate.
Dose: Most indications 0.25–1 g qds po, 500 mg qds im/iv[SPC/BNF] (meningitis 2 g 4-hrly ivi[1]). **NB: ↓dose in RF.**

ANTABUSE see Disulfiram; adjunct to alcohol withdrawal.

ANTACIDS see Alginates (e.g. Acidex, Gastrocote, Gaviscon or Peptac) or Co-magaldrox.

AQUEOUS CREAM Emulsifying ointment (phenoxyethanol in purified water). Topical cream used as emollient in dry skin conditions and as a soap-substitute.

▼ ARIPIPRAZOLE/ABILIFY
Atypical (third generation) antipsychotic; *partial* D_2 (and $5HT_{1A}$) agonist ⇒ ↓dopaminergic neuronal activity. Also potent $5HT_{2A}$ antagonist.

Use: schizophrenia, mania (Px and acute Rx).

CI: Coma, CNS depression, phaeo **B**.

Caution: cerebrovascular disease, Hx or ↑risk of seizures, family Hx of ↑QT **L/P/E**.

SE: EPSE (esp akathisia/restlessness, although generally ⇒ ↓EPSE than other antipsychotics), dizziness, sedation (or insomnia), blurred vision, fatigue, headache, gastrointestinal upset, anxiety and ↑salivation. Rarely ↑HR, depression, orthostatic ↓BP. Very rarely skin/blood disorders, ↑QTc, DM, NMS, tardive dyskinesia, seizures and CVA.

Interactions: metab by P450 ∴ many; most importantly levels ↑ by itra-conazole, HIV protease/itra-conazole, HIV protease inhibitors and levels ↓ by carbamazepine, rifampicin, rifabutin, phenytoin, primodone, efavirenz, nevirapine and St John's wort.

Dose: 10–15 mg po od (max 30 mg/od); 5.25–15 (usually 9.75) mg im as single dose repeated after ≥2 h if required (max 3 injections/day or combined im/po dose of 30 mg/day). **NB:** ↓**dose in elderly.**

ARTHROTEC

Combination tablets of diclofenac with misoprostol (200 microgram/tablet) to ↓GI SEs (esp PU/bleeds).

CI/Caution/SE/Interactions: see Diclofenac and Misoprostol.

Dose: 50 mg bd/tds po or 75 mg bd (prescribed as dose of diclofenac).

ASACOL see Mesalazine: 'new' aminosalicylate for UC with ↓SEs. Available po (3–6 tablets of 400 mg per day in divided doses), as suppositories (0.75–1.5 g daily in divided doses) or as foam enemas (1–2 g daily).

ASPIRIN

NSAID. Inhibits COX-1 and COX-2 ⇒ ↓PG synthesis (∴ anti-inflammatory and antipyrexial) and ↓thromboxane A_2 (∴ anti-Pt aggregation).

Use: mild to moderate pain/pyrexia[1], IHD and thromboembolic CVA Px[2] and acute Rx[3].

CI: <16 years old, unless specifically indicated (can ⇒ Reye's syndrome), PU (**active or PHx of**), hypersensitivity to any NSAID, haemophilia, **R** (GFR<10 ml/min)/**L** (if severe)/**B**.
Caution: asthma, any allergic disease*, dehydration, uncontrolled HTN, gout, G6PD deficiency, **L/R**(avoid if either severe)/**P/E**.
SE: GI irritation, bleeding (esp GI: ↑↑risk if also anticoagulated)**. Rarely hypersensitivity* (anaphylaxis, bronchospasm, skin reactions), AKI, hepatotoxicity, ototoxic in OD.
Interactions: ↑GI bleeding with anticoagulants**, other NSAIDs (avoid), SSRIs & venlafaxine. **W +** Can ⇒ ↑levels of methotrexate, ↑fx anticonvulsants & ↓fx spironolactone.
Dose: 300–900 mg 4–6-hrly (max 4 g/day)[1], 75 mg od[2], 300 mg stat[3].

> Stop 7 days before surgery if significant bleeding is expected. If cardiac surgery or patient has ACS, consider continuing.

ATENOLOL

β-blocker: (mildly) cardioselective* ($β_1 > β_2$), ↑H_2O solubility ∴ ↓central fx** and ↑renal excretion***.
Use: HTN[1] (*for advice on stepped HTN Mx see p. 235*), angina[2], MI (w/in 12 h as early intervention)[3], arrhythmias[4].
CI/Caution/SE/Interactions: see Propranolol ⇒ ↓bronchospasm* (but avoid in all asthma/only use in COPD if no other choice) and ↓sleep disturbance/nightmares***.
Dose: 25–50 mg od po[1]; 100 mg od po[2]; 5 mg iv over 5 min, 50 mg po 15 min later, 50 mg po after 12 h, then 100 mg od po[3]; 50–100 mg od po[4] (for iv doses see SPC/BNF). **NB: consider ↓dose in RF***.

ATORVASTATIN/LIPITOR

H MG-CoA reductase inhibitor.
Use/CI/Caution/SE: see Simvastatin.

Interactions: ↑risk of myopathy includes with ☠ fibrates ☠, daptomycin, ciclosporin, nicotinic acid, itra-/posa-conazole. Levels ↑by clari-/teli-thromycin.

Dose: initially 10 mg nocte (↑if necessary, at intervals ⩾4 wks, to max 80 mg). Post ACS dose 80 mg daily.

ATRACURIUM

A mixture of 10 isomers. Benzylisoquinolinium neuromuscular blocker. Intermediate duration of action. Non-enzymatically metabolised (∴independent of liver / kidney function).
Use: neuromuscular blockade for surgery[1] or during intensive care (esp in LF or RF)[2]
CI: anaesthetist not confident of airway maintenance.
Caution: neuromuscular disease (MG, Eaton-Lambert syndrome, old polio), hypersensitivity to other neuromuscular blockers (allergic cross-reactivity), burns (resistance can develop).
SE: histamine release (skin flushing, ↓BP, ↑HR, bronchospasm, anaphylactoid reactions), seizures.
Monitor: cardiac and respiratory function.
Interactions: fx ↑by aminoglycosides, clindamycin and polymyxins. Can ⇒ haemolysis if given with blood transfusion.
Dose: initially 300–600 micrograms/kg iv then 100–200 micrograms/kg iv as required *or* initially 200–600 micrograms/kg iv then 300–600 micrograms/kg/hr ivi[1]; initially 300–600 micrograms/kg iv (optional) then 270–1770 micrograms/kg/hr ivi (usually 650–780 micrograms/kg/hr)[2]. *NB: if obese (weight 30% above ideal body weight (IBW; see p.296)) use IBW for dose calculation.*

☠ Specialist use only; respiration needs assistance / control until drug inactivated or antagonised and anaesthetic / sedative to prevent awareness. ☠

ATROPINE (SULPHATE) iv

Muscarinic antagonist: blocks vagal SAN and AVN stimulation, bronchodilates and ↓s oropharyngeal secretions.
Use: severe ↓HR (see algorithm on inside front cover) or HB[1], CPR [atropine NOT recommended for asystole], organophosphate/anticholinesterase* OD/poisoning[2] and specialist anaesthetic uses.

CI: (*don't apply if life-threatening condition/CPR!*): glaucoma (angle closure), MG (*unless anticholinesterase overdosage*, when atropine is indicated*), paralytic ileus, pyloric stenosis, bladder neck obstruction (e.g. ↑prostate).

Caution: Down's syndrome, gastro-oesophageal reflux, diarrhoea, UC, acute MI, HTN, ↑HR (esp 2° to ↑T$_4$, cardiac insufficiency or surgery), pyrexia, **P/B/E**.

SE: transient ↓HR (followed by ↑HR, palpitations, arrhythmias), antimuscarinic fx (see p. 276), N&V, confusion (esp in elderly), dizziness.

Dose: 0.3–0.6 mg iv[1]; 1–2 mg im/iv every 10–30 min[2] (every 5 min in severe cases) up to max 100 mg in 1st 24 h, until symptomatic response (skin flushes and dries, pupils dilate, HR↑s).

ATROVENT see Ipratropium; bronchodilator for COPD/asthma.

AUGMENTIN see Co-amoxiclav (amoxicillin + clavulanic acid) 375 or 625 mg tds po (1.2 g tds iv).

AZATHIOPRINE

Antiproliferative immunosuppressant: inhibits purine-salvage p'ways; prodrug for 6-mercaptopurine.

Use: prevention of transplant rejection, autoimmune disease (esp as steroid-sparing agent, but also maintenance Rx for SLE/vasculitis).

CI: hypersensitivity (to azathioprine *or mercaptopurine*), **P/B**.

Caution: **L/R/E**.

SE: myelosuppression (dose-dependent, ⇒ ↑infections, esp HZV), **hepatotoxicity**, **hypersensitivity reactions** (inc interstitial nephritis: *stop drug!*), N&V&D (esp initially), pancreatitis. Rarely cholestasis, alopecia, pneumonitis, risk of neoplasia, hepatic veno-occlusion.

Warn: immediately report infections or unexpected bruising/bleeding.

Monitor: FBC (initially ⩾wkly ↓ing to ⩾3-monthly), LFTs, U&Es.

Interactions: fx ↑ by **allopurinol**, ACE-i, ARBs, trimethoprim (and septrin). fx ↓ by rifampicin. **W–**.

Dose: Initially 1–3 mg/kg daily for ≤12 wks[SPC/BNF] (preferably po as iv very irritant). **NB: ↓dose in RF.**

☠ Before starting Rx, screen for common gene defect that ↓s TPMT enzyme (which metabolises azathioprine) activity: if homozygote for defect avoid thiopurine drugs; if heterozygote, ↓dose (esp if taking aminosalicylate derivatives, e.g. olsalazine, mesalazine or sulfasalazine) ☠.

AZITHROMYCIN

Macrolide antibiotic: see Erythromycin.
Use: see Erythromycin (but with ↑activity against Gram −ve and ↓activity against Gram +ve organisms). Also genital chlamydia and non-severe typhoid.
CI: as erythromycin, plus **L** (if severe).
Caution/SE/Interactions: as erythromycin (NB: ↑**P450** ∴ many interactions) but ⇒ ↓GI SEs.
Dose: 500 mg od po *for 3 days only* (continue for 7 days for typhoid); for GU infections 1 g od po *as single dose*.

AZOPT see Brinzolamide; eye drops for glaucoma.

AZT see Zidovudine; antiretroviral for HIV.

BACLOFEN

Skeletal muscle relaxant: ↓s spinal reflexes, general CNS inhibition at ↑doses.
Use: spasticity, if chronic/severe, (esp 2° to MS or cord pathology).
CI: PU, porphyria, hereditary galactose intolerance.
Caution: Ψ disorders, epilepsy, Hx of PU, Parkinson's, porphyria, DM, hypertonic bladder sphincter, respiratory/cerebrovascular disease, **L/R/P/E.**
SE: sedation, ↓muscle tone, nausea, urinary dysfunction, GI upset, ↓BP. Others rare: ↑spasticity (*stop drug!*), multiple neurological/Ψ symptoms, cardiac/hepatic/respiratory dysfunction.
Warn: may ↓skilled tasks (esp driving), ↑s fx of alcohol.

Interactions: fx ↑by TCAs. May ↑fx of antihypertensives.
Dose: 5 mg tds po (after food) ↑ing, if required, to max of 100 mg/day. **NB ↓dose in RF**. In severe cases, can give by intrathecal pump (see SPC/BNF).

Stop gradually over ≥1–2 wks to avoid withdrawal symptoms: confusion, ↑spasticity, Ψ reactions, fits, ↑HR.

BACTROBAN see Mupirocin; topical antibiotic (esp for nasal MRSA). See local policy for infection control.

BECLOMETASONE
Inh corticosteroid: ↓s airway oedema and mucous secretions.
Use: chronic asthma not controlled by short-acting β_2 agonists alone.
Caution: TB (inc quiescent).
SE: oral candidiasis (2° to immunosuppression: ↓d by rinsing mouth with H_2O after use), **hoarse voice**. Rarely glaucoma, hypersensitivity. ↑Doses may ⇒ adrenal suppression, Cushing's, ↓bone density, lower RTI, ↓growth (controversial).
Dose: 200–2000 microgram daily inh (normally start at 200 microgram bd). Use high-dose inhaler if daily requirements are >800 microgram[SPC/BNF]. Specify named product for CFC metered disc inhalers as dose ranges from 50 to 400 microgram/delivery. CFC-free pressurized metered dose inhalers are not interchangeable.

Rarely ⇒ paradoxical bronchospasm: can be prevented by switching from aerosol to dry powder forms or by using inh β_2 agonists.

BECOTIDE see Beclometasone.

BENDROFLUMETHIAZIDE
Thiazide diuretic: ↓s Na^+ (and Cl) reabsorption from DCT ⇒ Na^+ and H_2O loss and stimulates K^+ excretion.
Use: oedema[1] (2° to HF or low-protein states), HTN[2] (in short term by ↓ing fluid volume and CO; in long term by ↓ing TPR; *for advice on stepped HTN Mx see p. 235*), Px against renal stones in hypercalciuria[3].

L/H = Liver, Renal and Heart failure (full key see p. xv)

CI: $\downarrow K^+$ (refractory to Rx), $\downarrow Na^+$, $\uparrow Ca^{2+}$, Addison's disease, $\uparrow$ urate (if symptoms), **L/R** (if either severe, otherwise caution).

Caution: porphyria, and can worsen gout, DM or SLE, **P/B/E**.

SE: dehydration (esp in elderly), $\downarrow BP$ (esp postural), $\downarrow K^+$, **impotence**, $\downarrow Na^+$, alkalosis (with $\downarrow Cl$), $\downarrow Mg^{2+}$, $\uparrow Ca^{2+}$, $\uparrow$ urate/gout, $\uparrow$ glucose, lipid metabolism (esp $\uparrow$ cholesterol), rash, photosensitivity, blood disorders (inc $\downarrow Pt$, $\downarrow N\emptyset$), pancreatitis, intrahepatic cholestasis, hypersensitivity reactions (inc severe respiratory and skin reactions), arrhythmias.

Interactions: $\uparrow$s lithium levels. fx $\downarrow$by **NSAIDs** and oestrogens. If $\downarrow K^+$ can $\uparrow$toxic fx of many drugs (esp digoxin, NSAIDs, corticosteroids and many antiarrhythmics). $\uparrow$risk of $\downarrow Na^+$ with carbamazepine $\uparrow$risk of $\downarrow K^+$ with amphotericin.

Dose: initially 5–10 mg mane po[1], then $\downarrow$dose *frequency* (i.e. omit days) if possible; 2.5 mg od po[2,3] (little benefit from $\uparrow$doses).

BENZYLPENICILLIN (= PENICILLIN G)

Penicillin with poor po absorption $\therefore$ only given im/**iv**: used mostly against streptococcal (esp *S. pneumoniae*) and neisserial (esp *N. gonorrhoeae*, *N. meningitidis*) infections.

Use: (usually in conjunction with other agents) severe skin infections (esp cellulitis, wound infections, gas gangrene) (see p. 287), meningitis, endocarditis, ENT infections, pneumococcal pneumonia.

CI: penicillin hypersensitivity (NB: cross-reactivity with cephalosporins common).

Caution: Hx of allergy, false +ve glycosuria, **R***.

SE: hypersensitivity (inc fever, arthralgia, rashes, urticaria, angioedema, anaphylaxis, serum sickness-like reactions, haemolytic $\downarrow Hb$, interstitial nephritis), **diarrhoea** (rarely AAC). Rarely blood disorders ($\downarrow Pt$, $\downarrow N\emptyset$, coagulation disorders), CNS toxicity (inc convulsions, esp at $\uparrow$doses or if RF*). $\uparrow$doses can $\Rightarrow \downarrow K^+$(and $\downarrow Na^+$).

Interactions: levels $\uparrow$d by probenecid. $\uparrow$risk of rash with allopurinol. Can $\downarrow$fx of OCP.

Dose: 0.6–1.2 g qds iv (or im/ivi). If very severe, give 2.4 g every 4 h (only as iv/ivi). **NB:** $\downarrow$dose in RF.

BETAHISTINE/SERC

Histamine analogue (H1 antagonism and H3 antagonism): ↑s middle-ear microcirculation ⇒ ↓endolymphatic pressure.

Use: Ménière's disease (if tinnitus, vertigo or hearing loss).

CI: phaeo.

Caution: asthma, Hx of PU, **P/B**.

SE: GI upset. Rarely headache, rash, pruritus.

Dose: 16 mg tds po (maintenance usually 24–48 mg/day).

BETAMETHASONE CREAM (0.1%)/OINTMENT

'Potent' strength topical corticosteroid (rarely used as weaker 0.05% or 0.025% preparations).

Use: inflammatory skin conditions, in particular eczema.

CI: untreated infection, rosacea, acne.

SE: skin atrophy, worsening of infections, acne.

Dose: apply thinly 1–2 times per day. Use 'ointment' in dry skin conditions.

BETNOVATE see Betamethasone cream 0.1% (potent strength). Available as Betnovate RD (moderate strength) 0.025%.

BEZAFIBRATE

Fibrate (lipid-lowering): ⇒ ↓**TG**, ↓**LDL**, ↑**HDL** by stimulating lipoprotein lipase (⇒ ↓conversion of VLDL/TG to LDL and ⇒ ↑LDL clearance from circulation). Also ⇒ (mild) ↓cholesterol.

Use: hyperlipidaemias (esp if ↑TG ∴ types IIa/b, III, IV, V).

CI: gallbladder disease, PBC, ↓albumin (esp nephrotic syndrome), **R***/ **L** (if either severe; otherwise caution), **P/B**.

Caution: ↓T_4 (needs to be corrected).

SE: GI upset, ↓appetite, ↑**gallstones**, **myositis** (rarer but important: ↑risk if RF*). Also impotence, rash (inc pruritus, urticaria), headache. Rarer: dizziness, vertigo, fatigue, hair loss, blood disorders (↓Hb, ↓WCC, ↓Pt).

Interactions: 💀 'statins' ⇒ ↑**risk of myositis** 💀. ↑s fx of anti-diabetics. ↑risk of hepatotoxicity with MAOIs. Can ↑renal toxicity of ciclosporin. **W +.**

Dose: 200 mg tds po (after food). MR 400 mg od preps available[BNF].
NB: ↓dose in RF.

BICARBONATE see Sodium bicarbonate.

BIMATOPROST EYE DROPS/LUMIGAN
Topical PG analogue for glaucoma; see Latanoprost.
Use/CI/Caution/SE: see Latanoprost.
Dose: 1 drop od.

BISOPROLOL
β-blocker, cardioselective ($β_1 > β_2$).
Use: HTN[1] (*for advice on stepped HTN Mx see p. 235*), angina[2], HF[3].
CI/Caution/SE/Interactions: as propranolol, but also CI in HF needing inotropes or if SAN block; caution if psoriasis.
Dose: 10 mg od po[1,2] (maintenance 5–20 mg od); initially 1.25 mg od po[3](↑ing slowly to max 10 mg od)[SPC/BNF]. NB: ↓dose in LF or RF.

BOSENTAN/TRACLEER
Endothelin receptor antagonist: relaxes vascular smooth muscle.
Use: pulmonary arterial HTN[1], Rx of digital ulcers in systemic sclerosis.[2]
CI: SBP <85 mmHg, acute porphyria, **P/B**.
Caution: ↓BP, L (avoid if severe).
SE: Δ LFTs, ↓BP, palpitations, oedema, headache, flushing, bleeding/↓Hb, ↓NO (O needs forward diagonal strike-through symbol for neutrophils), ↓Pt, hypersensitivity reactions, dyspepsia, D,.
Warn: avoid sudden withdrawal and report symptoms of LF.
Monitor: LFTs monthly (and 2 wks after dose ↑) and Hb monthly for 1st 4 wks then 3-monthly. INR at start or change in dose.
Interactions: metab by *and* ↑P450. Levels ↑by ciclosporin, keto-/flu-/itra-conazole. Levels ↓by rifampicin. ↓s fx of OCP and simvastatin. ↑risk of hepatoxicity with glibenclamide.

Dose: *specialist use only*: initially 62.5 mg po bd for 4 wks then ↑to 125 mg bd[1,2] (can ↑to 250 mg bd[1])[SPC/BNF].

BOWEL PREPARATIONS
Bowel-cleansing solutions for preparation for GI surgery/Ix.
CI: GI obstruction/ulceration/perforation, ileus, gastric retention, toxic megacolon/colitis, **H**.
Caution: UC, DM, heart disease, reflux oesophagitis, ↑risk of regurgitation/aspiration (e.g. ↓swallow/gag reflex/GCS), **R/P**.
SE: nausea, **bloating**, abdominal pains, vomiting.
Dose: see Citramag, Fleet (Phospho-soda), Klean-prep, Picolax.

BRICANYL see Terbutaline (inh β₂ agonist for asthma). Various delivery devices available[SPC/BNF].

BRIMONIDINE EYE DROPS/ALPHAGAN
Topical α₂ agonist: ↓s aqueous humour production ∴ ↓s IOP.
Use: open-angle glaucoma, ocular HTN (esp if β-blocker or PG analogue CI or fails to ↓IOP).
Caution: postural ↓BP/HR, Raynaud's, cardiovascular disease (esp IHD), cerebral insufficiency, depression*, **P/B R/L**.
SE: sedation, headache, dry mouth, HTN, blurred vision, **local reactions** (esp discomfort, pruritus, hyperaemia, follicular conjunctivitis). Rarely, palpitations, depression*, hypersensitivity.
Interactions: ☠ MAOIs, TCAs, mianserin (or other antidepressants affecting NA transmission) are CI ☠.
Dose: 1 drop bd of 0.2% solution. Also available as od combination drop with timolol 0.5% (Combigan).

BRINZOLAMIDE/AZOPT
Topical carbonic anhydrase inhibitor for glaucoma. Similar to dorzolamide (↓s aqueous humour production).
CI: Hyperchloraemic acidosis, **R** (GFR <30 ml/min)
Caution: **P/B**

Dose: 1 drop bd/tds. Also available as od combination drop with timolol 0.5% (Azarga).

BROMOCRIPTINE

DA agonist; ↓s pituitary release of prolactin and growth hormone.

Use: endocrine disorders[1] (e.g. prolactinoma, galactorrhoea, acromegaly) and NMS. Rarely used for Parkinsonism if L-dopa insufficient/not tolerated.

CI: cardiac valvulopathy, hypersensitivity to ergot alkaloids, uncontrolled HTN. Also HTN/IHD postpartum or in puerperium.

Caution: cardiovascular disease, PU, porphyria, Raynaud's disease, serious Ψ disorders (esp psychosis), **P/B**.

SE: GI upset, postural ↓BP (esp initially and if ↑alcohol intake), **behavioural Δs** (confusional states, Ψ disorders), ↑**sleep** (sudden onset/daytime). Rarely but seriously **fibrosis***: pulmonary**, cardiac, retroperitoneal*** (can ⇒ AKI).

Warn: of ↑sleep. Report persistent cough** or chest/abdo pain.

Monitor: BP, ESR*, U&Es***, CXR**; pituitary size and visual fields (pregnancy and[1])**.

Interactions: levels ↑by ery-/clari-thromycin and octreotide.

Dose: 1–30 mg/day[SPC/BNF]. **NB: consider ↓dose in LF.**

BUCCASTEM Prochlorperazine (antiemetic) buccal tablets: absorbed rapidly from under top lip ∴ don't need to be swallowed and retained in stomach for absorption if N&V.

Caution: See Prochlorperazine **L**.

Dose: 3–6 mg bd.

▼ BUDESONIDE

Inh corticosteroid for asthma[1]; similar to beclometasone but stronger (approximately double the strength per microgram). Also available po or as enemas for IBD[2] (see BNF).

Caution: **L**.

Dose: 200–800 microgram bd inh (aerosol or powder) or 1–2 mg bd neb[1].

BUMETANIDE

Loop diuretic: inhibits Na^+/K^+ pump in ascending loop of Henle.

Use/CI/Caution/SE/Monitor/Interactions: as furosemide; also headaches, gynaecomastia and at ↑doses can ⇒ myalgia.

Dose: 1 mg mane po (500 microgram may suffice in elderly), ↑ing if required (5 mg/24 h usually sufficient; ↑by adding a lunchtime dose, then ↑ing each dose). 1–2 mg im/iv (repeat after 20 min if required). 2–5 mg ivi over 30–60 min.

> NB: give iv in severe oedema; bowel oedema ⇒ ↓po absorption.

BUPROPION (= AMFEBUTAMONE)/ZYBAN

NA and to lesser extent DA reuptake inhibitor (NDRI) developed as antidepressant, but also ↑s success of giving up smoking.

Use: (adjunct to) smoking cessation[NICE].

CI: CNS tumour, acute alcohol/benzodiazepine withdrawal, Hx of seizures*, eating disorders, bipolar disorder, **L** (if severe cirrhosis)/**P/B**.

Caution: if ↑risk of seizures*: alcohol abuse, Hx of head trauma and DM, **R/E**.

SE: seizures*, insomnia (and other CNS reactions, e.g. anxiety, agitation, depression, fever, headaches, tremor, dizziness). Also ↑HR, AV block, ↑or ↓BP**, chest pain, hypersensitivity (inc severe skin reactions), GI upset, ↑Wt, mild antimuscarinic fx (esp **dry mouth**; see p. 276 for others).

Monitor: BP**.

Interactions: ↓P450 ∴ many interactions, but importantly **CNS drugs**, esp if ↓seizure threshold*, e.g. antidepressants (☠ MAOIs; avoid together, including <2 wks after MAOI ☠), antimalarials, antipsychotics (esp risperidone), quinolones, sedating antihistamines, systemic corticosteroids, theophyllines, tramadol. Ritonavir ⇒ ↓plasma level of bupropion. ↓dose of CYP2B6 mod anti-arrhythmics

L/R/H = Liver, Renal and Heart failure (full key see p. xv)

Dose: 150 mg od for 6 days then 150 mg bd for max 9 wks (↓dose if elderly or ↑seizure risk$^{SPC/BNF}$). Start 1–2 wks before target date of stopping smoking. **NB: max 150 mg/day in LF or RF.**

BURINEX Bumetanide 1-mg tablets.

BUSCOPAN see Hyoscine butylbromide; GI antispasmodic.

CACIT see Calcium carbonate.

CACIT D3 Calcium carbonate + low dose vitamin D_3.
Use: Px of vitamin D deficiency.
Caution: L.
Dose: 1 tablet od (= 12.5 mmol Ca^{2+} + 11 microgram cholecalciferol).

CALCICHEW see Calcium carbonate.

CALCICHEW D3 Calcium carbonate + low dose vitamin D_3.
Use: Px of vitamin D deficiency.
Dose: 1 tablet od. Each tablet = 12.5 mmol Ca^{2+} + 5 microgram vit D_3 (cholecalciferol) or 10 microgram vit D_3 in 'forte' preparations.

CALCIPOTRIOL OINTMENT AND CREAM
Vitamin D analogue for plaque psoriasis.
SE: local skin reactions (itching, redness).
Caution: Avoid excessive sunlight exposure use <100 g/wk, **E.**
CI: patients with disorders of Ca^{2+} metabolism.
Use: apply od or bd. Also used as ointment or gel combined with betamethasone (Dovobet) od ≤4 wks.

CALCITONIN
Synthetic hormone (normally produced by C cells of thyroid): binds to specific osteoclast receptors ⇒ ↓resorption of bone and ↓Ca^{2+}. Its fx are specific to abnormal (high-turnover) bone.

Use: ↑Ca^{2+} (esp dt malignancy; also ↓s bone metastases pain), Paget's disease (↓s pain and neurological symptoms, e.g. deafness). Rarely for Px/Rx of postmenopausal osteoporosis.

CI: ↓Ca^{2+} **P/B**.

Caution: Hx of *any* allergy, **R/H**.

SE: GI upset (esp N&V), **flushing**, ↑**urinary frequency**, taste, vision/sensory Δ, hypersensitivity (inc anaphylaxis), myalgia, local inflammation, oedema, rash, malignancy (long term use), tremor.

Dose: see BNF/SPC.

CALCIUM CARBONATE

Use: osteoporosis, ↓Ca^{2+}, ↑PO_4 (esp 2° to RF; binds PO_4 in gut ⇒ ↓absorption).

CI: conditions assoc with ↑Ca^{2+} (in serum or urine).

Caution: sarcoid, Hx of kidney stones, phenylketonuria, **R**.

SE: GI upset, ↑Ca^{2+} (serum or urine), ↓HR, arrhythmias.

Interactions: fx ↑by thiazides, fx ↓by corticosteroids, ↓s absorption of tetracyclines (give ≥2 h before or 6 h after) and bisphosphonates.

Dose: as required up to 40 mmol/day in osteoporosis if ↓dietary intake, e.g. Calcichew (standard 12.5-mmol or 'forte' 25-mmol tablets), Cacit (12.5-mmol tablets), Calcium 500 (12.5-mmol tablets) or Adcal (15-mmol tablets).

CALCIUM CHLORIDE

Ca^{2+} for emergency iv

Use: mostly CPR as ⇒ ↑venous irritation cf calcium gluconate. Can also use for severe ↓Ca^{2+} or ↑K^+.

CI: VF, conditions assoc with ↑Ca^{2+} (in serum or urine).

SE: GI upset, ↑Ca^{2+}, ↓HR, ↓BP, arrhythmias.

Dose: available as syringes of 10 ml of 10% solution (= total of 6.8 mmol Ca^{2+}). Give iv no quicker than 1 ml/min (otherwise can ⇒ arrhythmias) as per indication and clinical/e'lyte response.

E.g. Min-i-jet: often in crash trolleys if iv Ca^{2+} needed urgently.

CALCIUM + ERGOCALCIFEROL tablets of 2.4 mmol Ca^{2+} low-dose (10 microgram) ergocalciferol (= calciferol = vitamin D_2).

L/R/H = Liver, Renal and Heart failure (full key see p. xv)

Use: Px of vitamin D deficiency.
CI/Caution/SE: see Ergocalciferol.
Dose: 1 tablet od$^{SPC/BNF}$.

CALCIUM GLUCONATE

iv preparation of Ca^{2+} (also available po, but used rarely).
Use: $\downarrow Ca^{2+}$ (if severe)[1], $\uparrow K^+$ ($\downarrow$s arrhythmias: 'cardioprotective', see p. 269)[2], $\uparrow mg^{2+}$.
CI/SE: as calcium chloride.
Dose: 10 ml of 10% iv over 3 min (= total of 2.2 mmol Ca^{2+})[1,2], repeating if necessary according to clinical and electrolyte response; consider following with ivi[1].

CALCIUM RESONIUM

Polystyrene sulphonate ion-exchange resin.
Use: chronic $\uparrow K^+$ with oligo-anuria (not for *initial** Mx of acute $\uparrow K^+$).
CI: obstructive bowel disease, diseases likely to $\uparrow Ca^{2+}$ ($\uparrow$PTH, multiple myeloma, sarcoid, metastatic cancer), $K^+ < 5$ mmol/l.
Caution: Use sodium resin if HTN, oedema or **H. P/B**.
SE: GI upset (inc ulceration, GI necrosis, severe constipation; often need Px of 10–20 ml lactulose), $\downarrow K^+$, $\downarrow Mg^{2+}$, $\uparrow Ca^{2+}$.
Interactions: $\uparrow$risk GI obstruction with aluminium hydroxide, $\uparrow$risk of alkalosis with aluminium carbonate and magnesium hydroxide. May $\downarrow$lithium and levothyroxine levels. Avoid sorbitol (GI necrosis).
Dose: 15 g tds/qds po. NB: takes 24–48 h to work*. Also available as 30-g enemas (rarely $\Rightarrow$ rectal ulceration and colonic necrosis: needs cleansing enema first and washout afterwards; see SPC).

CALCIUM SANDOZ Ca^{2+} supplement syrup; 108.3 mg (2.7 mmol) Ca^{2+}/5 ml.

CALPOL Paracetamol (paediatric) suspension.

Dose: according to age; all doses up to 4-hrly, max qds < 3 mths^{BNF}: 3–6 months 60 mg, 6–24 months 120 mg, 2–4 yrs 180 mg, 6–8 yrs 250 mg, 8–10 yrs 375 mg, 10–12 yrs 500 mg, 12–16 yrs 480–750 mg

NB: Two strengths available: 'standard' INFANT (120 mg/5 ml) and stronger SIX Plus (250 mg/5 ml).

CANDESARTAN/AMIAS
Angiotensin II antagonist.
Use: HTN[1] (*for advice on stepped HTN Mx see p. 235*) or HF[2] (when ACE-i not tolerated).
CI: cholestasis, **L** (if severe)/**P/B**.
Caution/SE/Interactions: see Losartan.
Dose: initially 8 mg od[1] (4 mg if LF, 4 mg if RF/intravascular volume depletion) ↑ing at 4-wk intervals if necessary to max of 32 mg od; initially 4 mg od[2] ↑ing at intervals ≥2 wks to 'target dose' of 32 mg od (or max tolerated). NB: ↓**dose in LF**.

CANESTEN
Clotrimazole 1% cream: antifungal, esp for vaginal candida infections (thrush). Also available as powder, solution and spray for hairy areas.
Dose: apply bd/tds.

CAPTOPRIL
ACE-i: short-acting; largely replaced by longer-acting drugs.
Use: HTN (*for advice on stepped HTN Mx see p. 235*), HF, post-MI, and diabetic nephropathy (i.e. consistent proteinuria).
CI: renovascular disease* (known or suspected bilateral RAS), angioedema/other hypersensitivity 2° to ACE-i, porphyria, **P**.
Caution: symptomatic aortic stenosis, Hx of idiopathic or hereditary angioedema, if taking drugs that ↑K+***, **L/R/B/E**.
SE: ↓BP (esp with 1st dose, if HF, dehydrated or on diuretics, dialysis or ↓Na+ diet ∴ *take at night*), RF*, **dry cough**, ↑K+, acidosis, **hypersensitivity** (esp rashes and **angioedema**), photosensitivity, Δ taste, upper respiratory tract symptoms (inc sore throat/sinusitis/rhinitis), GI upset, Δ LFTs (rarely cholestatic jaundice/hepatitis), pancreatitis, blood disorders, many non-specific neuro symptoms.
Monitor: U&Es, esp baseline and *2 wks after starting**.

Interactions: fx ↓d by NSAIDs (also ⇒ ↑risk RF*). Diuretics, TCAs and antipsychotics ⇒ risk of ↓↓BP. ↑s fx of **lithium** (and antidiabetics). **Dose:** 6.25–75 mg bd po[SPC/BNF]. **NB:** ↓**dose in RF.**

☠ ****Beware if on other drugs that ↑K⁺, e.g. amiloride, spironolactone, triamterene, ARBs and ciclosporin. Don't give with oral K⁺ supplements – inc dietary salt substitutes** ☠.

CARBAMAZEPINE/TEGRETOL

Antiepileptic, mood stabiliser, analgesic; ↓s synaptic transmission.
Use: epilepsy[1] (generalised tonic-clonic and partial seizures, but may exacerbate absence/myoclonic seizures), Px bipolar disorder[2] (if unresponsive to lithium), neuralgia[3] (esp post-herpetic, trigeminal and DM-related).
CI: unpaced AV conduction dfx, Hx of BM suppression, acute porphyria.
Caution: cardiac disease, Hx skin disorders (HLA-B*1502 in Han Chinese or Thai origin have ↑risk of SE – esp SJS), Hx haematological drug reactions, glaucoma, **L/R, P** (⇒ neural tube dfx* ∴ ⇒ folate Px and screen for dfx), **B**.
Dose-related SEs: N&V, headache, drowsiness, dizziness, vertigo, ataxia, visual Δ (esp double vision): control by ↓ing dose, Δ dose times/spacing or use of MR preparations**.
Other SEs: skin reactions (**transient erythema common**), **blood disorders** (esp ↓WCC*** – often transient, ↓Pt, aplastic anaemia), ↑gamma-GT (usually not clinically relevant), oedema, ↓Na⁺ (inc SIADH), HF, arrhythmias. Many rarer SEs[SPC/BNF], including suicidal thoughts/behaviour.
Monitor: U&Es, LFTs, FBC*** ± serum levels (optimum therapeutic range = 4–12 mg/l). Vit D level.
Warn: driving may be impaired, and watch for signs of liver/skin/haematological disease.
Interactions: ↑**P450** ∴ many (see [SPC/BNF]) – may cause failure of OCP; fx are ↑d by **ery-/clari-thromycin**, isoniazid, verapamil and diltiazem; and fx are ↓d by phenytoin, phenobarbitone. ☠ CI with MAOIs ☠. **W–**.

Dose: initially 100–200 mg od/bd ($\uparrow$slowly to max of 1.6 g/day[2,3] or 2 g/day[1]). (MR forms** available[SPC/BNF])

CARBIMAZOLE

Thionamide antithyroid: peroxidase inhibitor; stops $I^- \Rightarrow I_2$ and $\therefore$ $\downarrow$s T_3/T_4 production. Possibly also immunosuppressive fx.

Use: $\uparrow T_4$.

CI: severe blood disorders. Severe **L**.

Caution: L, **P/B** (can cause fetal/neonatal goitre/$\downarrow T_4$ $\therefore$ use min dose to control symptoms and monitor neonatal development closely – 'block-and-replace' regimen $\therefore$ not suitable).

SE: hypersensitivity: rash and **pruritus** (if symptoms not tolerated or not eased by antihistamines, switch to propylthiouracil), fever, arthralgia. Also GI disturbance (esp nausea), headache. Rarely hepatic dysfunction, alopecia, blood disorders – esp **agranulocytosis*** (0.5%) and $\downarrow$WCC (often transient and benign).

Warn/monitor: see box below.

Dose: 15–60 mg/day in 2–3 divided doses ($\downarrow$dose once euthyroid; maintenance dose usually 5–15 mg od, unless on 'block-and-replace' regimen, where $\uparrow$d doses are maintained). *Normally give for only 12–18 months.* Remission often occurs; if not, other Rx (e.g. surgery/radioiodine) may be needed.

> ☠ Agranulocytosis: warn patient to report immediately signs/symptoms of infection (esp sore throat, but also fever, malaise, mouth ulcers, bruising and non-specific illness). If suspect infection, do FBC (routine screening unhelpful as can occur rapidly). Stop drug if clinical or laboratory evidence of $\downarrow$NØ* ☠.

CARVEDILOL

β-blocker: non-selective but also blocks α_1 $\therefore$ $\Rightarrow$ arterial vasodilation.

Use: HF[1] (added to stable treatment). Less commonly for angina[2] and HTN[3] (*for advice on stepped HTN Mx see p. 235*).

CI/Caution: as propranolol, plus **L**. Also **H** if severe *and chronic* HF (caution in severe *and non-chronic* HF, and avoid if acute or decompensated HF needing iv inotropes).

SE: as propranolol, but worse postural ↓BP.

Interactions: as propranolol, but can ↑levels of ciclosporin.

Dose: initially 3.125 mg bd[1] (↑at intervals ≥2 wks to max of 25–50 mg bd); initially 12.5 mg bd[2]/od[3] (can ↑to 50 mg/day).

Before ↑ing dose, check HF and renal function not worsening.

CEFACLOR

Oral 2nd-generation cephalosporin.

Use: mild respiratory infections, UTIs, external infections (skin/soft tissue infections, sinusitis, otitis media), esp in pregnancy* (is one of the safest antibiotics) or dt *H. influenzae*.

CI: cephalosporin hypersensitivity.

Caution: if at ↑risk of **AAC** (e.g. recent other antibiotic use, ↑age, severe underlying disease, ↑hospital/nursing home stay, GI surgery, conditions/drugs that ↓gastric acidity (esp PPIs)), penicillin hypersensitivity (10% also allergic to cephalosporins), **R/P/B** (but appropriate to use*).

SE: GI upset (esp N&D, but also **AAC**), **allergy** (anaphylaxis, fever, arthralgia, skin reactions (inc severe)), **AKI, interstitial nephritis** (reversible), hepatic dysfunction, blood disorders, CNS disturbance (inc headache).

Interactions: levels ↑by probenecid, mild **W +**.

Dose: 250 mg tds po (500 mg tds in severe infections; max 4 g/day). **NB:** ↓dose in RF.

Cephalosporins can ⇒ false-positive Coombs' and urine glucose tests.

CEFALEXIN

Oral 1st-generation cephalosporin.

Use/CI/Caution/SE/Interactions: see Cefaclor and AAC warning.

Dose: 250 mg qds or 500 mg bd/tds po (↑in severe infections to max 1.5 g qds). For Px of UTI, give 125 mg po nocte. **NB:** ↓dose in RF.

CEFOTAXIME

Parenteral 3rd-generation cephalosporin. Good Gram-neg activity, except *Pseudomonas*.

Use: severe infections, esp meningitis and typhoid, UTI, pyelonephritis, soft-tissue infections, gonorrhoea.
CI/Caution/SE/Interactions: see Cefaclor and **AAC warning**, but can also rarely ⇒ arrhythmias if given as rapid iv injection.
Dose: 1 g bd im/iv/ivi (↑ing to max of 3 g qds if needed). **NB:** ↓**dose in RF.**

CEFRADINE

Oral or parenteral 1st-generation cephalosporin.
Use: as cefaclor.
CI/Caution/SE/Interactions: see Cefaclor and **AAC warning**.
Dose: po: 250–500 mg qds *or* 0.5–1 g bd (max 1 g qds). **NB:** ↓**dose in RF.**

CEFTAZIDIME

Parenteral 3rd-generation cephalosporin: good against *Pseudomonas*.
Use: see Cefotaxime (often reserved for ITU setting).
CI/Caution/SE/Interactions: see Cefaclor and **AAC warning**.
Dose: 1 g tds im/iv/ivi, ↑ing (with care in elderly) to 2 g tds or 3 g bd iv (not im, where max single dose is 1 g) if life-threatening, e.g. meningitis, immunocompromised. **NB:** ↓**dose in RF.**

CEFTRIAXONE

Parenteral 3rd-generation cephalosporin.
Use: as cefotaxime, plus pre-operative Px[1].
CI/Caution/SE/Interactions: as Cefaclor and **AAC warning**, plus **L** (if coexistent RF), **R** (if severe), caution if dehydrated, young or immobile (can precipitate in urine or gallbladder). Rarely ⇒ pancreatitis and ↑PT.
Dose: 1 g od im/iv/ivi (max 4 g/day); 1–2 g im/iv/ivi at induction[1]. **NB:** ↓**dose in RF.**
Max im dose = 1 g per site; if total >1 g, give at divided sites.

CEFUROXIME

Parenteral and oral 2nd-generation cephalosporin: good for some Gram-negative infections (*H. influenzae*, *N. gonorrhoeae*) and better than 3rd-generation cephalosporins for Gram-positive infections (esp *S. aureus*).

Use: po: respiratory infections[1], UTIs[2], pyelonephritis[3]; **iv:** severe infections[4], pre-operative Px[5].

CI/Caution/SE/Interactions: see Cefaclor and AAC warning.

Dose: 250–500 mg bd po[1]; 125 mg bd po[2]; 250 mg bd po[3]; 750 mg tds/qds iv/im[4] (1.5 g tds/qds iv in very severe infections and 3 g tds if meningitis); 1.5 g iv at induction (+750 mg iv/im tds for 24 h if high-risk procedure)[5]. **NB: ↓dose in RF.**

CELECOXIB/CELEBREX

NSAID which selectively inhibits COX-2 ∴ ↓GI SEs (COX-1 mediated).

Use: osteoarthritis/RA[NICE], ankylosing spondylitis. Beneficial GI fx (↓bleeding) lost if on aspirin ∴ don't use together.

CI: **IHD, cerebrovascular disease**, *active* bleeding/PU, PVD, hypersensitivity to aspirin or any other NSAID (inc asthma, angioedema, urticaria, rhinitis), *sulphonamide* hypersensitivity, IBD, **L** (if severe)/**R** (GFR<30)/**H** (moderate-severe)/**P/B**.

Caution: Hx of PU/GI bleeding, left ventricular dysfunction, HTN (monitor BP), ↑cardiovascular risk (e.g. DM, ↑lipids, smokers), oedema **H** (mild), asthma. **R*/L**(if either mild-moderate)/**E**.

SE/Interactions: as ibuprofen, but ⇒ ↓PU/GI bleeding (but only if not in combination with aspirin) & ⇒ ↑risk of MI/CVA. Very rarely ⇒ seizures. Also, fluconazole ⇒ ↑serum levels & rifampicin ⇒ ↓serum levels. Mild **W +**.

Dose: 100–200 mg bd po. ↓dose in RF*. Consider gastroprotective Rx.

> **COX-2 inhibitors and ↑risk of cardiovascular complications:** CSM advises assessment of cardiovascular risk and use in preference to other NSAIDs only if at ↑↑risk of GI ulcer, perforation or bleeding. Use lowest effective dose and duration.

CEPH- see CEF-

CETIRIZINE/ZIRTEK

Non-sedating antihistamine: selective peripheral H_1 antagonist; antimuscarinic.

Use: symptomatic relief from allergy (esp hay fever, urticaria).

CI: acute porphyria, **P/B**.

Caution: epilepsy, ↑prostate/urinary retention, glaucoma, pyloroduodenal obstruction, **R/L**.

SE: mild antimuscarinic fx (see p. 276), very mild sedation, headache.

Warn: may impair driving.

Dose: 10 mg od (or 5 mg bd) po. ↓**dose in severe RF.**

CHARCOAL

Binds and ↓s absorption of tablets/poisons.

Use: ODs (up to 1 h post-ingestion; longer if MR/SR preparations or antimuscarinic drugs. See p. 276).

Caution: corrosive poisons, ↓GI motility (can ⇒ obstruction), ↓GCS (risk of aspiration, unless endotracheal tube in situ).

Dose: 50 g po. Give once for paracetamol and most drugs apart from alcohols or metal ions. Repeated doses (every 4 h) often needed for barbiturates, carbamazepine, phenytoin, digoxin, dapsone, paraquat, quinine, salicylates, theophylline and MR/SR preparations.

CHLORAMPHENICOL iv (and po)

Broad-spectrum antibiotic: inhibits bacterial protein synthesis; very potent action, but SEs limit use.

Use: severe infections inc *H. influenzae* and typhoid, esp where other drugs CI, e.g. due to allergy.

CI: porphyria, **L** (avoid if possible)/**P/B**.

Caution: avoid repeated courses **R/E**.

SE: blood disorders (inc aplastic ↓Hb), neuritis (peripheral, optic), GI upset, hepatotoxicity, hypersensitivity, stomatitis, glossitis.

Monitor: FBC, serum drug levels* pre-dose (trough) and 1-h post-dose (peak).

Interactions: ↑s fx of sulphonylureas, phenytoin, ciclosporin and tacrolimus. ↑risk of agranulocytosis with clozapine. Phenobarbital and primidone ↓ its fx. **W +**.
Dose: 50 mg/kg/day in 4 divided doses iv (or rarely po), ↑ing to 100 mg/kg/day if life-threatening infection. **NB:** ↓**dose/check levels*** in **RF and elderly**.

CHLORAMPHENICOL EYE DROPS

Topical antibiotic, with no significant systemic fx, for superficial bacterial eye infections (e.g. conjunctivitis), or as prophylaxis, e.g. postoperatively or for corneal abrasions. Can rarely ⇒ aplastic anaemia.
Dose: 1 drop of 0.5% qds. Can give as 1% ointment qds (or nocte only if using drops in daytime as well).

CHLORDIAZEPOXIDE

Benzodiazepine, long-acting.
Use: anxiety - short term use (esp in alcohol withdrawal).
CI/Caution/SE/Interactions: see Diazepam.
Dose: 10 mg tds po, ↑ing if required to max of 100 mg/day. **NB:** ↓**dose in RF, LF and elderly**. ↑dose if benzodiazepine-resistant or in initial Rx of alcohol withdrawal (see p. 272 for reducing regimen).

CHLORHEXIDINE

Disinfectant mouthwash or solution for skin cleansing before invasive procedures and bladder washout.
CI: avoid contact with eye, middle ear, brain, meninges, body cavities.

CHLOROQUINE

Antimalarial: inhibits protein synthesis and DNA/RNA polymerases.
Use: malaria Px[1] (only as Rx[2] if 'benign' spp (i.e. *P. ovale/vivax/malariae*); *P. falciparum* often resistant. Rarely for RA, SLE.
Caution: G6PD deficiency, severe GI disorders, can worsen psoriasis and MG, neurological disorders (esp epilepsy*), **L** (avoid other hepatotoxic drugs), **R/P**.

SE: GI upset, headache (mild, transient), **visual Δ** (rarely retinopathy**), **seizures***, hypersensitivity/skin reactions (inc pigment Δs), hair loss. Rarely **BM suppression**, cardiomyopathy. Arrhythmias common in OD.

Monitor: FBC, vision** (ophthalmology review if long-term Rx).

Interactions: absorption ↓by antacids. ↑risk of arrhythmias with amiodarone and moxifloxacin. ↑risk of convulsions with mefloquine. ↑s levels of digoxin and ciclosporin. ↓s levels of praziquantel.

Dose: Px[1]: 300 mg once wkly **as base** (*specify on prescription: don't confuse with* **salt** *doses*). Used mostly in conjunction with other drugs, depending on local resistance patterns[SPC/BNF]. **Rx[2]:** see p. 268. NB: ↓**dose in RF.**

CHLORPHEN(IR)AMINE/PIRITON

Antihistamine: H[1] antagonist (peripheral *and central* ∴ sedating).

Use: allergies[1] (esp drug reactions, hay fever, urticaria), anaphylaxis[2] (inc blood transfusion reaction[3]).

CI: hypersensitivity to any antihistamine.

Caution: pyloroduodenal obstruction, urinary retention/↑prostate, thyrotoxicosis, asthma, bronch-itis/-iectasis, severe HTN/ cardiovascular disease, glaucoma, epilepsy, **R/L/P/B.**

SE: drowsiness (rarely paradoxical stimulation), **antimuscarinic fx** (esp dry mouth; see p. 276), GI upset, arrhythmias, ↓BP, skin and hypersensitivity reactions (inc bronchospasm, photosensitivity). If given iv can cause transient CNS stimulation.

Warn: driving may be impaired.

Interactions: can ↑phenytoin levels. ☠ **MAOIs** can ⇒ ↑↑antimuscarinic fx (SPC says chlorphenamine CI if MAOI given w/ in 2 wks but evidence unclear)☠.

Dose: 4 mg 4–6-hrly po[1](max 24 mg/24 h)↓**E**; 10 mg iv over 1 min[2] (can ↑to 20 mg, max 40 mg/24 h); 10–20 mg sc[3] (max 40 mg/24 h).

CHLORPROMAZINE

Phenothiazine ('typical') antipsychotic: dopamine antagonist (D[1 and 3] > D[2 and 4]). Also blocks serotonin ($5HT_{2A}$), histamine (H[1]), adrenergic ($\alpha_{1>2}$) and muscarinic receptors, causing many SEs.

L/R/H = Liver, Renal and Heart failure (full key see p. xv)

Use: schizophrenia, acute sedation (inc mania, severe anxiety, violent behaviour), resistant migraine headache[1], intractable hiccups.

CI: CNS depression (inc coma), elderly patients with dementia, Hx of blood dyscrasias, severe cardiovascular disease.

Caution: Parkinson's, drugs that ↑QTc, epilepsy, MG, phaeo, glaucoma (angle-closure), ↑prostate, severe respiratory disease, jaundice, blood disorders, predisposition to postural ↓BP, ↑or ↓temperature. Avoid direct sunlight (⇒ photosensitivity), **L/R/H/P/B/E.**

Class SE: sedation, extrapyramidal fx (see p. 278), **antimuscarinic fx** (see p. 276), **seizures**, **↑Wt**, **↓BP** (esp postural), ECG Δs (↑QTc), arrhythmias, endocrine fx (menstrual Δs, galactorrhoea, gynaecomastia, sexual dysfunction), ΔLFTs/jaundice, blood disorders (inc agranulocytosis, ↓WCC), ↓ or ↑temperature (esp in elderly), rash/↑pigmentation, **neuroleptic malignant syndrome**. Don't crush tablets (contact hypersensitivity; also possible from iv solution).

Warn: avoid alcohol/direct sunlight, ↓s skilled tasks (e.g. driving).

Monitor: FBC, BP.

Interactions: May ↑sedation caused by alcohol and sedative medications. May ↑hypotension caused by other medications, fx ↑d by TCAs (esp antimuscarinic fx), lithium (esp extrapyramidal fx ± neurotoxicity), ritonavir, cimetidine and β-blockers (esp arrhythmias with sotalol; propranolol fx also ↑d by chlorpromazine). ↑risk of CNS toxicity with sibutramine. Avoid artemether/lumefantrine and drugs that ↑QTc or risk of ventricular arrhythmias (e.g. disopyramide, moxifloxacin).

Dose: 25–300 mg tds po[SPC/BNF]; 25–50 mg tds/qds im (painful, and may ⇒ ↓BP/↑HR); 0.2 mg/kg iv[1]. **NB:** **↓dose in elderly (approx 1/3–1/2 adult dose but 10 mg od po may suffice) or if severe RF.**

CICLESONIDE/ALVESCO

Inh corticosteroid for asthma Px, similar to beclomethasone but od.

Caution: L.

Dose: 80–160 microgram od inh (aerosol).

CICLOSPORIN

Calcineurin inhibitor: $\Rightarrow \downarrow$IL-2-mediated LØ proliferation.

Use: immunosuppression (esp nephrotic syndrome and post-transplant), atopic dermatitis, psoriasis, RA.

CI: *only apply if given for nephrotic syndrome*: uncontrolled infection or HTN, malignancy. Avoid co-treatment with sirolimus.

Caution: HTN, $\uparrow$urate, porphyria, drugs that $\uparrow$K⁺, **L/R/P/B/E.**

SE: nephrotoxicity and tremor (both dose-related), $\uparrow$BP, hepatotoxicity, GI upset, biochemical Δs ($\uparrow$K⁺, $\uparrow$urate/gout, $\downarrow$Mg²⁺, $\uparrow$cholesterol, $\uparrow$glucose), pancreatitis. Rarely neuromuscular symptoms, HUS, neoplasms (esp lymphoma), BIH, encephalopathy, demyelination (esp if liver transplant).

Warn: hypertrichosis, gingival hypertrophy, avoid XS sun exposure (photosensitivity); burning sensation in hands and feet.

Monitor: levels, LFTs, U&Es, Mg²⁺, lipids, BP.

Interactions: metab by **P450**, ∴ many, particularly antibacterials and antifungals[SPC/BNF] (cephalosporins and penicillins OK). Levels esp $\downarrow$by phenytoin, carbamazepine, phenobarbital, St John's wort, rifampicin, orlistat, ticlopidine and octreotide. Levels esp $\uparrow$by ery-/clari-thromycin, keto-/flu-/itra-conazole, protease inhibitors, diltiazem, nicardipine, verapamil, metoclopramide, amiodarone, allopurinol, danazol, ursodeoxycholic acid, corticosteroids and OCP. Can $\uparrow$levels of digoxin and diclofenac. Nephrotoxic and myotoxic drugs can become more so.

Dose: specialist use[SPC/BNF]. Must prescribe by brand name (**Neoral, Sandimmun** or **SangCya**) as have different bioavailabilities and changing brands can ∴ $\downarrow$immunosuppression or $\uparrow$toxicity. **NB: dose adjustment needed if LF or RF.**

> 🐝 Check all new drugs for interactions before prescribing if on ciclosporin: $\uparrow$d levels $\Rightarrow$ toxicity; $\downarrow$d levels may $\Rightarrow$ rejection. 🐝

CIMETIDINE

As ranitidine, but $\uparrow\uparrow$interactions ($\downarrow$ P450 and **W +**) and $\uparrow$gynaecomastia ∴ prescribed rarely. **Dose:** 400 mg bd (can $\uparrow$to 4-hrly[SPC/BNF]). NB: $\downarrow$dose if LF or RF.

CIPROFLOXACIN

(Fluoro)quinolone antibiotic: inhibits DNA gyrase; 'cidal' with broad spectrum, but particularly good for Gram-negative infections.

Use: GI infections[1] (esp salmonella, shigella, campylobacter), **respiratory infections** (non-pneumococcal pneumonias[2], esp *Pseudomonas*). Also GU infections (esp UTIs[3], acute uncomplicated cystitis in women[4], gonorrhoea[5]), 1st-line initial Rx of anthrax.

CI: hypersensitivity to any quinolone, **P/B**.

Caution: seizures (inc Hx of, or predisposition to), MG (can worsen), G6PD deficiency, children/adolescents (theoretical risk of arthropathy), avoid ↑urine pH or dehydration*, **R**.

SE: GI upset (esp N&D, sometimes AAC), pancreatitis, **neuro-Ψ fx** (esp confusion, **seizures**; also headache, dizziness, hallucinations, sleep and mood Δs), **tendinitis ± rupture** (esp if elderly or taking steroids), chest pain, oedema, **hypersensitivity** (rash, pruritis, fever). Rarely hepatotoxicity, RF/interstitial nephritis, crystalluria*, blood disorders, ↑glucose, skin reactions (inc photosensitivity**, SJS, TEN).

Warn: avoid UV light**, avoid ingesting Fe- and Zn-containing products (e.g. antacids***). May impair skilled tasks/driving.

Interactions: ↑s levels of theophyllines; NSAIDs ⇒ ↑risk of seizures; ↑s nephrotoxicity of ciclosporin; FeSO$_4$ and antacids*** ⇒ ↓ciprofloxacin absorption (give 2 h before or 6 h after ciprofloxacin), **W +**.

Dose: 250–750 mg bd po, 100–400 mg bd ivi (each dose over 1 h) according to indication[SPC/BNF] (100 mg bd po for 3 days for cystitis); 500 mg po single dose[4]; 100 mg iv single dose[5]. **NB: ↓dose if severe RF.**

☠ Stop if tendinitis, severe neuro-Ψ fx or hypersensitivity ☠.

CITALOPRAM/CIPRAMIL

SSRI antidepressant.

Use: depression[1] (and panic disorder). Useful if polypharmacy, as ↓interactions and ↓cardio-/hepato-toxicity cf other SSRIs.

CI/Caution/SE/Warn: as fluoxetine, but ↑risk of withdrawal syndrome if stopped abruptly. Can also ↑QT_c (dose dependent); CI if ↑QT_c (or congenital ↑QT_c syndrome or taking other drugs that can ↑QT_c) and caution if ↑risk torsades de pointes (e.g. congestive HF, recent MI, bradyarrhythmias, predisposition to ↓K^+ or ↓Mg^{2+} dt concomitant illness or medicines), epilepsy.

Interaction: ☠ Never give with, or <2 wks after, MAOIs ☠.
Dose: 20 mg od[1] ↑ing if necessary to max 40 mg (max 20 mg **if** elderly or **LF**).

CITRAMAG see Bowel preparations
CI: GI obstruction or perforation. **R** (if severe).
Caution: risk of ↑ Mg^{2+} in RF.
Dose: 1 sachet at 8 am and 3 pm the day before GI surgery or Ix.

CLARITHROMYCIN

Macrolide antibiotic: binds 50S ribosome.
Use: as erythromycin; (see p. 65), part of triple therapy for *H. pylori*.
CI/Caution/SE/Interactions: as erythromycin, but ⇒ ↓GI SEs.
Dose: 250–500 mg bd po or 500 mg bd iv. **NB:** ↓**dose if RF.**

CLEXANE see Enoxaparin; low-molecular-weight heparin.

CLINDAMYCIN

Antibiotic; same action (but different structure and ∴ class) as clarithromycin; good against staphylococci, streptococci and anaerobes (esp bacteroides); penetrates bone well.
Use: cellulitis, osteomyelitis, intra-abdominal sepsis, endocarditis Px, falciparum malaria. Alternative to penicillin in case of allergy. *Use limited due to SEs (esp AAC).*
CI: diarrhoea.
Caution: GI disease, porphyria, atopy, **L/R/P/B**.
SE: GI upset (often ⇒ **AAC**), hepatotoxicity, blood disorders, local reactions at injection site, arthralgia, myalgia, hypersensitivity.
Monitor: U&Es, LFTs.

Interactions: ↑s fx of neuromuscular blocking agents.
Dose: 150–450 mg qds po; 0.6–4.8 g daily in divided doses im/ivi (doses >600 mg must be as ivi), max single dose iv is 1.2 g.

> 🐝 Stop drug if diarrhoea develops: AAC common and potentially very severe.

CLOBETASOL PROPIONATE 0.05% CREAM OR OINTMENT/DERMOVATE
Very-potent-strength topical corticosteroid.
Use: short-term Rx of severe inflammatory skin conditions (esp discoid lupus, lichen simplex and palmar plantar psoriasis).
CI: untreated infection including H. zoster, rosacea, acne.
SE: skin atrophy, worsening of infections, acne (↑SEs cf less potent topical steroids).
Dose: apply thinly od/bd, usually under specialist supervision.

CLOBETASONE BUTYRATE 0.05% CREAM OR OINTMENT/EUMOVATE
Moderately-potent-strength topical corticosteroid.
Use: inflammatory skin conditions, esp eczema, dermatitis.
CI: untreated infection, rosacea, acne.
SE: skin atrophy, worsening of infections, acne.
Dose: apply thinly od/bd.

CLONAZEPAM
Benzodiazepine; long-acting
Use: epilepsy (all forms[1] inc status epilepticus[2]). Not licensed, but often used, for Ψ disorders[3] (esp psychosis and mania).
CI/Caution/SE/Warn/Interactions: see Diazepam.
Dose: 0.5–1 mg ↑ing according to response to max 20 mg/day[1/3] in divided doses; 1 mg iv (over ≥2 min) or as ivi[2].

CLOPIDOGREL/PLAVIX
Antiplatelet agent: ADP receptor antagonist. ↑antiplatelet fx cf aspirin (but also ↑SEs).

Use: Px of atherothrombotic events if STEMI or NSTEMI (for 12 months in combination with aspirin, aspirin continued indefinitely), MI (within 'a few' to 35 days), ischaemic CVA (within 7 days to 6 months) or peripheral arterial disease. For use in ACS (see p. 226).
CI: active bleeding, **L** (if severe – otherwise caution), **B**.
Caution: ↑bleeding risk; trauma, surgery, drugs that ↑bleeding risk (*avoid with* **warfarin**), ↓fx by omeprazole, esomeprazole. **R/P**.
SE: haemorrhage (esp GI or intracranial), **GI upset**, PU, pancreatitis, headache, fatigue, dizziness, paraesthesia, rash/pruritus, hepatobiliary/respiratory/blood disorders (↓NØ, ↑EØ, very rarely, TTP).
Monitor: FBC and for signs of occult bleeding (esp after invasive procedures).
Dose: 75 mg od. If not already on clopidogrel, usually load with 300 mg for ACS then 75 mg od starting next day. If pre-PCI, load with 300–600 mg usually on morning of procedure.

Stop 7 days before operations if antiplatelet fx not wanted (e.g. major surgery); discuss with surgeons doing operation.

CLOTRIMAZOLE/CANESTEN

Imidazole antifungal (topical).
Use: external candida infections (esp vaginal thrush).
Caution: can damage condoms and diaphragms.
Dose: 2–3 applications/day of 1% cream, continuing for 14 days after lesion healed. Also available as powder/solution/spray for hairy areas, as pessary, and in 2% strength. See more[BNF/SPC]

CLOZAPINE

Atypical antipsychotic: blocks dopamine ($D_4 > D_1 > D_{2 \text{ and } 3}$) and $5HT_{2A}$ receptors. Also mild blockade of muscarinic and adrenergic receptors.
Use: schizophrenia, but only if resistant or intolerant (e.g. severe extrapyramidal fx) to other antipsychotics[NICE].
CI: severe cardiac disorders (inc Hx of circulatory collapse, myocarditis, cardiomyopathy), coma/severe CNS depression, alcoholic/toxic psychosis, drug intoxication, Hx of agranulocytosis or ↓NØ,

bone marrow disorders, paralytic ileus, uncontrolled epilepsy, **R/H** (if severe, otherwise caution), **L** (inc active liver disease), **B**.
Caution: Hx of epilepsy, cardiovascular disease, ↑prostate, glaucoma (angle-closure), **P/E**.
SE: as olanzapine, but also can ⇒ ↓NØ* (3% of patients) and 💀 **agranulocytosis** 💀 (1%). Also commonly ⇒ ↑**salivation** (Rx with hyoscine hydrobromide), ↓**BP** (esp during initial titration), **constipation** (can ⇒ ileus/obstruction: have low threshold for giving laxatives), ↑Wt, sedation. Less commonly seizures, urinary incontinence, priapism, **myocarditis/cardiomyopathy** (*stop immediately!*), ↑HR, arrhythmias, hyperglycaemia, N&V, ↑BP, delirium, RF, ↓Pt. Rarely hepatic dysfunction (*stop immediately!*), ↑TG, neuroleptic malignant syndrome.
Monitor: FBC*, BP (esp during start of Rx), serum levels (pre-dose) and cardiac function (get baseline ECG/watch for persistent ↑HR).
Warn: to report symptoms of infection, e.g. fever, sore throat.
Interactions: as chlorpromazine, plus care with all drugs that constipate, ↑QT threshold or ↓leucopoiesis (e.g. cytotoxics, sulphonamides/co-trimoxazole, chloramphenicol, penicillamine, carbamazepine, phenothiazines, esp depots). Caffeine, risperidone, SSRIs, cimetidine and erythromycin ↑clozapine levels. Smoking, carbamazepine and phenytoin ↓clozapine levels.
Dose: initially 12.5 mg nocte, ↑ing to 200–450 mg/day^{SPC/BNF} usually given bd (max 900 mg/day). ↓doses if elderly.

If >2 days' doses missed, restart at 12.5 mg od and ↑gradually.

Monitoring: primarily to avoid fatal agranulocytosis, is done by the manufacturers: in the UK Clozaril Patient Monitoring Service (tel: 0845 7698269), Denzapine Monitoring Service (tel: 01635 568500) or Zaponex Treatment Access System (tel: 0207 3655842). Register and then authorise/monitor baseline and subsequent FBCs* and serum levels*. *These are very useful resources for all clozapine questions.*

CO-AMILOFRUSE

Diuretic combination preparation for oedema that keeps K^+ stable: amiloride (K^+-sparing) + furosemide (K^+-wasting) in 3 strengths of tablet as 2.5/20, 5/40 and 10/80 (reflecting amiloride mg/furosemide mg).
Monitor: BP, U&Es.
Dose: 1 tablet mane (NB: *specify strength!*).

CO-AMILOZIDE

Diuretic combination preparation for HTN (*for advice on stepped HTN Mx see p. 235*), CCF and oedema. Keeps K^+ stable: amiloride (K^+-sparing) + hydrochlorothiazide (K^+-wasting) in 2 strengths of tablet as 2.5/25 and 5/50 (reflecting amiloride mg/ hydrochlorothiazide mg).
Caution: crystalluria esp if ↑dose or RF.
Monitor: BP, U&Es.
Dose: 1/2–4 tablets daily, according to tablet strength and indication[SPC/BNF].

CO-AMOXICLAV/AUGMENTIN

Combination of amoxicillin + clavulanic acid (β-lactamase inhibitor) to overcome resistance.
Use: UTIs, respiratory/skin/soft-tissue (plus many other) infections. Reserve for when β-lactamase-producing strains known/strongly suspected or other Rx has failed.
CI/Caution/SE/Interactions: as ampicillin, plus caution if anticoagulated, **L** (↑risk of cholestasis), **P**.
Dose: as amoxicillin Dose: 250 mg tds po (500 mg tds po if severe); 1 g tds/qds iv/ivi. Non-proprietary and as **Augmentin**. NB: ↓**dose if LF**.

CO-BENELDOPA/MADOPAR

L-dopa + benserazide (peripheral dopa-decarboxylase inhibitor).
Use: Parkinsonism.
CI/Caution/SE/Warn/Interactions: see Levodopa.

Dose: (*expressed as levodopa only*) initially 50 mg tds/qds, ↑ing total dose and number of doses, according to response, to usual maintenance of 400–800 mg/day (↓in elderly)$^{BNF/SPC}$. Available in dispersible form.

CO-CARELDOPA/SINEMET
L-dopa + carbidopa (peripheral dopa-decarboxylase inhibitor).
Use: Parkinsonism.
CI/Caution/SE/Warn/Interactions: see Levodopa.
Dose: (*expressed as levodopa only*) initially 100 mg tds, ↑ing total dose and number of doses, according to response, to usual maintenance of 400–800 mg/day (↓in elderly)$^{BNF/SPC}$. Available in dispersible form.

CO-CODAMOL (30/500) = codeine 30 mg + paracetamol 500 mg per tablet.
Use/CI/Caution/SE/Interactions: see Paracetamol and Codeine.
Warning: prescribe by dose as also available as 8/500 and 15/500.
Dose: 2 tablets qds prn. NB: ↓dose if LF, RF or elderly.

CO-DANTHRAMER see Dantron; stimulant laxative - palliative care.
Dose: 1–2 capsules or 5–10 ml suspension nocte (available in regular and strong formulations).

CO-DANTHRUSATE see Dantron; stimulant laxative - palliative care.
Dose: 1–3 capsules or 5–15 ml suspension nocte.

CODEINE (PHOSPHATE)
Weak opiate analgesic. Mainly metabolised to morphine.
Use: mild/moderate pain, diarrhoea, anti-tussive.
CI: acute respiratory depression, risk of ileus, ↑ICP/head injury/coma.
Caution: all other conditions where morphine is either contraindicated or cautioned.
SE: as morphine, but milder. **Constipation** is the major problem: dose and length of Rx-dependent; anticipate this and give laxative Px as appropriate, esp in elderly. Also sedation, esp if LF.

Interactions: ☠ MAOIs: don't give within 2 weeks of ☠. As morphine, but does not interact with baclofen, gabapentin and ritonavir.
Dose: 30–60 mg up to 4-hrly po/im (max 240 mg/24 h). Genetic ultrarapid metabolisers (3% of Europeans, 8% of Americans, 40% of North Africans) risk serious toxicity & poor metabolisers obtain little analgesia. Watch closely when initiating & adjust dose/change drug accordingly. NB: ↓dose if LF, RF or elderly.

CO-DYDRAMOL Dihydrocodeine 10/20/30 mg + paracetamol 500 mg per tablet (10/500, 20/500, 30/500).
Dose: 1–2 tablets 4–6 hrly, max qds po. Usually prescribed 2 tablets qds (prn). NB: ↓dose if LF, RF or elderly.

COLCHICINE

Anti-gout: binds to tubulin of leucocytes and stops their migration to uric acid deposits ∴ ⇒ ↓inflammation. NB: slow action (needs >6 h to work).
Use: gout: Rx of acute attacks or Px when starting allopurinol* (which can initially ↑symptoms) or awaiting other drugs to work.
CI: blood dyscrasias, P-glycoprotein and strong CYP3A4 inhibitors. **P**
Caution: GI diseases, **L/H/R/B/E**.
SE: GI upset (N&V&D and **abdominal pain** – all common and dose-related). Rarely GI haemorrhage, hypersensitivity, renal/hepatic impairment, peripheral neuritis, myopathy, alopecia, ↓spermatogenesis (reversible), blood disorders (if prolonged Rx).
Interactions: ↑s nephro-/myo-toxicity of ciclosporin and myopathy of simvastatin. fx ↓by thiazide diuretics. Toxicity ↑by erythromycin and tolbutamide.
Dose: 0.5 mg bd/qds until relief (start ASAP after symptom onset). Max. 6 mg. More aggressive regimens exist[SPC/BNF] but ⇒ ↑GI upset w/o significant ↑in response. Continue 0.5 mg bd when starting allopurinol*. Do not repeat course within 3 days. NB: ↓dose if RF.

COLESTYRAMINE

Anion exchange resin. Binds bile acids in gut preventing reabsorption; ⇒ ↑hepatic cholesterol ⇒ bile acids; ⇒ ↑hepatic LDL receptors ⇒ ↑LDL cholesterol plasma clearance.

Use: pruritus (2° to PBC or partial biliary obstruction)[1], diarrhoeal disorders[2]. *If diet and other measures insufficient*: hyperlipidaemia[3] (esp type IIa), Px of IHD[4], 1° hypercholesterolaemia[5].
CI: ineffective in complete biliary obstruction.
Caution: Risk of ↓ fat soluble vitamins. Sachets contain sucrose or aspartame. DM. **P/B**.
SE: ↓Vits A/D/K, ↑bleeding risk, taste Δ, GI upset/obstruction, ↑Cl⁻ acidosis.
Warn: take other drugs >1 h before or > 4–6 h after colestyramine*.
Monitor: for vitamin deficiency (and INR if on warfarin).
Interactions: delay or ↓drug absorption* inc digoxin, tetracycline, chlorothiazide, thyroxine. **W +** *or* **W–**.
Dose: initially 4 g od, ↑ing if required by 4 g/wk to 8 g/day[1] (max 36 g/day[2,3,4,5])
NB: take with ⩾150 ml suitable liquid/4 g sachet.

CO-MAGALDROX antacid (AlOH + MgOH).
Dose: 10–20 ml 20–60 min after meals, and at bedtime or prn.

COMBIVENT Compound bronchodilator (salbutamol + ipratropium bromide).
Dose: 2.5 ml (one vial: ipratropium 500 microgram + salbutamol 2.5 mg) tds/qds neb[SPC/BNF].

CORSODYL Chlorhexidine mouthwash for Rx/Px of mouth infections (inc MRSA eradication); see local infection protocol.

CO-TRIAMTERZIDE

Diuretic for HTN[1](*for advice on stepped HTN Mx see p. 235*), or oedema[2]: triamterene (↑s K⁺) combined with hydrochlorothiazide (↓s K⁺) to keep K⁺ stable.
Monitor: BP, U&Es.
Dose: initially 1 tablet[1] (or 2 tablets[2]) mane of 50/25 strength (= 50 mg triamterene + 25 mg hydrochlorothiazide), ↑ing if necessary to max of 4 tablets/day.

CO-TRIMOXAZOLE/SEPTRIN

Antibiotic combination preparation: 5 to 1 mixture of sulfamethoxazole (a sulphonamide) + trimethoprim ⇒ synergistic action.

Use: PCP; other uses limited due to SEs (also rarely used for toxoplasmosis and nocardiosis).

CI: porphyria, **L/R** (if either severe, otherwise caution).

Caution: blood disorders, asthma, G6PD deficiency, risk factors for ↓folate **P/B/E**.

SE: skin reactions (inc SJS, TEN), **blood disorders** (↓NØ, ↓Pt, ↓Glucose, BM suppression, agranulocytosis) relatively common, esp in elderly. Also N&V&D (inc AAC), nephrotoxicity, hepatotoxicity, hypersensitivity, anorexia, abdo pain, glossitis, stomatitis, pancreatitis, arthralgia, myalgia, SLE, pulmonary infiltrates, seizures, ataxia, myocarditis.

Interactions: ↑s phenytoin levels. ↑s risk of arrhythmias with amiodarone, crystalluria with methenamine, antifolate fx with pyrimethamine, agranulocytosis with clozapine and toxicity with ciclosporin, azathioprine, mercaptopurine and methotrexate. **W +.**

Dose: PCP Rx: 120 mg/kg/day po/ivi in 2–4 divided doses (PCP Px 480–960 mg od po). PCP Px[BNF/SPC]. **NB:** ↓dose if RF.

☠ Stop immediately if rash or blood disorder occurs ☠

CYCLIZINE

Antihistamine antiemetic.

Use: N&V Rx/Px (esp 2° to iv/im opioids, but not 1st choice in angina/MI/LVF*), vertigo, motion sickness, labyrinthine disorders.

CI/Caution/SE/Warn: as chlorphenamine, but also avoid in severe HF* (may undo haemodynamic benefits of opioids). Antimuscarinic fx (see p. 276) are most prominent SEs.

Dose: 50 mg po/im/iv tds.

CYCLOPENTOLATE 0.5%/1% EYE DROPS/MYDRILATE

For pupil dilation (for pain relief and prevention of complications in uveitis). Also cycloplegic (paralyses accommodation); useful for refracting children.

SE: blurred vision.
Dose: 1 drop (tds for prolonged use). 30 min to work, lasts several hours.

CYCLOPHOSPHAMIDE

Cytotoxic[1] and immunosuppressant[2]: alkylating agent (cross-links DNA bases, ↓ing replication).
Use: cancer[1], autoimmune diseases[2]: esp vasculitis (inc rheumatoid arthritis, ANCA-associated vasculitis and SLE (esp if renal/cerebral involvement)), systemic sclerosis, Wegener's, nephrotic syndrome in children.
CI: haemorrhagic cystitis, **P/B**.
Caution: BM suppression, severe infections, **L/R**.
SE: GI upset, alopecia (reversible). Others rare but important: hepatotoxicity, blood disorders, malignancy (esp acute myeloid leukaemia), ↓fertility (can be permanent), cardiac toxicity, pulmonary fibrosis (at high doses), haemorrhagic cystitis (only if given iv: ensure good hydration, give 'mesna' as Px; can occur months after Rx).
Warn: ↓fertility may be permanent (bank sperm if possible) – need to counsel and obtain consent regarding this before giving.
Monitor: FBC.
Interactions: can ↑fx of oral hypoglycaemics. ↑risk of agranulo-cytosis with clozapine and toxicity with pentostatin.
Dose: specialist use only. NB: ↓dose if LF or RF.

☠ Stop immediately if rash or blood disorder occurs ☠.

CYCLOSPORIN see Ciclosporin

CYPROTERONE ACETATE

Anti-androgen; blocks androgen receptors. Also ↑s progestogens.
Use: Ca prostate[1] (as adjunct), acne[2] (esp 2° to PCOS, where often used with ethinylestradiol as co-cyprindiol), rarely for hypersexuality/sexual deviation[3] (*males only!*).
CI: (*none apply if for Ca prostate*) advanced DM (if vascular disease), sickle cell, malignancy/wasting diseases, Hx of TE, age

<18 years (can ⇒ ↓bone/testicular development), severe depression, **L/P/B**.
SE: fatigue, gynaecomastia, ↑or ↓Wt, hepatotoxicity, blood disorders, hypersensitivity, osteoporosis, ↓spermatogenesis (reversible), TE, depression, carbohydrate metabolism and hair Δs.
Monitor: FBC, LFTs, adrenocortical function.
Warn: driving and other skilled tasks may be impaired.
Dose: 200–300 mg po daily in divided doses[1], 50 mg bd po[3].

▼ DABIGATRAN (ETEXILATE)/PRADAXA

Oral anticoagulant; direct thrombin inhibitor. Rapid onset and doesn't require therapeutic monitoring (unlike warfarin).
Use: Px of VTE (after THR/TKR)[1]; and non-valve AF embolism[BNF,2].
CI: active bleeding, impaired haemostasis, **L** (if severe) **P/B**.
Caution: bleeding disorders, active GI ulceration, recent surgery, bacterial endocarditis, anaesthesia with postoperative indwelling epidural catheter (risk of paralysis; give initial dose ≥2 h after catheter removal and monitor for neurological signs), weight <50 kg, **R** (avoid if creatinine clearance <30 ml/min) **H/E**.
SE: haemorrhage, hepatobiliary disorders.
Monitor: for ↓Hb or signs of bleeding (stop drug if severe).
Interactions: NSAIDs ↑risk of bleeding. Levels ↑by amiodarone*.
Dose: 110 mg (75 mg if >75 years old) 1–4 h after surgery then 220 mg od (150 mg if >75 years old) for 9 days after knee replacement or 27–34 days after hip replacement[1]; 150 mg po bd[2].
NB: ↓dose in RF, elderly or if taking amiodarone*.

▼ DALTEPARIN/FRAGMIN

Low-molecular-weight heparin (LMWH).
Use: DVT/PE Rx[1] and Px[2] (inc pre-operative), ACS (with aspirin)[3].
CI/Caution/SE/Monitor/Interactions: see Heparin.
Dose: *all sc:* 200 units/kg (max 18000 units) od[1]; 2500–5000 units od[2] (according to risk[SPC/BNF]) for ≥5 days; 120 units/kg bd[3] for ≥5 days (max 10000 units bd) reviewing dose if >8 days needed[SPC/BNF].

Consider monitoring anti Xa (3–4 h post dose) $\pm$ ↓dose if RF (i.e. creatinine >150), pregnancy, Wt >100 kg or <45 kg; see p. 209.

DANTRON
Stimulant laxative; theoretical risk of **carcinogenicity***.
Use: constipation (often limited to the terminally ill*).
Caution/SE: see Senna; possible carcinogenic risk. (CI if GI obstruction, **P/B**)
Dose: see Co-danthramer and Co-danthrusate.

DARBEPOETIN see Erythropoietin (recombinant form for ↓Hb).

DERMOVATE see Clobetasol propionate (steroid) cream 0.05%.

DESFERRIOXAMINE
Chelating agent; binds Fe (and Al) in gut ↓ing absorption/↑ing clearance.
Use: ↑Fe: acute (OD/poisoning[1]), chronic (e.g. xs transfusions for blood disorders, haemochromatosis when venesection CI). Also for ↑Al (e.g. 2° to dialysis).
Caution: Al-induced encephalopathy (may worsen), ↑risk of *Yersinia*/mucormycosis infection **R/P/B**.
SE: ↓BP (related to rate of ivi), lens opacities, retinopathy, GI upset, blood disorders, hypersensitivity. Also neurological/respiratory/renal dysfunction. ↑doses can ⇒ ↓growth and bone Δs.
Monitor: vision and hearing during chronic **Rx**.
Dose: acutely up to 15 mg/kg/h ivi (max 80 mg/kg/day)[1]. Otherwise according to degree of Fe or Al overload[SPC/BNF].

DEXAMETHASONE 0.1% EYE DROPS/MAXIDEX
Topical corticosteroid.
Use: uveitis, Px of post-eye surgery anterior segment inflammation.
CI: ocular infection.
SE: ocular infection (aggravation of existing or ↑susceptibility) or ocular HTN. If prolonged use, glaucoma and cataract possible.
Dose: 1 drop qds (max 1-hrly); specialist use only.

DEXAMETHASONE PHOSPHATE

Glucocorticoid; minimal mineralocorticoid activity, long duration of action (see p. 217).

Use: cerebral oedema (from malignancy), spinal cord compression, Dx of Cushing's, N&V (2° to chemotherapy or surgery), allergy/inflammation (esp if unresponsive shock), congenital adrenal hyperplasia, rheumatic disease.

CI/Caution/SE/Warn/Interactions: see Prednisolone and steroids section (p. 217).

Dose: cerebral oedema: acutely 10 mg iv, then 4 mg im qds 2–4 days (if not life-threatening, some go straight to 4 mg qds iv then switch to po a few days later, stopped gradually over 5–7 days). For other indications, see SPC/BNF.

> ☠ Doses given here are for dexamethasone phosphate and must be prescribed as such: other forms have different doses ☠ !

DF118 (suffix FORTE often omitted) Dihydrocodeine 40 mg.
Dose: 40–80 mg tds po.

> NB: tablets are different dose to non-proprietary dihydrocodeine.

DIAMORPHINE (HEROIN HYDROCHLORIDE)

Strong opiate (1.5 × strength of morphine if both given iv).
Use: severe pain (acute and chronic)[1], AMI[2], acute LVF[3].
CI/Caution/SE/Interactions: as morphine, but less nausea/↓BP, and does not interact with baclofen, gabapentin and ritonavir.

☠ Respiratory depression ☠ (esp elderly)

Dose: 5–10 mg sc/im (or 1/4–1/2 this dose iv) up to 4-hrly[1]; 5 mg iv (at 1–2 mg/min) followed by further 2.5–5 mg if necessary[2]; 0.5–1 mg iv (at 0.5 mg/min)[3]. Can give via sc pump in chronic pain/palliative care. **NB: ↓dose if elderly, LF or RF**[BNF/SPC].

DIAZEMULS iv diazepam emulsion: ⇒ ↓venous irritation.

DIAZEPAM

Benzodiazepine, long-acting.

Use: seizures (esp status epilepticus[1], febrile convulsions), *short-term* Rx of acute alcohol withdrawal[2], anxiety[3], insomnia[4] (if also anxiety; if not, then shorter-acting forms preferred as $\Rightarrow$ $\downarrow$hangover sedation). Also used for muscle spasm[5].

CI: respiratory depression, marked neuromuscular respiratory weakness inc unstable myasthenia gravis, sleep apnoea, acute pulmonary insufficiency, chronic psychosis, depression (don't give diazepam alone), **L** (if severe).

Caution: respiratory disease, muscle weakness (inc MG), Hx of drug/alcohol abuse, personality disorder, porphyria, **R/P/B/E**.

SE: **respiratory depression (rarely apnoea), drowsiness, dependence.** Also ataxia, amnesia, headache, vertigo, GI upset, jaundice, $\downarrow$BP, $\downarrow$HR, visual/libido/urinary disturbances, blood disorders, paradoxical disinhibition in Ψ disorder.

Warn: sedation $\uparrow$by alcohol and $\Rightarrow$ $\downarrow$driving/skilled task ability.

Interactions: metab by **P450** $\therefore$ many: ery-/clari-/-teli-thromycin, quinu-/dalfo-pristin and flu-/itra-/keto-/posa-conazole can $\uparrow$levels. Sedative fx $\uparrow$by antipsychotics, antidepressants, antiepileptics and antiretrovirals. Can $\uparrow$fx of zidovudine and sodium oxybate. $\uparrow$risk of $\downarrow$HR/BP and respiratory depression with im olanzapine.

Dose: for status epilepticus[1] and alcohol withdrawal[2], see p. 260 and p. 271, respectively; 2 mg tds po ($\uparrow$up to 30 mg/day)[3,5]; 5–15 mg nocte po[4]. **NB: $\downarrow$dose if elderly, LF or RF.** If chronic exposure to benzodiazepines, $\uparrow$doses may be needed; don't stop suddenly, as can $\Rightarrow$ withdrawal.

> 🐛 **Respiratory depression:** if $\uparrow$doses used (esp iv/im), monitor O_2 sats and have O_2 ($\pm$ intubation equipment) at hand, caution with flumazenil – see p. 284 for Mx 🐛.

DICLOFENAC

Medium-strength NSAID; non-selective COX inhibitor.

Use: pain/inflammation, esp musculoskeletal; RA, osteoarthritis, acute gout, migraine, post-op and dental pain.

CI/Caution/SE/Interactions: as ibuprofen, but somewhat ↑risk PU/GI bleeds & thrombotic events (↓risk PU/GI bleeds if given with misoprostol as Arthrotec). Doses ≥ 150 mg daily associated with ↑thrombotic risk. Avoid in acute porphyria. Ciclosporin ⇒ ↑serum levels. No known interaction with baclofen. Mild **W +**.

Dose: 25–50 mg tds po or 75 mg bd po (or im, but for max of 2 days); 75–150 mg/day pr (**divided doses**). Rarely used iv[BNF/SPC]. MR and top preparations available[BNF/SPC]. **NB: Avoid/↓dose in RF & consider gastroprotective Rx.**

DIFFLAM Benzydamine: topical NSAID for painful inflammatory conditions of oropharynx (e.g. mouth ulcers, radio-/chemo-therapy-induced mucositis). Available as spray (4–8 sprays 1.5–3-hrly) or oral rinse (15 ml 1.5–3-hrly, diluting in 15 ml water if stinging). Rarely ⇒ hypersensitivity reactions.

DIGIBIND Anti-digoxin Ab for digoxin toxicity/OD unresponsive to supportive Rx. See SPC for dose.

DIGOXIN

Cardiac glycoside: ↓s HR by slowing AVN conduction and ↑ing vagal tone. Also weak inotrope.

Use: AF (and other SVTs), HF.

CI: HB (intermittent complete), 2nd-degree AV block, VF, VT, HCM (can use with care if also AF and HF), SVTs 2° to WPW.

Caution: recent MI, ↓K+*/↓T₄ (both ⇒ ↑digoxin sensitivity*), SSS, rhythms resembling AF (e.g. atrial tachycardia with variable AV block), **R/E** (↓dose), **P**.

SE: generally mild unless rapid ivi, xs Rx or OD: **GI upset** (esp nausea), **arrhythmias/HB, neuro-Ψ disturbances** (inc visual Δs, esp blurred vision and yellow/green halos), fatigue, weakness, confusion, hallucinations, mood Δs. Also gynaecomastia (if chronic Rx), rarely ↓Pt, rash, ↑EØ.

Monitor: U&Es, digoxin levels (ideally take 6 h post-dose: therapeutic range = 1–2 microgram/l).

Interactions: digoxin fx/toxicity ↑d by Ca^{2+} antagonists (esp verapamil), amiodarone, propafenone, quinidine, antimalarials, itraconazole, amphotericin, ciclosporin, St John's wort and diuretics (mostly via ↓K^{+*}), but also ACE-i/ARBs and spironolactone (despite potential ↑K^+). Cholestyramine and antacids can ↓digoxin absorption.

Dose: *non-acute AF/SVTs*: load with 125–250 microgram bd po (maintenance dose 62.5–250 microgram od). For HF: 62.5–125 microgram od. NB: ↓dose if RF, elderly or digoxin given <2 wks ago.

Digoxin loading for acute AF/SVTs: *either* 0.75–1 mg as ivi over 2 h *or* 500 microgram po repeated 12 h later. Then follow non-acute schedule.

DIHYDROCODEINE see Codeine: similar-strength opioid.
Dose: 30 mg 4–6 hourly po (or up to 50 mg 4–6 hourly im/sc) with or after food. ↑doses can be given under close supervision. ↓dose if RF.

DILATING EYE DROPS (for funduscopy). Generally safe but rarely ⇒ angle closure glaucoma (suspect if develops red painful eye with ↓vision and nausea; *ophthalmic emergency*). Dilation blurs vision. Driving unsafe for at least 4 hours when both eyes dilated. Apply 1 drop and allow 15 mins for effect.

1 **Tropicamide 1%** Most common; CI in children <1 yr old (use 0.5%).
2 **Phenylephrine 2.5% or 10%** Frequently used in combination with tropicamide. 2.5% most common. 10% ↑s systemic SEs. CI if cardiac disease, HTN, ↑HR, aneurysms, ↑T_4.

Consider cycloplegic forms (e.g. cyclopentolate 1%) for refraction in children or if analgesia required, e.g. corneal abrasions & uveitis (↓s ciliary spasm).

DILTIAZEM
Rate-limiting benzothiazepine Ca^{2+} channel blocker: ↓s HR and contractility* (but < verapamil) and ↓s BP. Also dilates peripheral/coronary arteries.
Use: Rx/Px of angina[1] (esp if β-blockers CI) and HTN[2] (*for advice on stepped HTN Mx see p. 235*).

CI: LVF* with pulmonary congestion, ↓↓HR, 2nd/3rd-degree AV block (without pacemaker), SSS, acute porphyria **P/B**.

Caution: 1st-degree AV block, ↓HR, ↑PR interval, **L/R/H**.

SE: headache, flushing, GI upset (esp N&C), oedema (esp ankle), ↓HR, ↓BP, gum hyperplasia. Rarely SAN/AVN block, arrhythmias, rash, hepatotoxicity, gynaecomastia.

Interactions: β-blockers and verapamil (can ⇒ asystole, AV block, ↓↓HR, HF). ↑s fx of digoxin, ciclosporin, theophyllines, carbamazepine and phenytoin. 💀 ↑risk of VF with iv dandrolene 💀.

Dose: 60 mg tds (↑ing to max of 360 mg/day)[1]; 180–480 mg/day in 1 or 2 doses[2] (suitable for HTN only as MR preparation: no non-proprietary forms exist and brands vary in clinical fx ∴ specify which is required[SPC/BNF]). NB: Consider ↓ing doses if LF or RF.

DIPROBASE Paraffin-based emollient cream/ointment for dry skin conditions (e.g. eczema, psoriasis).

DIPYRIDAMOLE/PERSANTIN

Antiplatelet agent: inhibits Pt aggregation, adhesion and survival (also ⇒ arterial dilation: inc coronaries).

Use: 2° prevention of ischaemic TIA/CVA[1], Px of TE from prosthetic valves (as adjunct to warfarin)[2].

Caution: recent MI, angina (if unstable), aortic stenosis, coagulation disorders, ↓BP, MG*, migraine (may worsen), **H/B**.

SE: GI upset, dizziness, myalgia, headache, ↓BP, ↑HR, hot flushes, rarely worsening of IHD, hypersensitivity (rash, urticaria, broncho-spasm, angioedema), ↑postoperative bleeding, ↓Pt.

Interactions: ↓s fx (but ↑s hypotensive fx) of cholinesterase inhibitors*, ↑s fx of adenosine. **W +**.

Dose: 200 mg bd po as MR preparation (Persantin Retard)[1,2]; 100–200 mg tds po[2]. All doses to be taken with food.

DISODIUM ETIDRONATE see Pamidronate.

DISODIUM PAMIDRONATE see Pamidronate.

DISULFIRAM/ANTABUSE

Alcohol dehydrogenase inhibitor: $\Rightarrow$ ↑systemic acetaldehyde $\Rightarrow$ unpleasant SE when alcohol ingested (inc small amounts ∴ care with alcohol-containing medications, foods, toiletries).

Use: alcohol withdrawal (maintenance of).

CI: Hx of IHD or CVA, HTN, psychosis, ↑suicide risk, severe personality disorder, **H/P/B**.

Caution: DM, epilepsy, respiratory disease, **L/R**.

SE: only if alcohol ingested – N&V, flushing, headache, ↑HR, ↓BP ($\pm$ collapse if xs alcohol intake).

Interactions: ↑s fx of phenytoin, ↑toxicity with paraldehyde **W +**.

Dose: initially 200 mg od, ↑dose if needed: max. 500 mg po od Review if >6 months.

> NB: Must have consumed no alcohol within at least 24 h of 1st dose. Prescribe under specialist supervision.

DOBUTAMINE

Inotropic sympathomimetic: mostly β_1 fx $\Rightarrow$ ↑contractility. ↓fx on HR compared with dopamine.

Use: shock (cardiogenic, septic).

Caution: Avoid in phaeo. severe ↓BP, arrhythmias, AMI.

SE: ↑HR, ↑BP (if xs Rx), phlebitis, ↓Pt.

Interactions: risk of ↑BP crisis with β-blockers (esp if 'non-selective').

Dose: 2.5–10 microgram/kg/min ivi, titrating to response (via central line, preferably with invasive cardiac monitoring). Often given with dopamine; seek expert help.

DOCUSATE SODIUM

Stimulant laxative: $\Rightarrow$ ↑GI motility (also a softening agent).

Use/Caution/SE: see Senna (**CI if GI obstruction**).

Dose: 50–100 mg up to tds po (max 500 mg/day). Also available as enemas[SPC/BNF].

DOMPERIDONE

Antiemetic: D_2 antagonist – inhibits central nausea chemoreceptor trigger zone. Poor BBB penetration ∴ ↓central SEs (extrapyramidal fx, sedation) cf other dopamine antagonists.

Use: N&V, esp 2° to chemotherapy or 'morning-after pill', and in Parkinson's disease or migraine. Rarely for gastro-oesophageal reflux and dyspepsia.

CI: prolactinoma, when GI obstruction harmful, drugs that ↑QTc **L**.

Caution: GI obstruction **R/P/B**.

SE: ↑QTc, rash, allergy, ↑prolactin (can ⇒ gynaecomastia, galactorrhoea and hyperprolactinoma). Rarely ↓libido, dystonia and extrapyramidal fx.

Dose: 10 mg tds po (can ↑to max 20 mg qds); 60 mg bd pr. Not available im/iv. **NB:** ↓dose if RF.

DONEPEZIL/ARICEPT

Acetylcholinesterase inhibitor (reversible); see Rivastigmine.

Use: Alzheimer's disease: mild or moderate[NICE].

CI: P/B.

Caution: supraventricular conduction dfx (esp SSS), ↑risk of PU (e.g. Hx of PU or NSAID), COPD/asthma, extrapyramidal symptoms can worsen, **L**.

SE: cholinergic fx (see p. 276), **GI upset** (esp initially), **insomnia** (if occurs, change dose to mane), **headache**, fatigue, dizziness, syncope, rash, Ψ disturbances. Rarely ↓ or ↑BP, seizures, PU/GI bleeds, SAN/AVN block, hepatotoxicity.

Interactions: metab by **P450** ∴ inhibitors and inducers on p. 279 could ↑ or ↓ levels, respectively; check BNF/SPC.

Dose: 5 mg nocte (↑to 10 mg after 1 month if necessary); specialist use only – need review for clinical response and tolerance. Continue only if MMSE remains 10–20[NICE].

DOPAMINE

Inotropic sympathomimetic: dose-dependent fx on receptors: low doses (2–3 microgram/kg/min) stimulate peripheral DA receptors but little else ∴ ⇒ ↑renal perfusion*; higher doses (>5 microgram/kg/min) also have β_1 fx ($\Rightarrow$ ↑contractility); even higher doses have α fx ($\Rightarrow$ vasoconstriction, but can worsen HF).

Use: shock, esp if AKI* or cardiogenic (e.g. post-MI or cardiac surgery).

CI: tachyarrhythmias, phaeo, ↑T_4.

Caution: correct hypovolaemia before giving.

SE: N&V, ↓ or ↑BP, ↑HR, peripheral vasoconstriction.

Interactions: fx ↑by cyclopropane and halogen hydrocarbon anaesthetics (are CI) or MAOIs (can $\Rightarrow$ ↑↑BP; consider ↓↓dose of dopamine).

Dose: initially 2–5 microgram/kg/min ivi (via central line, preferably with invasive cardiac monitoring), then adjust to response; seek specialist help.

DORZOLAMIDE/TRUSOPT

Topical carbonic anhydrase inhibitor: as acetazolamide (oral preparation, which is more potent but has ↑SEs*).

Use: glaucoma (esp if β-blocker or PG analogue CI or fails to ↓IOP).

CI: ↑Cl^- acidosis, **R** (severe only), **P/B**.

Caution: Hx of renal stones[†], **L**.

SE: local irritation & allergic reactions, blurred vision, bitter taste, rash. Rarely* systemic SEs (esp urolithiasis[†]) and interactions; see Acetazolamide.

Dose: apply 2% drop tds (bd with topical β-blocker). Available as combination drop with timolol 0.5% (Cosopt).

DOXAPRAM

Respiratory stimulant: ↑s activity of respiratory and vasomotor centres in medulla $\Rightarrow$ ↑depth (and, to lesser extent, rate) of breathing. Also indirect fx by stimulation of chemoreceptors in aorta and carotid artery.

Use: hypoventilation, life-threatening respiratory failure – usually only if dt transient/reversible cause, e.g. post-operative/-general anaesthetic or acute deterioration with known precipitant. Mostly used in preventing respiratory depression 2° to ↑FiO_2 used in severe respiratory acidosis (can be harmful if CO_2 ↓ or normal).

CI: severe asthma or HTN, IHD, $\uparrow T_4$, epilepsy, physical obstruction of respiratory tract.

Caution: if taking MAOIs, phaeo **L/H/P**.

SE: headache, flushing, chest pains, arrhythmias, vasoconstriction, $\uparrow$BP, $\uparrow$HR, laryngo-/broncho-spasm, cough, salivation, GI upset, dizziness, seizures.

Dose: specialist use only (mostly in ITU).

▼ DOXAZOSIN/CARDURA

α_1-Blocker $\Rightarrow$ systemic vasodilation and relaxation of internal urethral sphincter $\therefore \Rightarrow \downarrow$TPR[1] and $\uparrow$bladder outflow[2].

Use: HTN[1] *(for advice on stepped HTN Mx see p. 235)*, BPH[2].

CI: postural $\downarrow$BP, anuria **B**.

Caution: postural $\downarrow$BP, micturition syncope, **L/H/P/E**.

SE: postural $\downarrow$BP (esp after 1st dose*), **dizziness, headache, urinary incontinence** (esp women), GI upset (esp N&V), drowsiness/fatigue, syncope, mood Δs, dry mouth, oedema, somnolence, blurred vision, rhinitis. Rarely erectile dysfunction, $\uparrow$HR, arrhythmias, hypersensitivity/rash. Chronic Rx $\Rightarrow$ beneficial lipid Δs ($\uparrow$HDL, $\downarrow$LDL, $\downarrow$VLDL, $\downarrow$TG, $\downarrow$Pt, $\downarrow$NØ).

Interactions: $\uparrow$s hypotensive fx of diuretics, β-blockers, Ca^{2+} antagonists, silden-/tadal-/varden-afil, general anaesthetics, moxisylyte and antidepressants.

Dose: initially 1 mg od (give 1st dose before bed*), then slowly $\uparrow$according to response (max 16 mg/day[1] or 8 mg/day[2]). 4 mg or 8 mg od if MR preparation, as Cardura XL.

DOXYCYCLINE

Tetracycline antibiotic: inhibits ribosomal (30S) subunit. Has longest $t_{1/2}$ of all tetracyclines $\therefore$ od dosing.

Use: genital infections, esp syphilis, chlamydia, PID, salpingitis, urethritis (non-gonococcal). Also *Rickettsia* (inc Q fever), *Brucella*, Lyme disease (*Borrelia burgdorferi*), malaria (Px/Rx, not 1st-line), mycoplasma (genital/respiratory), COPD infective exac (*H. influenzae*), **MRSA** infection (if mild, sensitive strain).

CI/Caution/SE/Interactions: as tetracycline, but can give with caution if RF, although is also CI in SLE and achlorhydria. Can ⇒ anorexia, flushing, tinnitus and can ↑ciclosporin levels.

Warn: avoid UV light and Zn-/Fe-containing products (e.g. antacids).

Dose: 100–200 mg od/bd[SPC/BNF]. NB: ↓dose in RF.

▼ DULOXETINE/CYMBALTA[1,2,3] or YENTREVE[4]

5HT and noradrenaline reuptake inhibitor.

Use: depression[1], generalised anxiety disorder[2], diabetic neuropathy[3] (review need ≤3 monthly and stop if inadequate response after 2 months), stress urinary incontinence[4] (assess benefit/tolerability after 2–4 wks).

CI: R (avoid if creatinine clearance <30 ml/min) **L/P/B**.

Caution: cardiac disease, Hx of mania or seizures, ↑IOP, susceptibility to angle closure glaucoma, bleeding disorders/on drugs ↑ing bleeding risk, **H/P/B/E**.

SE: N&V&C, abdominal pain, dyspepsia, WtΔ, ↓appetite, palpitations, hot flushes, insomnia, sexual dysfunction, suicidal behaviour.

Interactions: metabolism ↓by ciprofloxacin, fluvoxamine. ↑5HT fx with St John's wort and antidepressants (esp moclobemide and MAOIs; avoid concomitant use and don't start for 1 wk after stopping duloxetine). Avoid with artemether/lumefantrine. ↑risk CNS toxicity with sibutramine.

Warn: patient not to stop suddenly*.

Dose: 60 mg od[1]; initially 30 mg od (↑to max 120 mg/day if required)[2]; 60 mg od (↑to bd if required)[3]; 40 mg bd[4]. NB: stop gradually over 1–2 wks to ↓risk of withdrawal fx*.

EDROPHONIUM

Short-acting cholinesterase antagonist, given iv during Tensilon test for Dx of MG: look for ↓signs (e.g. ↑power, ↓ptosis).

ENALAPRIL/INNOVACE

ACE-i.

Use: HTN[1] *(for advice on stepped HTN Mx see p. 235)*, LVF[2].

CI/Caution/SE/Interactions: as Captopril, plus **L**.
Dose: initially 5 mg od[1] (2.5 mg od[2]) ↑ing according to response max 40 mg/day. NB: ↓dose elderly, taking diuretics or RF.

ENOXAPARIN/CLEXANE

Low-molecular-weight heparin (LMWH).
Use: DVT/PE Rx[1] and Px[2] (inc pre-operative), ACS (with aspirin)[3].
CI/Caution/SE/Monitor/Interactions: as Heparin, plus **B**.
Dose: (all sc; 1 mg = 100 units) 1.5 mg/kg od[1], 40 mg od (20 mg od if not high risk)[2], 1 mg/kg bd[3].

Consider monitoring anti-Xa (3–4 h post dose) and ↓dose if RF (i.e. creatinine >150), pregnancy, Wt >100 kg or <45 kg; see p. 209.

ENSURE Protein and calorie supplement drinks.

EPADERM Paraffin-based emollient ointment for very dry skin (and as soap substitute).

EPILIM see Valproate.

EPINEPHRINE see Adrenaline.

EPOETIN see Erythropoietin (recombinant form for ↓Hb).

EPROSARTAN/TEVETEN

Angiotensin II antagonist; see Losartan.
Use: HTN (*for advice on stepped HTN Mx see p. 235*)
CI: L (if severe), **P/B**.
Caution/SE/Interactions: see Losartan.
Dose: 600 mg od (max 800 mg od). Start at 300 mg and then ↑as required if elderly, RF or LF.

EPTIFIBATIDE/INTEGRILIN

Antiplatelet agent: glycoprotein IIb/IIIa receptor inhibitor – stops binding of fibrinogen and inhibits platelet aggregation.
Use: Px of MI in unstable angina or NSTEMI (if last episode of chest pain w/in 24 h), esp if high risk and awaiting PCI[NICE] (see p. 233).

L/R/H = Liver, Renal and Heart failure (full key see p. xv)

CI: haemorrhagic diathesis, severe trauma or major surgery w/in 6 wks, abnormal bleeding or CVA w/in 30 days, Hx of haemorrhagic CVA or intracranial disease (AVM, aneurysm or neoplasm), ↓Pt, ↑INR, severe HTN, **L** (if significant), **R** (if severe), **B**.

Caution: drugs that ↑bleeding risk (esp thrombolysis), **P**.

SE: bleeding.

Monitor: FBC (baseline, w/in 6 h of giving, then at least daily) plus clotting and creatinine (baseline at least).

Dose: initially 180 microgram/kg iv bolus followed by ivi of 2 microgram/kg/min for up to 72 h (or 96 h if PCI during treatment). **NB: needs concurrent heparin and ↓dose if RF**[SPC/BNF].

Specialist use only: get senior advice or contact on-call cardiology.

ERGOCALCIFEROL (= CALCIFEROL)

Vit D_2: needs renal (1) and hepatic (25) hydroxylation for activation.

Use: vitamin D deficiency.

CI: ↑Ca^{2+}, metastatic calcification.

Caution: **R** (if high 'pharmacological'* doses used), **B**.

SE: ↑Ca^{2+}. If over-Rx: **GI upset**, weakness, headache, polydipsia/polyuria, anorexia, RF, arrhythmias.

Monitor: Ca^{2+} (esp if N&V develops or ↑doses in RF*).

Interactions: fx ↓by anticonvulsants and ↑by thiazides.

Dose: 10–20 microgram (400–800 units) od as part of multivitamin preparations or combined with calcium lactate or phosphate as 'calcium + ergocalciferol': non-proprietary preparations available but is often prescribed by trade name (e.g. Cacit D3, or Calcichew D3). ↑doses of 0.25–1.0 mg od (of 'pharmacological strength' preparations*) used for GI malabsorption and chronic liver disease (up to 5 mg daily for ↓PTH or renal osteodystrophy).

*Specify strength of tablet required to avoid confusion[SPC/BNF].

ERYTHROMYCIN

Macrolide antibiotic: binds 50S ribosome.

Use: atypical pneumonias (with other agents; see p. 244), rarely *Chlamydia*/other GU infections, *Campylobacter* enteritis. Often used if allergy to penicillin.

CI: macrolide hypersensitivity or if taking terfenadine, pimozide, ergotamine or dihydroergotamine.

Caution: ↑QTc (inc drugs that predispose to), porphyria, **L/R/P/B**.

SE: GI upset (rarely AAC), **dry itchy skin**, hypersensitivity (inc SJS, TEN), arrhythmias (esp VT), chest pain, reversible hearing loss (dose-related, esp if RF), cholestatic jaundice.

Interactions: ↓P450 ∴ many; most importantly ↑s levels of ciclosporin, digoxin, theophyllines and carbamazepine, **W +**.

Dose: 500 mg qds po (250 mg qds if mild infection, 1 g qds if severe); 50 mg/kg daily iv in 4 divided doses.

> **NB:** venous irritant ∴ give po if possible.

ERYTHROPOIETIN

Recombinant erythropoietin.

Use: ↓Hb 2° to CRF or chemotherapy (AZT or platinum-containing). Also unlicensed use for myeloma, lymphoma and certain myelodysplasias. 3 types: α (Eprex), β (NeoRecormon) and longer-acting darbepoetin (Aranesp).

SE: ↑BP, ↑K⁺, headache, arthralgia, oedema, TE. ☠ Rarely ⇒ red cell aplasia (esp subcutaneous Eprex if RF, which is now CI) ☠.

CI/Caution/Dose: specialist use only^SPC/BNF; given subcutaneously (self-administered) or iv (as inpatient). ↓Fe/folate (monitor), ↑Al, infections and inflammatory disease can ↓response. **NB:** *transfusion is 1st-line Rx for ↓Hb 2° to cancer chemotherapy.*

ESCITALOPRAM/CIPRALEX

SSRI (active enantiomer of citalopram).

Use: Depression, OCD, anxiety disorders.

CI/Caution/SE/Warn/Interactions: as citalopram.

Dose: initially 10 mg od, ↑ing if necessary to 20 mg od. **NB: max dose 10 mg in elderly and halve doses in LF and for most anxiety disorders.**

ESMOLOL

β-blocker: cardioselective (β₁ > β₂) and short-acting*.

Use: SVTs (inc AF, atrial flutter, sinus ↑HR), HTN (esp peri-operatively), acute MI (*safer than long-acting preparations).

CI/Caution/SE/Interactions: see Propranolol.

Dose: usually 50–200 microgram/kg/min ivi, preceded by loading dose if perioperative[SPC].

ESOMEPRAZOLE/NEXIUM

PPI; as Omeprazole, plus **R** (if severe).
Dose: 20 mg od po (40 mg od for 1st 4 wks, if for gastro-oesophageal reflux); 20–40 mg/day iv[SPC/BNF](▼).
NB: Max 20 mg/day if severe LF.

ETANERCEPT/ENBREL

Monoclonal Ab against TNF-α (an inflammatory cytokine).
Use: severe arthritis (rheumatoid[NICE], juvenile idiopathic[NICE] and psoriatic), severe plaque psoriasis[NICE] and ankylosing spondylitis[NICE].
CI/Caution/Interactions: See SPC.
SE: blood disorders, severe infections, CNS demyelination, GI upset, exac of HF, headache. *Specialist use only.*

☠ Don't give live vaccines during Rx. Risk of infections (e.g. TB, inc extrapulmonary) and theoretical malignancy risk ☠.

ETHAMBUTOL

Anti-TB antibiotic: inhibits cell-wall synthesis ('static').
Use: TB initial Rx phase (1st 2 months) *if isoniazid resistance known or suspected* (see pp. 267) as part of combination drugs.
CI: optic neuritis, ↓vision.
Caution: **R** (monitor levels* and ↓dose if creatinine clearance <30 ml/min), **P/E**.
SE: neuritis; peripheral and optic (can ⇒ ↓visual acuity**, colour-blindness, ↓visual fields ∴ ⇒ baseline and regular ophthalmology review). Rarely GI upset, skin reactions, ↓Pt.
Warn: patient to report immediately any visual symptoms – use alternative drug if unable to do this (e.g. very young, ↓IQ).
Monitor: visual acuity** (inc baseline before Rx), plasma levels*.
Dose: 15 mg/kg od (30 mg/kg 3 times a week if 'supervised' Rx)[SPC/BNF].
NB: ↓dose if RF.

ETOMIDATE

Intravenous anaesthetic.

Use: induction of anaesthesia.

CI: anaesthetist not confident of airway maintenance

Caution: acute porphyria, produces fx in one arm-brain circulation, hypovolaemia cardiovascular disease. Can cause apnoea & ↓BP **L/P/E**

SE: N&V, apnoea, ↓BP (esp on induction), hyperventilation, stridor, rash, dyskinesia, extraneous muscle movements (minimised with opiod or benzodiazepine just before induction), pain on injection, ↓s adrenocortical function (not for maintenance anaesthesia or in sepsis), seizure, ☠ cardiac arrest ☠.

Warn: injection painful, don't drive for 24h.

Monitor: cardiac and respiratory function.

Interactions: ↑s hypotensive effect with adrenergic neurone blockers, α-blockers, antipsychotics, verapamil. Alfentanyl ↑s levels.

Dose: titrated to effect except during 'rapid sequence induction'; PREPARATION DEPENDENT: Etomidate-Lipuro: 150–300 micrograms/kg iv (slow). Hypnomidate: 300 micrograms/kg (max. total dose 60 mg) iv slow. ↓ **Dose if elderly (150–200 micrograms/kg)** or LF.

> ☠ Should only be administered by, or under the direct supervision of, personnel experienced in their use, with adequate training in anaesthesia and airway management, and when resuscitation equipment is available. ☠

▼ ETORICOXIB/ARCOXIA

NSAID which selectively inhibits COX-2 ∴ ↓GI SEs (COX-1 mediated). *Provides no Px against IHD/CVA* (unlike aspirin).

Use: osteo[1]/rheumatoid[2] arthritis[NICE], ankylosing spondylitis[2], acute gout[3].

CI/Caution/SE/Interactions: as celecoxib (except fluconazole interaction), plus CI in uncontrolled HTN (persistently >140/90 mmHg) – monitor BP w/in 2 wks of starting & regularly thereafter. Also ↑s ethinylestradiol levels. *Not* CI in *sulphonamide* hyper-sensitivity. Mild [**W +**].

Dose: 30–60 mg od[1]; 90 mg od[2]; 120 mg od[3] for max 8 days.
NB: ↓**dose if LF**.

EUMOVATE see Clobetasone butyrate 0.05%; steroid cream.

FANSIDAR
Antimalarial: combination tablet of pyrimethamine (25 mg) +
sulfadoxine (500 mg).
Use: Rx of falciparum malaria (with or following quinine).
CI: sulphonamide or pyrimethamine allergy, porphyria.
Caution: blood disorders, asthma, G6PD deficiency, **L/R/P/B/E**.
SE: blood disorders, skin reactions*, pulmonary infiltrates,
insomnia, GI upset, nephrotoxicity, hepatotoxicity,
hypersensitivity.
Monitor: FBC (if chronic Rx) and for rash* or cough/SOB (stop drug).
Dose: see BNF/SPC.

FELODIPINE/PLENDIL
Ca^{2+} channel blocker (dihydropyridine): as amlodipine but ⇒ ↓HF/
–ve inotropic fx.
Use: HTN[1] (for advice on stepped Mx see p. 235), angina Px[2].
CI: IHD (if unstable angina or w/in 1 month of MI), significant
aortic stenosis, acute porphyria, **H** (if uncontrolled)/**P**.
Caution: stop drug if angina/HF worsen, **L/B**.
SE: as nifedipine but ↑ankle swelling and possibly ↓vasodilator fx
(headache, flushing and dizziness).
Interactions: metab by **P450** ∴. levels ↑by cimetidine, erythro-
mycin, ketoconazole and **grapefruit juice**. Hypotensive fx ↑by
α-blockers. Levels ↓by primidone. ↑s fx of tacrolimus.
Dose: initially 5 mg od, ↑if required to 10 mg (max 20 mg[1]).
NB: ↓dose if LF or elderly.

FENTANYL
Strong opioid; used in severe chronic/palliative pain (top/sl/buccal/
nasal spray) and in anaesthesia (iv).

CI: acute respiratory depression, risk of ileus, ↑ICP/head injury/coma.

Caution: all other conditions where morphine is CI or cautioned, but better tolerated in RF. Also DM, cerebral tumour.

SE: as morphine but generally ↓N&V/constipation.

Interactions: as morphine but levels ↑(not ↓) by ritonavir, levels ↑by itra-/flu-conazole & no known interaction with gabapentin. May ↑levels of midazolam.

Warn: patients/carers of signs/symptoms of opiate toxicity.

Dose: Patches: last 72 h and come in 5 strengths: 12, 25, 50, 75 and 100, which denote release of microgram/h (to calculate initial dose, these are approx equivalent to daily oral morphine requirement of 45, 90, 180, 270 and 360 mg, respectively).

Lozenges (buccal) for 'breakthrough' pain as Actiq: initially 200 microgram over 15 min, repeating after 15 min if needed and adjusting dose to give max 4 lozenges daily (available as 200, 400, 600, 800, 1200 or 1600 microgram).

Tablets: for 'breakthrough' pain as ▼ Effentora (buccal) or ▼ Abstral(sl) 100, 200, 400, 600 and 800 microgram^SPC/BNF.
Only use if taking regular opioids (fatalities reported otherwise).
If >4 doses/day needed, adjust background analgesia.

Nasal spray: for 'breakthrough' pain as ▼ Instanyl or ▼ PecFent ^SPC/BNF.

NB: ↓dose if LF or elderly. No initial ↓dose needed in RF, but may accumulate over time. Unless given iv has prolonged onset/offset; use only when opioid requirements stable & cover 1st 12 hrs after initial Rx with prn short acting opioid. Only for use if have previously tolerated opioids. If serious adverse reactions remove patch immediately and monitor for up to 24 h. Fever/external heat can ⇒ ↑absorption (∴ ↑fx) from patches.

FERROUS FUMARATE

As ferrous sulphate, but ↓GI upset; available in UK as Fersaday (322-mg tablet od as Px or bd as Rx), Fersamal (1–2 tablets of 210 mg tds) or Galfer (305 mg capsule od/bd).

FERROUS GLUCONATE

As ferrous sulphate, but ↓GI upset. Px: 600 mg od; Rx: 1.2–1.8 g/day in 2–3 divided doses.

FERROUS SULPHATE

Oral Fe preparation.

Use: Fe-deficient ↓Hb Rx/Px.

Caution: P.

SE: dark stools (can confuse with melaena, which smells worse (!) and is always unformed), **GI upset** (esp **nausea;** consider switching to ferrous gluconate/fumarate or take with food, but latter can ⇒ ↓absorption), Δ bowel habit (dose-dependent).

Dose: Rx: 200 mg bd/tds. Px: 200 mg od.

FINASTERIDE

Antiandrogen: 5-α-reductase inhibitor; ↓s testosterone conversion to more potent dihydrotestosterone.

Use: BPH[1] (↓s prostate size and symptoms), male-pattern baldness[2].

Caution: Ca prostate (can ⇒ ↓PSA and ∴ mask), obstructive uropathy, **P** (teratogenic; although not taken by women, partners of those on the drug can absorb it from handling crushed tablets and from semen, in which it is excreted ∴ *females must avoid handling tablets, and sexual partners of those on the drug must use condoms if, or likely to become, pregnant*).

SE: sexual dysfunction, testicular pain, gynaecomastia, hypersensitivity (inc swelling of lips/face).

Dose: 5 mg od[1] (Proscar), 1 mg od[2](Propecia).

FLAGYL see Metronidazole; antibiotic for anaerobes

FLECAINIDE

Class Ic antiarrhythmic; local anaesthetic; ↓s conduction.

Use: VT[1] (if serious and symptomatic), SVT[2] (esp junctional re-entry tachycardias and paroxysmal AF).

CI: SAN dysfunction, atrial conduction dfx, HB (not 1st-degree), BBB, AF post-cardiac surgery, chronic AF (with no attempts at cardioversion), Hx of MI plus asymptomatic VEs or non-sustained VT, valvular heart disease (if haemodynamically compromised), **H.**

Caution: pacemakers, ensure e'lytes normalised before use, **L/R/P/B/E.**

SE: GI upset, syncope, dyspnoea, oedema, vision/mood disturbances. Rarely **arrhythmias.**

Monitor: pre-dose plasma levels in LF or RF (keep at 0.2–1 mg/l), ECG if giving iv.

Interactions: levels ↑d by amiodarone, ritonavir, fluoxetine and quinine. ↑s digoxin levels. Myocardial depression may occur with β-blockers/verapamil. ↑risk of arrhythmias with antipsychotics, TCAs, artemether/lumefantrine and dolasetron.

Dose: initially 100 mg bd po, ↓ing after 3–5 days if possible (max 400 mg/day)[1]; 50 mg bd po, ↑ing if necessary to 300 mg/day[2]. Acutely, 2 mg/kg iv over 10–30 min (max 150 mg), then (if required) 1.5 mg/kg/h ivi for 1 h, then ↓ing to 100–250 microgram/kg/h for up to 24 h, then give po (max cumulative dose in 1st 24 h = 600 mg). With ECG monitoring. **NB:** ↓dose if LF/RF. Drug initiated under consultant supervision.

FLEET (PHOSPHO-SODA) see Bowel preparations.

Dose: 45 ml (mixed with 120 ml water, then followed by 240 ml water) taken twice: for morning procedures, at 7 am and 7 pm the day before; for afternoon procedures, at 7 pm the day before and at 7 am on the day of procedure.

FLIXOTIDE see Fluticasone (inh steroid). 50, 100, 250 or 500 microgram/puff as powder. 50, 125 or 250 microgram/puff as aerosol.
Dose: 100–2000 microgram/day[SPC/BNF] (aerosol doses ?<powder doses).

FLOMAXTRA XL see Tamsulosin; α₁-blocker for ↑prostate.

FLUCLOXACILLIN

Penicillin (penicillinase-resistant).

Use: penicillin-resistant (β-lactamase-producing) staphylococcal infections, esp skin[1] (surgical wounds, iv sites, cellulitis, impetigo, otitis externa), rarely as adjunct in pneumonia[1]. Also osteomyelitis[2], endocarditis[3].

CI/Caution/SE/Interactions: as benzylpenicillin, plus CI if Hx of flucloxacillin-associated jaundice/hepatic dysfunction and caution if LF, as rarely ⇒ hepatitis or **cholestatic jaundice** (may develop up to 2 months after Rx stopped).

Dose: 250–500 mg qds po/im (or up to 2 g qds iv)[1]; up to 2 g qds iv[2]; 2 g qds (4-hrly if Wt > 85 kg) iv[3].

NB: ↓dose in severe RF.

FLUCONAZOLE

Triazole antifungal: good po absorption and CSF penetration.

Use: fungal meningitis (esp cryptococcal), candidiasis (mucosal, vaginal, systemic), other fungal infections (esp tinea, pityriasis).

Caution: susceptibility to ↑QTc, **L/R/P/B**.

SE: GI upset, **hypersensitivity** (can ⇒ angioedema, TEN, SJS, anaphylaxis: if develops rash, stop drug or monitor closely), **hepatotoxicity**, headache. Rarely blood/metabolic (↑lipids, ↓K^+) disorders, dizziness, seizures, alopecia.

Monitor: LFTs; stop drug if features of liver disease develop.

Interactions: ↓**P450** ∴ many; most importantly, ↑s fx of theophyllines, ciclosporin, phenytoin and tacrolimus. Also ↓ clopidogrel fx. **W +.**

Dose: 50–400 mg/day po or iv according to indication[SPC/BNF].

NB: ↓dose in RF.

FLUDROCORTISONE

Mineralocorticoid (also has glucocorticoid actions).

Use: adrenocortical deficiency, esp Addison's disease[1].

CI/Caution/Interactions: See Prednisolone.

SE: H_2O/Na^+ retention, ↓K^+ (monitor U&Es). Also can ⇒ immunosuppression (and other SEs of corticosteroids; see p. 217).

Dose: 50–300 microgram/day po[1].

FLUMAZENIL

Benzodiazepine antagonist (competitive).

Use: benzodiazepine OD/toxicity (only if respiratory depression and ventilatory support not immediately available).

CI: life-threatening conditions controlled by benzodiazepines (e.g. ↑ICP, status epilepticus).

Caution: mixed ODs (esp TCAs), benzodiazepine dependence (may ⇒ withdrawal fx), Hx of panic disorder (can ⇒ relapse), head injury, epileptics on long-term benzodiazepine Rx (may ⇒ fits), **L/P/B/E**.

SE: N&V, dizziness, flushing, rebound anxiety/agitation, transient ↑BP/HR. Very rarely anaphylaxis.

Dose: initially 200 microgram iv over 15 sec, then, if required, further doses of 100 microgram at 1 min intervals. *Max total dose 1 mg (2 mg in ITU).* Can also give as ivi at 100–400 microgram/h adjusting to response. NB: see p. 284 for Rx of acute OD.

NB: short $t_{1/2}$ (40–80 min); observe closely after Rx and consider further doses or ivi (at 0.1–0.4 mg/h adjusted to response).

> 😩 *Flumazenil is not recommended as a diagnostic test and should not be given routinely in overdoses as risk of inducing:*
>
> - fits (esp if epileptic, or if co-ingested drugs that predispose to fits)
> - withdrawal syndrome (if habituated to benzodiazepines)
> - arrhythmias (esp if co-ingested TCA or amphetamine-like drug).
>
> If in any doubt get senior opinion and exclude habituation to benzodiazepines and get ECG before giving unless life-threatening respiratory depression and benzodiazepine known to be cause 💀.

FLUOXETINE/PROZAC

SSRI antidepressant: long $t_{1/2}$ compared with others*.

Use: depression[1], other Ψ disorders (inc bulimia[2], OCD[3]).

CI: active mania.

L/R/H = **L**iver, **R**enal and **H**eart failure (full key see p. xv)

Caution: epilepsy, receiving ECT, Hx of mania or bleeding disorder (esp GI), heart disease, DM†, glaucoma (angle closure), ↑risk of bleeding, age <18 yrs **L/R/H/P/B/E**.

Class SEs: GI upset, ↓Wt, insomnia**, agitation**, headache, hypersensitivity. Can ⇒ withdrawal fx when stopped (see p. 277) ∴ *stop slowly*; more important for SSRIs with ↓t$_{1/2}$*. Rarely extrapyramidal (see p. 278) and antimuscarinic fx (see p. 276), sexual dysfunction, convulsions, ↓Na$^+$ (inc SIADH), blood disorders, GI bleed, serotonin syndrome (see p. 277) and suicidal thoughts/behaviour.

Specific SEs: rarely hypoglycaemia†, **vasculitis** (**rash** may be 1st sign).

Warn: can ↓performance at skilled tasks (inc driving). Don't stop suddenly (not as important as for other SSRIs).

Interactions: ↓**P450** ∴ many, but most importantly ↑s levels of TCAs, benzodiazepines, clozapine and haloperidol. ↑s lithium toxicity and ⇒ HTN and ↑CNS fx with sele-/rasa-giline (and other dopaminergics). ↑risk of CNS toxicity with drugs that ↑5HT (e.g. tramadol, sibutramine, sumatriptan, St John's wort). ↑risk of bleeding with aspirin and NSAIDs. Levels ↑by ritonavir. Antagonises antiepileptics (but ↑s levels of carbamazepine and phenytoin). Avoid with artemether/lumefantrine and tamoxifen. ☠ *Never give with, or ≤2 wks after, MAOIs* ☠. (Mild **W +**.)

Dose: initially 20 mg^{1,3} (↑to max 60 mg) od; 60 mg od^2 – give mane as can ↓sleep**.
NB: ↓dose in LF.

FLUTICASONE/FLIXOTIDE (various delivery devices available^{BNF})
Inhaled corticosteroid for asthma: see Beclometasone.
Dose: 100–2000 microgram/day inh (or 0.5–2 mg bd as nebs).

1 microgram equivalent to 2 microgram of beclometasone or budesonide.

FOLIC ACID (= FOLATE)
Vitamin: building block of nucleic acids. Essential co-factor for DNA synthesis ⇒ normal erythropoiesis.

Use: megaloblastic ↓Hb Rx/Px if haemolysis/dialysis[1] (or GI malabsorption where ↑doses may be needed), Px against neural-tube dfx in pregnancy[2] (esp if on antiepileptics), Px of mucositis and GI upset if on methotrexate[3].

CI: malignancy (unless megaloblastic ↓Hb due to ↓folate is an important complication).

Caution: undiagnosed megaloblastic ↓Hb (i.e. ↓B_{12}, as found in pernicious anaemia) – never give alone if B_{12} *deficiency as can precipitate subacute combined degeneration of spinal cord.*

SE: GI disturbance (rare).

Dose: 5 mg od[1] (in maintenance, ↓frequency of dose, often to wkly); 400 microgram od from before conception until wk 12 of pregnancy[2] (unless mother has neural-tube defect herself or has previously had a child with a neural-tube defect, when 5 mg od needed); 5 mg once wkly[3].

FOMEPIZOLE Antidote for toxic alcohols.

▼ **FONDAPARINUX**/ARIXTRA

Anticoagulant; activated factor X inhibitor.

Use: ACS (UA, NSTEMI or STEMI), Px of VTE, Rx of DVT/PE.

CI: active bleeding, bacterial endocarditis.

Caution: bleeding disorders, active PU, other drugs that ↑risk of bleeding, recent intracranial haemorrhage, recent brain/ophthalmic/spinal surgery, spinal/epidural anaesthesia (avoid Rx doses), Wt <50 kg. **R** (avoid or ↓dose according to indication and creatinine clearance[SPC/BNF]), **L/P/B/E**.

SE: bleeding, ↓Hb, ↓(or ↑)Pt, coagulopathy, purpura, oedema, LFT Δs, GI upset. Rarely ↓K^+, ↓BP, hypersensitivity.

Dose: UA/NSTEMI/Px of VTE 2.5 mg sc od (start 6-h post-op); STEMI 2.5 mg iv/ivi od for 1st day then sc; Rx of PE/DVT by Wt (<50 kg = 5 mg sc od, 50–100 kg = 7.5 mg sc od, >100 kg = 10 mg sc od). NB: Length of Rx depends on indication[SPC/BNF], timing of doses post-op critical if Wt <50 kg or elderly. **Consider** ↓dose in RF.

Specialist use only: get senior advice or contact on-call cardiology/haematology.

FORMOTEROL (= EFORMOTEROL)/FORADIL, OXIS

Long-acting β₂ agonist 'LABA'; as Salmeterol plus **L**.
Dose: 6–48 microgram daily (mostly bd regime)$^{SPC/BNF}$ inh (min/max doses vary with preparations$^{SPC/BNF}$).

FOSPHENYTOIN

Antiepileptic: prodrug of phenytoin; allows safer rapid loading.
Use: epilepsy (esp 'status' & seizures assoc with neurosurgery/head injury).
CI/Caution/SE/Monitor/Warn/Interactions: as phenytoin, but ↓SEs (esp ↓arrhythmias and 'purple glove syndrome').
Dose: as phenytoin, but prescribe as 'phenytoin sodium equivalent' and note ☠ **fosphenytoin 1.5 mg = phenytoin 1 mg** ☠.
NB: consider ↓dose in LF or RF.

FOSTAIR

Combination asthma inhaler: each puff contains 100 microgram beclomethasone (steroid) + 6 microgram formoterol (long-acting β₂-agonist) in a metered dose inhaler.
Dose: 1–2 puffs bd inh.

▼ FRAGMIN see ▼ Dalteparin; low-molecular-weight heparin.

FRUMIL see Co-amilofruse; tablets are 5/40 (5 mg amiloride + 40 mg furosemide) unless stated as LS (2.5/20) or generic (10/80).

FRUSEMIDE now called Furosemide.

FUROSEMIDE (previously Frusemide).

Loop diuretic: inhibits Na⁺/K⁺ pump in ascending loop of Henle ⇒ ↓resorption and ∴ ↑loss of Na⁺/K⁺/Cl/H₂O.
Use: LVF (esp in acute pulmonary oedema, but also in chronic LVF/CCF or as Px during blood transfusion), resistant HTN (*for advice on stepped HTN Mx see p. 235*), oliguria secondary to AKI (after correcting hypovolaemia first).
CI: ↓↓K⁺, ↓Na⁺, Addison's, cirrhosis (if precomatose), **R** (if anuria).
Caution: ↓BP, ↑prostate, porphyria, diabetes, **L/P/B**.

SE: ↓BP (inc postural), ↓K⁺, ↓Na⁺, ↓Ca²⁺, ↓ Mg²⁺, ↓Cl alkalosis. Also ↑urate/gout, GI upset, ↑glucose/impaired glucose tolerance, ↑cholesterol/TGs (temporary). Rarely **BM suppression** (stop drug), RF, skin reactions, pancreatitis, tinnitus/deafness (if ↑doses or RF: reversible).
Interactions: ↑s toxicity of digoxin, flecainide, sotalol, NSAIDs, vancomycin, gentamicin and lithium. ↓s fx of antidiabetics. NSAIDs may ↓diuretic response.
Monitor: U&Es; if ↓K⁺, add po K⁺ supplements/K⁺-sparing diuretic or change to combination tablet (e.g. co-amilofruse).
Dose: usually 20–80 mg po/im/iv daily in divided doses. ↑doses used in acute LVF (see p. 234) and oliguria. If HF or RF, ivi (max 4 mg/min) can ⇒ smoother control of fluid balance$^{SPC/BNF}$. For blood transfusions, a rough guide is to give 20 mg with every unit if *existing LVF*, and with every 2nd unit if *at risk of LVF*. **NB: may need ↑dose in RF.**
Give iv if severe oedema: as bowel oedema ⇒ ↓po absorption.

FUSIDIC ACID/FUCIDIN

Antibiotic; good bone penetration and activity against *S. aureus*.
Use: osteomyelitis, endocarditis (2° to penicillin-resistant staphylococci) – needs 2nd antibiotic to prevent resistance.
Caution: biliary disease or obstruction (⇒ ↓elimination), **L/P/B**.
SE: GI upset, hepatitis*. Rarely: skin/blood disorders, AKI.
Monitor: LFTs* (esp if chronic Rx, ↑doses or LF).
Dose: 500 mg tds po (equivalent to 750 mg tds if using suspension) – in severe infection to ↑1 g tds po; 500 mg tds iv (6–7 mg/kg tds if Wt <50 kg). **NB: ↓dose in LF.**

FUSIDIC ACID 1% EYE DROPS/FUCITHALMIC

Topical antibiotic (esp vs. *Staphylococcus*); commonly used for blepharitis.
Dose: 1 drop bd.

FYBOGEL

Laxative: bulking agent (ispaghula husk) for constipation (inc IBS).
CI: ↓swallow, GI obstruction, faecal impaction, colonic atony.
Dose: 1 sachet or 10 ml bd after meals with water.

GABAPENTIN

Antiepileptic: similar structure to GABA but mechanism of action is different from drugs affecting GABA receptors.

Use: neuropathic pain, epilepsy (adjunctive Rx of partial seizures ± 2° generalisation).

Caution: Hx of psychosis or DM, R/P/B/E.

SE: fatigue/somnolence, dizziness, cerebellar fx (esp ataxia; see p. 278), dipl-/ambly-opia, headache, rhinitis. Rarely ↓WCC, GI upset, arthra-/my-algia, skin reactions, suicidal ideation.

Interactions: fx ↓by antidepressants and antimalarials (esp mefloquine). Antipsychotics reduce seizure threshold.

Dose: initially 300 mg od, ↑ing by 300 mg/day to max 3.6 g daily in 3 divided doses (*NB: stop drug over ≥1 wk*). NB: ↓dose in RF.

Can give false-positive urinary dipstick results for proteinuria.

GASTROCOTE Compound alginate for acid reflux.
Dose: 5–15 ml or 1–2 tablets after meals and at bedtime
(NB: 2.13 mmol Na^+/5 ml and 1 mmol Na^+/tablet).

GAVISCON (ADVANCE) Alginate raft-forming oral suspension for acid reflux.
Dose: 5–10 ml or 1–2 tablets after meals and at bedtime
(NB: 2.3 mmol Na^+ and 1 mmol K^+/5 ml and 2.25 mmol Na^+ and 1 mmol K^+/tablet).

Ensure good hydration, esp if elderly, GI narrowing or ↓GI motility.

GELOFUSINE

Colloid plasma substitute (gelatin-based) for iv fluid resuscitation (see p. 201). 1 l contains 154 mmol Na^+(but no K^+).

GENTAMICIN

Aminoglycoside: broad-spectrum 'cidal' antibiotic; inhibs ribosomal 30S subunit. Good Gram-negative aerobe/staphylococci cover; other organisms often need concurrent penicillin ± metronidazole.

Use: severe infections, esp sepsis, meningitis, endocarditis. Also pyelonephritis/prostatitis, biliary tract infections, pneumonia.

CI: MG*.

Caution: obesity, **R/P/B/E**.

SE: **ototoxic, nephrotoxic** (dose- and Rx length-dependent), **hypersensitivity**, rash. Rarely AAC, N&V, seizures, encephalopathy, blood disorders, myasthenia-like syndrome* (at ↑doses; reversible), ↓ Mg^{2+} (if prolonged Rx).

Monitor: serum levels** after 3 or 4 doses (earlier if RF).

Interactions: fx (esp toxicity) ↑by loop diuretics (esp **furosemide**), cephalosporins, vancomycin, amphotericin, ciclosporin, tacrolimus and cytotoxics; if these drugs must be given, space doses as far from time of gentamicin dose as possible. ↑s fx of muscle relaxants and anticholinesterases. **W +**.

Dose: **once daily regimen:** initially 5–7 mg/kg ivi adjusting to levels (NB: consult local protocol; od regimen not suitable if endocarditis, >20% total body surface burns or creatinine clearance <20 ml/min). **Multiple daily regimen:** 3–5 mg/kg/day in 3 divided doses im/iv/ivi (if endocarditis give 1 mg/kg tds iv).

NB: ↓doses if RF (and consider if elderly or ↑↑BMI), otherwise adjust according to serum levels*: call microbiology department if unsure.

Gentamicin levels: Measure peak at 1 h post-dose (ideally = 5–10 mg/l) and trough immediately predose (ideally ≤2 mg/l). Halve ideal peak levels if for endocarditis. If levels high, can ↑*spacing* of doses (as well as ↓ing *amount* of dose); as ⇒↑risk of ototoxicity, monitor auditory/vestibular function. *NB: od regimens usually only require **pre-dose level.***

GLIBENCLAMIDE

Oral antidiabetic (long-acting sulphonylurea): ↑s pancreatic insulin release – stimulates β islet cell receptors (and inhibits gluconeogenesis).

Use: type 2 DM; requires endogenous insulin to work. Not recommended for obese* (use metformin) or elderly** (use short-acting preparations, e.g. gliclazide).

CI: ketoacidosis, acute porphyria, **L/R** (if either severe, otherwise caution), **P/B**.

L/R/H = Liver, Renal and Heart failure (full key see p. xv)

Caution: may need to replace with insulin during intercurrent illness/surgery, porphyria, **E**.

SE: **hypoglycaemia** (esp in elderly**), **GI upset**, ↑Wt*. Rarely hypersensitivity (inc skin) reactions, blood disorders, hepatotoxicity and transient visual Δs (esp initially).

Interactions: fx ↑d by chloramphenicol, sulphonamides (inc co-trimoxazole), sulfinpyrazone, antifungals (esp flu-/mic-onazole), warfarin, fibrates and NSAIDs. Levels ↓by rifampicin/rifabutin. ↑Risk of hepatotoxicity with bosentan.

Dose: initially 5 mg mane (with food), ↑ing as necessary (max 15 mg/day).

NB: ↓dose in severe LF.

GLICLAZIDE

Oral antidiabetic (short-acting sulphonylurea).

Use/CI/Caution/SE/Interactions: as glibenclamide, but shorter action* and hepatic metabolism** mean ↓d risk of hypoglycaemia (esp in elderly* and RF**).

Dose: initially 40–80 mg mane (with food), ↑ing as necessary (max 320 mg/day). MR tablets available (Diamicron MR) of which 30 mg has equivalent effect to 80 mg of normal release (dose initially is 30 mg od, ↑ing if necessary to max 120 mg od). **NB: ↓dose in RF or severe LF.**

GLIMEPIRIDE

Oral antidiabetic (short-acting sulphonylurea).

Use/CI/Caution/SE/Interactions: as gliclazide, plus manufacturer recommends monitoring of FBC and LFTs. CI in severe LF. May need to substitute with insulin; seek specialist advice.

Dose: initially 1 mg mane (with food), ↑ing as necessary (max 6 mg/day).

GLIPIZIDE

Oral antidiabetic (short-acting sulphonylurea).

Use/CI/Caution/SE/Interactions: as gliclazide, plus avoid if both **L** and **R**.

Dose: initially 2.5–5.0 mg mane (with food), ↑ing as necessary (max single dose 15 mg; max daily dose 20 mg).

NB: ↓dose in severe LF and RF.

GLUCAGON

Polypeptide hormone: ↑s hepatic glycogen conversion to glucose.

Use: hypoglycaemia: if acute and severe, esp if no iv access or if 2° to xs insulin (see p. 251).

CI: phaeo.

Caution: glucagonomas/insulinomas. Will not work if hypoglycaemia is chronic (inc starvation) or 2° to adrenal insufficiency.

SE: N&V&D, ↓BP, ↓K$^+$, rarely hypersensitivity, **W +.**

Dose: 1 mg (= 1 unit) im (or sc/iv)$^{SPC/BNF}$.

Often stocked in cardiac arrest ('crash') trolleys.

GLYCEROL (= GLYCERIN) SUPPOSITORIES

Rectal irritant bowel stimulant.

Use: constipation: 1st-line suppository if oral methods such as lactulose and senna fail.

Dose: 1–2 pr prn.

GLYCERYL TRINITRATE see GTN.

GRANISETRON

Antiemetic: 5HT$_3$ antagonist.

Use: N&V; see Ondansetron.

Caution: GI obstruction (inc subacute), ↑QTc, **P/B.**

SE: constipation (or diarrhoea), headache, sedation, fatigue, dizziness. Rarely seizures, chest pain, ↓BP, Δ LFTs, rash, hypersensitivity.

Dose: 1 mg bd or 2 mg od po/iv/ivi for non-specialist use. 2–3 mg loading doses often given before chemotherapy$^{SPC/BNF}$ (max 9 mg/24 h).

GTN (= GLYCERYL TRINITRATE)

Nitrate: $\Rightarrow$ coronary artery + systemic vein dilation $\Rightarrow$ $\uparrow O_2$ supply to myocardium and $\downarrow$preload, $\therefore$ $\downarrow O_2$ demand of myocardium.

Use: Angina, LVF.

CI: $\downarrow$BP, $\downarrow\downarrow$Hb, aortic/mitral stenosis, constrictive pericarditis, tamponade, HCM, glaucoma (closed-angle), hypovolaemia, $\uparrow$ICP.

Caution: recent MI, $\downarrow T_4$, hypothermia, head trauma, cerebral haemorrhage, malnutrition, **L/R** (if either severe).

SE: $\downarrow$BP (inc postural), **headache**, dizziness, flushing, $\uparrow$HR.

Interactions: 💀 sildenafil, tadalafil and vardenafil (are CI as $\Rightarrow$ $\downarrow\downarrow$BP) 💀. $\downarrow$s fx of heparins (if given iv).

Warn: may develop tolerance with $\downarrow$therapeutic effect (esp if long-term transdermal patch use) and don't stop abruptly.

Dose: 2 sprays or tablets sl prn (also available as transdermal SR patches[SPC/BNF]). For acute MI/LVF: 10–200 microgram/min ivi, titrating to clinical response and BP (see p. 234).

HALOPERIDOL

Butyrophenone ('typical') antipsychotic: dopamine antagonist ($D_{2\ and\ 3} > D_{1\ and\ 4}$). Also blocks serotonin ($5HT_{2A}$), histamine (H_1), adrenergic ($\alpha_{1\ >\ 2}$) and muscarinic receptors, causing many SEs.

Use: acute sedation[1] (e.g. agitation and behavioural disturbance), schizophrenia/bipolar disorder[2], N&V[3].

CI/Caution/SE: as chlorpromazine, but $\Rightarrow$ $\uparrow$incidence of **extrapyramidal fx** (see p. 278), although $\Rightarrow$ $\downarrow$sedation, $\downarrow$skin reactions, $\downarrow$antimuscarinic fx, $\downarrow$BP fx, but can $\Rightarrow$ hypoglycaemia and SIADH. Also risk of CNS toxicity with lithium.

Interactions: metab by P450 [many, but most importantly: levels $\uparrow$by fluoxetine, venlafaxine, quinidine, buspirone and ritonavir]. Levels $\downarrow$by carbamazepine, phenytoin, rifampicin. $\uparrow$risk of arrhythmias with amiodarone and $\downarrow$s fx of anticonvulsants.

Dose: 1.5–5.0 mg bd/tds po (max 30 mg/day)[1,2]; 2–10 mg im/iv 4–8-hrly (max 18 mg/day)[1,2]; 0.5–2.0 mg tds im/sc/iv[3]. Also used im as a 4-wkly 'depot'[2] if concerns over compliance. **NB:** $\downarrow$dose in severe RF or elderly.

Start at bottom of dose range if naive to antipsychotics, esp if elderly.
See p. 219 for advice on acute sedation.

HARTMANN'S SOLUTION

Compound sodium lactate iv fluid. GIFTASUP guidelines
recommend this over 0.9% NaCl in surgical patients for
resuscitation or fluid replacement unless vomiting/gastric losses. 1 l
contains **5 mmol K$^+$**, 2 mmol Ca^{2+}, 29 mmol HCO$_3$, 131 mmol Na$^+$,
111 mmol Cl$^-$.

HEPARIN, standard/unfractionated (NB: ≠ LMWHs).

iv (and rarely sc) anticoagulant: potentiates protease inhibitor
antithrombin III, which inactivates thrombin. Also inhibits factors
IXa/Xa/XIa/XIIa.

Use: anticoagulation if needs to be immediate or quickly reversible
(only as inpatient); DVT/PE Rx/Px (inc preoperative), MI/
unstable angina Rx/Px, extracorporeal circuits (esp haemodialysis,
cardiopulmonary bypass).

CI: haemorrhagic disorders (inc haemophilia), ↓Pt (inc Hx of
HIT*), severe HTN, PU, acute bacterial endocarditis, recent cerebral
haemorrhage or major surgery/trauma to eye/brain/spinal cord,
epidural/spinal anaesthesia (but can give Px doses), **L** (if severe, esp
if oesophageal varices).

Caution: ↑K$^+$**, **R/P/E**.

SE: haemorrhage, ↓Pt* (HIT*), **hypersensitivity** (inc anaphylaxis,
urticaria, angioedema), ↑K$^+$ ** (inhibits aldosterone: ↑risk if DM,
CRF, acidosis or on K$^+$-sparing drugs), osteoporosis (if prolonged Rx).

Monitor: FBC* if >5 days Rx, U&E** if > 7 days Rx.

Interactions: fx may ↓by GTN ivi. NSAIDs ⇒ ↑bleeding risk.

Dose: see p. 210 (inc dose-adjustment advice).

🔔 HIT* Heparin Induced Thrombocytopenia: immune mediated ∴
delayed onset – ↑risk if Rx for >5 days (see p. 209) 🔔.

HUMALOG see Insulin lispro; short-acting recombinant insulin.
Also available as biphasic preparations (Mix 25, Mix 50), are
combined with longer-acting isophane suspension.

HUMULIN Recombinant insulin available in various forms:

1 HUMULIN S soluble, short-acting for iv/acute use.
2 HUMULIN I isophane (combined with protamine), long-acting.
3 HUMULIN M 'biphasic' preparations, combination of short-
   acting (S) and long-acting (I) forms to give smoother control
   throughout the day. Numbers denote 1/10% of soluble insulin
   (i.e. M3 = 30% soluble insulin).

HYDRALAZINE

Antihypertensive: vasodilates smooth muscle (arteries > veins).
Use: HTN[1] (inc severe[2], esp if RF or pregnancy), HF[3]. *For advice on
HTN Mx see p. 235.*
CI: severe ↑HR, myocardial insufficiency (2° to mechanical
obstruction, e.g. aortic/mitral stenosis or constrictive pericarditis),
cor pulmonale, dissecting aortic aneurysm, SLE*, porphyria, **H** (if
'high output', e.g. ↑T_4).
Caution: IHD, cerebrovascular disease, **L/R/P/B**.
SE: (*all SEs ↓if dose 100 mg/day*) ↑HR, GI upset, headache, **lupus-
like syndrome*** (watch for unexplained ↓Wt, arthritis, ill health
– measure ANA* and dipstick urine for protein if on high doses/
clinical suspicion). Also fluid retention (↓↓d if used with diuretics),
palpitations, dizziness, flushing, ↓BP (even at low doses), blood
disorders, arthr-/my-algia, rash and can worsen IHD.
Dose: 25–50 mg bd po[1]; 5–10 mg iv[2] (can be repeated after
20–30 min) or 50–300 microgram/min ivi[2]; 25–75 mg tds/qds po[3].
NB: ↓dose if LF or RF.

HYDROCORTISONE BUTYRATE CREAM (0.1%)

Potent-strength topical corticosteroid. NB: much stronger than
'standard' (i.e. non-butyrate) hydrocortisone cream; see below!

HYDROCORTISONE CREAM/OINTMENT (1%)

Mild-strength topical corticosteroid (rarely used as weaker 0.5%,
0.25% and 0.1% preparations).
Use: inflammatory skin conditions, in particular eczema.
CI: untreated infection, rosacea, acne.

SE: rare compared to more potent steroids: skin atrophy, worsening of infections, acne.
Dose: apply thinly 1 or 2 times per day.

HYDROCORTISONE iv/po

Glucocorticoid (with significant mineralocorticoid activity).
Use: acute hypersensitivity (esp anaphylaxis, angioedema), Addisonian crisis, asthma, COPD, $\downarrow T_4$ (and $\uparrow T_4$), IBD. Also used po in chronic adrenocortical deficiency.
CI/Caution/SE/Interactions: see p. 217.
Dose: *acutely*: 100–500 mg im or slowly iv up to qds if required. Exact dose recommendations vary: consult local protocol if unsure (see Medical emergencies section of this book for rational starting dose for some specific indications). *Chronic replacement*: usually 20–30 mg po daily in divided doses (usually 2/3 in morning and 1/3 nocte), often together with fludrocortisone.

▼ HYDROXOCOBALAMIN

Vitamin B_{12} replacement.
Use: pernicious anaemia (also macrocytic anaemias with neurological involvement, tobacco amblyopia, Leber's optic atrophy).
SE: skin reactions, nausea, 'flu-like symptoms, $\downarrow K^+$ (initially), rarely anaphylaxis.
Interactions: fx $\downarrow$ by OCP and chloramphenicol.
Dose: 1 mg im injection: frequently at first for Rx (3–7/wks: exact number depends on indication[SPC/BNF]) until no further improvement, then $\downarrow$ frequency (to once every 1–3 months) for maintenance.

HYDROXYCARBAMIDE (= HYDROXYUREA)

Antineoplastic agent for primary polycythaemia and essential thrombocythaemia (1st line Rx) and CML (initial Rx only). Also (unlicensed) use for severe psoriasis.
CI/Caution: see SPC.
SE: Nausea, blood disorders (esp **myelosuppression**), skin reactions.
Dose: 20–30 mg/kg daily titrated against full blood count. Specialist use only.

L/R/H = Liver, Renal and Heart failure (full key see p. xv)

HYDROXYCHLOROQUINE/PLAQUENIL

DMARD ($\downarrow$s activation of dendritic cells/inflammatory response) and antimalarial (action as chloroquine).
Use: RA, SLE, dermatological disorders aggravated/caused by sunlight.
CI/Caution/SE/Interactions/Monitor: see Chloroquine.
Dose: 200–400 mg/day.

Seek expert advice before commencing treatment.

HYOSCINE BUTYLBROMIDE/BUSCOPAN

Antimuscarinic: $\downarrow$s GI motility. Does not cross BBB (unlike hyoscine *hydrobromide*) $\therefore$ less sedative.
Use: GI (or GU) smooth-muscle spasm; esp biliary colic, diverticulitis and IBS. Rarely used for dysmenorrhoea.
CI: glaucoma (closed-angle), MG, megacolon, $\uparrow$prostrate.
Caution: GI obstruction, $\uparrow$prostate/urinary retention, $\uparrow$HR (inc $\uparrow T_4$) **H/P/B/E**.
SE: antimuscarinic fx (see p. 276), drowsiness, confusion.
Interactions: $\downarrow$s fx of metoclopramide (and vice versa) and sublingual nitrates. $\uparrow$s tachycardic fx of β-agonists.
Dose: 20 mg qds po (for IBS, start at 10 mg tds) or 20 mg im/iv (repeating once after 30 min, if necessary; max 100 mg/day).

Don't confuse with hyoscine *hydrobromide*: different fx and doses!

HYOSCINE HYDROBROMIDE (= SCOPOLAMINE)

Antimuscarinic: predominant fx on CNS ($\downarrow$s vestibular activity[1]). Also $\downarrow$s respiratory/oral secretions[2,3].
Use: motion sickness[1], terminal care/chronic $\downarrow$swallow[2] (e.g. CVA), hypersalivation 2° to antipsychotics[3] (unlicensed use).
CI: glaucoma (closed-angle).
Caution: GI obstruction, $\uparrow$prostate/urinary retention, cardiovascular disease, porphyria, Down's, MG, **L/R/P/B/E**.
SE: antimuscarinic fx (see p. 276), generally sedative (although rarely $\Rightarrow$ paradoxical agitation when given as sc infusion).
Warn: driving may be impaired, $\uparrow$s fx of alcohol.

Interactions: ↓s fx of sublingual nitrates (e.g. GTN).
Dose: 300 microgram 6-hrly po (max 3 doses/24 h)[1] (or as transdermal patches; release 1 mg over 72 h); 0.6–2.4 mg/24 h as sc infusion[2]; 300 microgram bd po[3] (can ↑to tds).

Don't confuse with hyoscine *butylbromide*: different fx and doses!

HYPROMELLOSE 0.3% EYE DROPS
Artificial tears for treatment of dry eyes.
Dose: 1 drop prn, max 4–6 times/day unless preservative free drops.

IBUGEL Ibuprofen topical gel, for musculoskeletal pain.

IBUPROFEN
Mild-moderate strength NSAID. Non-selective COX inhibitor; analgesic, anti-inflammatory and antipyrexial[†] properties.
Use: mild/moderate pain[1] (inc musculoskeletal, headache, migraine, dysmenorrhoea, dental, post-op; not 1st choice for gout/RA as ↓anti-inflammatory fx compared to other NSAIDs), mild local inflammation[2].
CI: Hx of hypersensitivity to aspirin or any other NSAID (inc asthma/angioedema/urticaria/rhinitis). **Active/Hx of PU/GI bleeding/ perforation, L/R/H** (if any of these 3 are severe)/**P** (3rd trimester).
Caution: Asthma, allergic disorders, uncontrolled HTN, IHD, PVD, cerebrovascular disease, cardiovascular risk factors, connective tissue disorders, coagulopathy, IBD. *Can mask signs of infection*[†].
L/R/H/P (1st/2nd trimester: preferably avoid)/**B/E**.
SE: GI upset/bleeding/PU (*less than other NSAIDs*). AKI, hypersensitivity reactions (esp bronchospasm and skin reactions, inc, very rarely, SJS/TEN), fluid retention/oedema, headache, dizziness, nervousness, depression, drowsiness, insomnia, tinnitus, photosensitivity, haematuria. >1.2 g/day ⇒ small ↑risk thrombotic events. Reversible ↓female fertility if long-term use. Very rarely, blood disorders, ↑BP, ↑K^+.
Interactions: ↑risk GI bleeding with aspirin, clopidogrel, anti-coagulants, corticosteroids, SSRIs, venlafaxine and erlotinib. ↑s

(toxic) fx of digoxin, quinolones, lithium, phenytoin, baclofen, methotrexate, AZT and sulphonylureas. ↑risk of RF with ACE-i, ARB, diuretics, tacrolimus and ciclosporin. ↑risk ↑K⁺ with K-sparing diuretics and aldosterone antagonists. ↓s fx of antihypertensives and diuretics. ↑levels with ritonavir and triazoles. Mild **W +**.

Dose: initially 300–400 mg tds po[1] (max 2.4 g/day); topically as gel[2].

NB: Avoid/↓dose in RF & consider gastroprotective Rx.

INDAPAMIDE

Thiazide derivative diuretic; see Bendroflumethiazide.

Use: HTN (*for advice on stepped HTN Mx see p. 235*).

CI: Hx of sulphonamide derivative allergy, ↓K⁺, ↓Na⁺, ↑Ca²⁺, **L/R** (if either severe).

Caution: ↑PTH (stop if ↑Ca²⁺), ↑aldosterone, gout, porphyria, **R/P/B/E**.

SE: as bendroflumethiazide, but reportedly fewer metabolic disturbances (esp less hyperglycaemia).

Monitor: U&Es, urate.

Interactions: ↑s lithium levels and toxicity of digoxin (if ⇒ ↓K⁺).

Dose: 2.5 mg od mane (or 1.5 mg od of SR preparation).

INDOMETACIN

High-strength NSAID; non-selective COX inhibitor.

Use: musculoskeletal pain[1], esp RA, ankylosing spondylitis, OA; acute gout[2]; dysmenorrhoea[3]. Use limited by SEs*. Specialist uses: PDA closure, premature labour[SPC/BNF].

CI/Caution/SE/Interactions: as ibuprofen, but ↑incidence of SEs*, inc PU/GI bleeds, thrombotic events, GI upset and headache. Light-headedness (impairing driving) is common. Rarely: Ψ disturbances, convulsions, syncope, blood disorders, ↑CBG, peripheral neuropathy, optic neuritis, intestinal strictures; pr doses may ⇒ rectal irritation/bleeding. Caution in epilepsy, Parkinsonism & Ψ disturbance. Probenecid ⇒ ↑serum levels. ↑risk of AKI with triamterene: avoid. Possible severe drowsiness with haloperidol. No known interaction with baclofen or triazoles. Mild **W +**.

Dose: 25–50 mg max qds po or 100 mg max bd pr[1]. 150–200 mg/day in divided doses, ↓ing dose once pain under control[2]. 75 mg/day in divided doses[3]. MR preparations available[SPC/BNF].
NB: Avoid/↓dose in RF & consider gastroprotective Rx.

INFLIXIMAB/REMICADE

Monoclonal Ab against TNF-α (inflammatory cytokine).
Use: Crohn's/UC[NICE], RA[NICE], psoriasis (for skin or arthritis)[NICE] or ankylosing spondylitis[NICE].
CI: TB or other severe infections, **H** (unless mild when only caution), **P/B**.
Caution: infections, demyelinating CNS disorders, **L/R**.
SE: severe infections, TB (inc extrapulmonary), CCF (exac of), **CNS demyelination**. Also GI upset, 'flu-like symptoms, cough, fatigue, headache. ↑incidence of hypersensitivity (esp transfusion) reactions.
Dose: specialist use only. Often prescribed concurrently with methotrexate.

INSULATARD Long-acting (isophane) insulin, either recombinant human or porcine/bovine.

INSULIN see p. 204 for different types and prescribing advice.

INTEGRILIN see Eptifibatide; anti-Pt agent for IHD.

IODINE and IODIDE see Lugol's solution; used for ↑↑T₄.

IPOCOL see Mesalazine; 'new' aminosalicylate for UC, with ↓SEs.

IPRATROPIUM

Inh muscarinic antagonist; bronchodilator and ↓s bronchial secretions.
Use: chronic[1] and acute[2] bronchospasm (COPD > asthma). Rarely used topically for rhinitis.
SE: antimuscarinic fx (see p. 276), usually minimal.
Caution: glaucoma (angle closure only; protect patient's eyes from drug, esp if giving nebs: use tight-fitting mask), bladder outflow obstruction (e.g. ↑prostate), **P/B**.
Dose: 20–40 microgram tds/qds inh[1] (max 80 microgram qds); 250–500 microgram qds neb[2] (↑ing up to 4-hrly if severe).

IRBESARTAN/APROVEL

Angiotensin II antagonist.

Use: HTN (*for advice on stepped HTN Mx see p. 235*), type 2 DM nephropathy.

CI: P/B.

Caution/SE/Interactions: see Losartan.

Dose: initially 150 mg od, ↑ing to 300 mg od if required (halve initial dose if age >75 years or on haemodialysis).

IRON TABLETS see Ferrous sulphate/fumarate/gluconate.

ISMN see Isosorbide mononitrate.

ISMO see Isosorbide mononitrate.

ISONIAZID

Antituberculous antibiotic; 'static'.

Use: TB (see p. 267).

CI: drug-induced liver disease.

Caution: Hx of psychosis/epilepsy/porphyria or if ↑d risk of neuropathy[†] (e.g. DM, alcohol abuse, CRF, malnutrition, HIV: give pyridoxine 10–20 mg od as Px), porphyria, **L/R/P/B**.

SE: optic neuritis, **peripheral neuropathy**[†], **hepatitis**[*], rash, gynaecomastia, GI upset. Rarely lupus, blood disorders (inc rarely agranulocytosis[**]), hypersensitivity, convulsions, psychosis.

Warn: patient of symptoms of liver disease and to seek medical help if they occur.

Monitor: LFTs[*], FBC[**].

Interactions: ↓ **P450** ∴ many, but most importantly ↑s levels of carbamazepine, phenytoin, ethosuximide and benzodiazepines **W +**.

Dose: by weight[SPC/BNF] or as combination preparation (see p. 267). Take on empty stomach (⩾30 min before or ⩾ 2 h after meal).

Acetylator-dependent metabolism: if slow acetylator ⇒ ↑risk of SEs.

ISOSORBIDE MONONITRATE (ISMN)

Nitrate; as GTN, but po rather than sl delivery.

Use/CI/Caution/SE/Interactions: as GTN, but ⇒ ↓headache.

Dose: 10–40 mg bd/tds po (od MR preparations available[SPC/BNF]).

ISTIN see Amlodipine; Ca^{2+} channel blocker for HTN/IHD.

ITRACONAZOLE/SPORANOX

Triazole antifungal: needs acidic pH for good po absorption*.
Use: fungal infections (candida, tinea, cryptococcus, aspergillosis, histoplasmosis, onychomycosis, pityriasis versicolor).
Caution: risk of HF: Hx of cardiac disease or if on negative inotropic drugs (risk ↑s with dose, length of Rx and age), **L/R/P/B**.
SE: HF, hepatotoxicity**, GI upset, headache, dizziness, peripheral neuropathy (if occurs, stop drug), cholestasis, menstrual Δs, skin reactions (inc angioedema, SJS). With prolonged Rx can ⇒ ↓K^+, oedema, hair loss.
Monitor: LFTs** if Rx >1 month or Hx of (or develop clinical features of) liver disease: stop drug if become abnormal.
Interactions: ↓ **P450** ∴ many; most importantly ↑s risk of myopathy with statins (avoid together) and ↑s risk of **HF with negative inotropes** (esp Ca^{2+} blockers). ↑s fx of 😴 **midazolam, quinidine, pimozide** 💀, ciclosporin, digoxin, indinavir and siro-/tacro-limus. fx ↓d by rifampicin, phenytoin and **antacids***, **W +**.
Dose: dependent on indication[SPC/BNF]. *Take capsules with food (or liquid on empty stomach).* NB: consider ↓dose in LF.

▼ IVABRADINE/PROCORALAN

↓s HR by selective cardiac pacemaker I_f channel current blockade ⇒ ↓SAN myocyte Na^+ and K^+ entry.
Use: angina (if sinus rhythm and β-blockers CI/not tolerated).
CI: severe ↓HR (<60 bpm) or ↓BP, cardiogenic shock, ACS (inc acute MI), acute CVA, 2nd or 3rd degree HB, SSS, pacemaker dependent, SAN block congenital ↑QT syndrome, strong **P450 3A4** inhibitors**, **L** (if severe)/**H** (if moderate/severe)/**P/B**.
Caution: retinitis pigmentosa, galactose intolerance*/Lapp lactase deficiency*/glucose-galactose malabsorption*, **R/E**.
SE: visual Δs (esp luminous phenomena*), ↓HR, HB, ectopics, VF, headaches, dizziness. Less commonly GI upset, cramps, dyspnoea, ↑EØ, ↑uric acid, ↓GFR.

Warn: tablets contain lactose*, may ↓vision if night driving/using machinery with rapid light intensity Δs.

Monitor: HR (maintain resting ventricular rate >50 bpm) and rhythm, BP.

Interactions: ☠ **metab by P450 3A4**; inhibitors ↑levels and strong inhibitors** (clari-/ery-/josa-/teli-thromycin, itra-/keto-conazole, nelfi-/rito-navir, nefazodone) are CI but ↓doses can be given with fluconazole. Inducers ↓levels (inc rifampicin, barbiturates, phenytoin, St John's wort). Levels also ↑by diltiazem and verapamil. ↑risk of VF with drugs that ↑QTc (inc amiodarone, disopyramide, mefloquine, pentamidine, pimozide, sertindole, sotalol) ☠.

Dose: initially 5 mg bd po; ↑ing if required after 3–4 wks to max 7.5 mg bd po.

NB: consider ↓dose if not tolerated, elderly or severe RF^{SPC/BNF}.

KAY-CEE-L

KCl syrup (1 mmol/ml) for ↓K⁺; see Sando-K.

Dose: according to serum K⁺: average 25–50 ml/day in divided doses if diet normal. Caution if taking other drugs that ↑K⁺.

NB: ↓dose if RF.

KETAMINE/KETALAR

IV anaesthetic (but can also be given im). NMDA receptor antagonist & inhibitor of nitric oxide synthase.

Use: induction and maintenance of anaesthesia (mainly paediatric use; esp if repeated administration required).

CI: anaesthetist not confident of airway maintenance, HTN, pre-eclampsia / eclampsia, severe coronary or myocardial disease, CVA, ↑ICP, head trauma, acute porphyria.

Caution: hypovolaemia / dehydration, cardiovascular disease, patients in whom ↑BP would constitute a serious hazard, respiratory tract infection (⇒ laryngospasm), ↑IOP, head injury / intracranial mass lesions, ↑CSF pressure, ↑seizure risk, Ψ disorders (esp psychosis), thyroid dysfunction, EtOH xs (acute or chronic). **L / H / P** (may ↓ neonatal respiration if used during delivery) / **B** (avoid for ≥ 12 hrs after last dose); **E** (↓ dose & rate of administration);

SE: nightmares, psychosis (can ↓ with benzodiazepines), N&V, ↑RR, ↑HR/BP, diplopia, nystagmus, rash, hypertonia, extraneous muscle movements. Can ⇒ delirium during recovery period.

Warn: don't drive or use hazardous machinery for 24 hrs.

Monitor: Cardiac, respiratory and motor function (recovery is relatively slow).

Interactions: memantine (⇒ CNS toxicity). ↑s fx of atracurium and tubocurarine (respiratory depression and apnoea). Theophylline ⇒ convulsions. ↓BP with adrenergic neurone blockers, α-blockers, antipsychotics, verapamil (also ⇒ AV delay). Thyroid hormones (⇒ HTN and ↑HR).

Dose: titrate to effect, except during 'rapid sequence induction'. **IM:** For short procedures; initially 6.5–13 mg/kg adjusting to response (10 mg/kg usually ⇒ 12–25 mins anaesthesia). For diagnostic manoeuvres / procedures not involving intense pain, initially 4 mg/kg. **IV** (over ≥60 secs): short procedures, initially 1 – 4.5 mg/kg (2 mg/kg usually ⇒ 5–10 mins anaesthesia). **IVI** (1 mg/mL solution): For longer procedures; induction total dose of 0.5–2 mg/kg then maintenance 10–45 micrograms/kg/min adjusting to response.

> ☠ Should only be administered by, or under direct supervision of, personnel experienced in its use, with adequate training in anaesthesia and airway management, and when resuscitation equipment is available. Can ⇒ apnoea and ↓BP within one arm-brain circulation time. ☠

KETOCONAZOLE/NIZORAL

Imidazole antifungal: good po absorption.

Use: fungal infection Rx (if systemic, severe or resistant to topical Rx) and Px if immunosuppression; use limited (due to hepatotoxicity) to dermatophytosis, *Malassezia* folliculitis and cutaneous or oropharyngeal candidosis and only when topical and oral agents can't be used.

CI: L/P/B.

Caution: porphyria.

SE: hepatitis*, **GI upset**, **skin reactions** (rash, urticaria, pruritus, photosensitivity, rarely angioedema), **gynaecomastia**, blood disorders, paraesthesia, dizziness, photophobia.

L/R/H = Liver, Renal and Heart failure (full key see p. xv)

Monitor: LFTs*, esp if Rx >14 days.

Warn: seek urgent medical attention if signs of LF (explain symptoms to patient).

Interactions: ↓ **P450** ∴ many; most importantly, ↑s risk of **myopathy with statins** (avoid together). ↑s fx of ☠ **midazolam, quinidine, pimozide** ☠, vardenafil, eplerenone, cilostazol, reboxetine, aripiprazole, sertindole, felodipine, ergot alkaloids, antidiabetics, buprenorphine, artemether/lumefantrine, indi-/ rito-navir and ciclosporin (and possibly theophyllines). ↓s fx of rifampicin (rifampicin can also ↓fx of ketoconazole, as can phenytoin and clopidogrel), **W +**.

Dose: 200 mg od po *with food* (400 mg od in severe/resistant cases).

KLEAN-PREP see Bowel preparations.

Dose: up to 2 powder sachets the evening before and repeated on the morning of GI surgery or Ix.

LABETALOL

β-blocker with arteriolar vasodilatory properties ∴ also ⇒ ↓TPR.

Use: uncontrolled/severe HTN (inc during pregnancy[1] or post-MI[2] or with angina). *For advice on HTN Mx see p. 235.*

CI/Caution/SE/Interactions: as propranolol, plus can ⇒ ☠ severe/postural ↓BP ☠ and hepatotoxicity* (**L**).

Monitor: LFTs* (if deteriorate stop drug).

Dose: initially 100 mg bd po (halve dose in elderly), ↑ing every fortnight if necessary to max of 600 mg qds po; if essential to ↓BP rapidly give 50 mg iv over ≥1 min repeating after 5 min if necessary (or can give 2 mg/min ivi), up to max total dose 200 mg; 20 mg/h ivi[1], doubling every 30 min to max of 160 mg/h; 15 mg/h ivi[2], ↑ing slowly to max of 120 mg/h. NB: consider ↓dose in RF.

LACRI-LUBE

Artificial tears for dry eyes.

SE: blurred vision ∴ usually used at bedtime (or if vision secondary consideration, e.g. Bell's palsy or blind eye).

Dose: 1 application prn.

LACTULOSE

Osmotic laxative[1]: bulking agent. Also ↓s growth of NH_4-producing bacteria[2].

Use: constipation[1], hepatic encephalopathy[2].

CI: GI obstruction, galactosaemia.

Caution: lactose intolerance.

SE: flatulence, distension, abdominal pains.

Dose: 15 ml od/bd[1] (↑dose according to response; NB: *can take 2 days to work*); 30–50 ml tds[2]. *Take with plenty of water.*

LAMISIL see Terbinafine.

▼ LAMOTRIGINE/LAMICTAL

Antiepileptic: ↓s release of excitatory amino acids (esp glutamate) via action on voltage-sensitive Na^+ channels.

Use: epilepsy (esp partial and 1° or 2° generalised tonic–clonic), Px depressive episode in bipolar disorder.

Caution: avoid abrupt withdrawal[†] (rebound seizure risk; taper off over ≥2 wks unless stopping due to serious skin reaction*), **L/R/P/B/E**.

SE: cerebellar symptoms (see p. 278), **skin reactions*** (often severe, e.g. SJS, TEN, lupus, esp in children, if on valproate, or high initial doses), **blood disorders**** (↓Hb, ↓WCC, ↓Pt), N&V. Rarely, ↓memory, sedation, Ψ disorders, sleep Δ, acne, pretibial ulcers, alopecia, worsening of seizures, poly-/an-uria, **hepatotoxicity**.

Monitor: U&Es, FBC, LFTs, clotting.

Warn: report rash* plus any 'flu-like symptoms, signs of infection/ ↓Hb or bruising**. Don't stop tablets suddenly[†]. Risk of suicidal ideation.

Interactions: fx are ↓d by OCP, phenytoin, carbamazepine, mefloquine, TCAs and SSRIs. fx ↑d by valproate.

Dose: 25–700 mg daily[SPC/BNF]; ↑dose slowly to ↓risk of skin reactions* (also need to restart at low dose). NB: ↓**dose in LF**.

LANSOPRAZOLE/ZOTON

PPI. As omeprazole, but ↓interactions.

Dose: 15–30 mg od po (↓to 15 mg od for maintenance).

LARIAM see Mefloquine; antimalarial (Px and Rx).

LASIX see Furosemide; loop diuretic.

▼ LATANOPROST 0.01%/XALATAN

Topical PG analogue: ↑s uveoscleral outflow.

Use: ↑IOP in glaucoma and *ocular* HTN (1st line agent).

Caution: asthma (if severe), aphakia, pseudophakia, uveitis, macular oedema **P/B**.

SE: iris colour Δ* (can ⇒ permanent ↑brown pigmentation, esp if uniocular use), blurred vision, local reactions (e.g. conjunctival hyperaemia in up to 30% initially). Also darkening of periocular skin and ↑eyelash length (both reversible). Rarely cystoid macular oedema (if aphakia), uveitis, angina.

Warn: can Δ iris colour*.

Dose: 1 drop od.

LEFLUNOMIDE/ARAVA

DMARD; inhibits pyrimidine synthesis (also anti-inflammatory fx).

Use: active rheumatoid or psoriatic arthritis if standard DMARDs (e.g. methotrexate or sulfasalazine) CI or not tolerated.

CI: severe immunodeficiency, BM suppression, severe hypoproteinaemia, serious infection, **L/R/P/B**.

Caution: blood disorders, recent hepato-/myelo-toxic drugs, TB (inc Hx of).

SE: BM toxicity, ↑risk of **infection/malignancy**, hepatotoxicity (potentially life-threatening in 1st 6 months), SJS, HTN.

Warn: teratogenic: must exclude pregnancy before starting Rx and use contraception during Rx (and until drug no longer active*).

Monitor: LFTs, FBC, BP.

Dose: specialist use only.

> Long $t_{1/2}$*: if serious SE discontinue treatment and needs prolonged washout period or active measures (e.g. cholestyramine 8 g tds or activated charcoal 50 g qds) to ↑elimination if wishing to conceive.

LEVOBUNOLOL

β-blocker eye drops: similar to timolol ⇒ ↓aqueous humour production. *Significant systemic absorption can occur.*
Use: chronic simple (wide-/open-angle) glaucoma.
CI/Caution/Interactions: as propranolol; interactions less likely.
SE: local reactions. Rarely anterior uveitis and anaphylaxis. Can ⇒ systemic fx, esp bronchoconstriction/cardiac fx; see Propranolol.
Dose: 1 drop of 0.5% solution od/bd.

LEVODOPA (= L-DOPA)

Precursor of dopamine: needs concomitant peripheral dopa decarboxylase inhibitor such as benserazide (see Co-beneldopa) or carbidopa (see Co-careldopa) to limit SEs.
Use: Parkinsonism.
CI: glaucoma (closed-angle), taking MAO-A inhibitors*, melanoma[†], **P/B.**
Caution: pulmonary/cardiovascular/Ψ disease, endocrine disorder, glaucoma (open angle), osteomalacia, Hx of PU or convulsions, ventricular arrhythmias, **L/R.**
SE: dyskinesias, abdominal upset, postural ↓BP/arrhythmias, drowsiness, aggression, Ψ disorders (confusion, depression, suicide, hallucinations, psychosis, hypomania), seizures, dizziness, headache, flushing, sweating, peripheral neuropathy, taste Δs, rash/pruritus, can reactivate melanoma[†], Δ LFTs, GI bleeding, blood disorders, dark body fluids (inc sweat).
Warn: can ⇒ daytime sleepiness (inc sudden-onset sleep) and ↓ability to drive/operate machinery.
Interactions: fx ↓d by neuroleptics, SEs ↑d by bupropion, **risk of ↑BP crisis with MAOIs*** (but can give with MAO-B inhibitors), risk of arrhythmias with halothane.
Dose: 125–500 mg daily, *after food*, ↑ing according to response.

Abrupt withdrawal can ⇒ neuroleptic malignant-like syndrome.

LEVOMEPROMAZINE (= METHOTRIMEPRAZINE)

Phenothiazine antipsychotic; as chlorpromazine, but used in palliative care as has good antiemetic[1] and sedative[2] fx, but little respiratory depression.

Use: refractory N&V[1] or restlessness/distress[2] in the terminally ill.

CI/Caution/SE/Interactions: as chlorpromazine, but ↑risk of postural ↓BP (esp in elderly: don't give if age >50 years and ambulant) and ↑risk of seizures (caution if epilepsy/brain tumour).

Dose: 6.25–25 mg po/sc/im/iv od/bd (can ↑to tds/qds), or 25–200 mg/24 h sc infusion. **Parenteral dose is half equivalent oral dose.**
NB: for N&V low doses may be effective and ⇒ ↓sedation. Doses >25 mg sc/24 hrs rarely needed except as major sedation.
NB: ↓dose in RF and elderly.

LEVOTHYROXINE see Thyroxine.

LIBRIUM see Chlordiazepoxide; long-acting benzodiazepine.

LIDOCAINE (previously Lignocaine)

Class Ib antiarrhythmic (↓s conduction in Purkinje and ventricular muscle fibres), local anaesthetic (blocks axonal Na⁺ channels).

Use: ventricular arrhythmias (esp post-MI), local anaesthesia.

CI: myocardial depression (if severe), SAN disorders, atrioventricular block (all grades), porphyria.

Caution: epilepsy, severe hypoxia/hypovolaemia/↓HR, **L/H/P/B/E.**

SE: **dizziness, drowsiness, confusion, tinnitus,** blurred vision, paraesthesia, GI upset, arrhythmias, ↓BP, ↓HR. Rarely respiratory depression, seizures, anaphylaxis.

Monitor: ECG during iv administration.

Interactions: ↑risk of arrhythmias with antipsychotics, dolasetron and quinu-/dalfo-pristin. ↑myocardial depression with other antiarrhythmics and β-blockers. Levels ↑by propranolol, ataza-/lopinavir and cimetidine. Prolongs action of suxamethonium.

Dose (for ventricular arrhythmias): 50–100 mg iv at rate of 25–30 mg/min followed immediately by ivi at 4 mg/min for

30 min then 2 mg/min for 2 h and 1 mg/min thereafter (↓dose further if drug needed for >24 h). NB: short $t_{1/2}$ ∴ if 15 min delay in setting up ivi, can give max 2 further doses of 50–100 mg iv ≥10 min apart. In emergencies, can often be found stocked in crash trolleys as Minijet syringes of 1% (10 mg/ml) or 2% (20 mg/ml) solutions.

☠ Local anaesthetic preparations must never be injected into veins or inflamed tissue, as can ⇒ systemic fx (esp arrhythmias) ☠.

LIGNOCAINE see Lidocaine.

LIOTHYRONINE (= L-TRI-IODOTHYRONINE) SODIUM

Synthetic T_3: quicker and more potent action than thyroxine (T_4).
Use: severe hypothyroidism (e.g. myxoedema coma*: see page 257).
CI/Caution/SE/Interactions: see Thyroxine.
Dose: 5–20 microgram iv slowly. Repeat every 4–12 h as necessary; seek expert help. Also available po, but thyroxine (T_4) often preferred. NB: 20 microgram liothyronine = 100 microgram (levo) thyroxine.

Concurrent hydrocortisone iv is often also needed*.

LISINOPRIL

ACE-i; see Captopril.
Use: HTN[1] (*for advice on stepped HTN Mx see p. 235*), HF[2], Px of IHD post-MI[3], DM nephropathy[4].
CI/Caution/SE/Interactions: as Captopril.
Dose: initially 10 mg od[1] (2.5–5.0 mg if RF or used with diuretic) ↑ing if necessary to max 80 mg/day; initially 2.5–5 mg od[2,4] adjusted to response to usual maintenance of 5–20 mg/day. Doses post-MI[3] depend on BP[SPC/BNF].
NB: ↓dose in LF or RF.

LITHIUM

Mood stabiliser: modulates intracellular signalling; blocks neuronal Ca^{2+} channels and changes GABA pathways.

Use: mania Rx/Px, bipolar disorder Px. Rarely for recurrent depression Px and aggressive/self-mutilating behaviour Rx.

CI: ↓T_4 (if untreated), Addison's, SSS, cardiovascular disease, **P** (⇒ Ebstein's anomaly: esp in 1st trimester), **R/H/B.** (NB: manufacturers don't agree on definitive list and all CI are **relative** – decisions should be made in clinical context and expert help sought if unsure.)

Caution: thyroid disease, MG, **E**.

SE: thirst, polyuria, GI upset (↑Wt, N&V&D), *fine* tremor* (NB: in toxicity ⇒ *coarse* tremor), tardive dyskinesia, muscular weakness, acne, psoriasis exacerbation, ↑WCC, ↑Pt. Rarer but serious: ↓(or ↑) T_4 ± goitre (esp in females), renal impairment (diabetes insipidus, interstitial nephritis), arrhythmias. Very rarely can ⇒ neuroleptic malignant syndrome.

Monitor: serum levels *12 h post-dose*: keep at 0.6–1 mmol/l (>1.5 mmol/l may ⇒ toxicity, esp if elderly), U&Es, TFTs.

Warn: report symptoms of ↓T_4, avoid dehydration.

Interactions: toxicity (± levels) ↑d by **NSAIDs, diuretics**** (esp thiazides), SSRIs, ACE-i, ARBs, amiodarone, methyldopa, carbamazepine and haloperidol. Theophyllines, caffeine and antacids may ↓lithium levels.

Dose: see SPC/BNF: 2 *types* (salts) available with different doses ('carbonate' 200 mg = 'citrate' 509 mg) and bioavailabilities of particular *brands* vary ∴ *must specify salt and brand required*. For 'carbonate' starting dose usually 200 mg nocte, adjusting to plasma levels (maintenance usually 600 mg – 1 g nocte).
NB: ↓dose in LF.

Consider stopping 24 h before major surgery or ECT; restart once e'lytes return to normal. Discuss with anaesthetist ± psychiatrist.

Lithium toxicity
Features: D&V, coarse tremor*, cerebellar signs (see p. 278), renal impairment/oliguria, ↓BP, ↑reflexes, convulsions, drowsiness ⇒ coma, arrhythmia. *Rx*: stop drug, control seizures, correct electrolytes (normally need saline ivi; high risk if ↓Na^+: avoid low-salt diets and diuretics**). Consider haemodialysis if RF.

LOCOID see Hydrocortisone butyrate 0.1% (potent steroid) cream.

LOFEPRAMINE
2nd generation TCA.

Use: depression

CI/Caution/SE/Warn/Monitor/Interactions: as amitriptyline but also **R** (if severe). Also ⇒ ↓**sedation** (sometimes alerting – don't give nocte if occurs) and ↓**anticholinergic and cardiac SEs** ∴ ↓*danger in OD*.

Dose: 140–210 mg daily in divided (bd/tds) doses.

LOPERAMIDE/IMODIUM
Antimotility agent: synthetic opioid analogue; binds to receptors in GI muscle ⇒ ↓peristalsis, ↑transit time, ↑H_2O/electrolyte resorption, ↓gut secretions, ↑sphincter tone. Extensive 1st-pass metabolism ⇒ minimal systemic opioid fx.

Use: diarrhoea.

CI: constipation, ileus, megacolon, bacterial enterocolitis 2° to invasive organisms (e.g. salmonella, *Shigella*, *Campylobacter*), abdominal distension, active UC/AAC, pseudomembranous colitis.

Caution: in young (can ⇒ fluid + electrolyte depletion), **L/P**.

SE: constipation, abdominal cramps, bloating, dizziness, drowsiness, fatigue. Rarely hypersensitivity (esp skin reactions), paralytic ileus.

Dose: initially 4 mg, then 2 mg after each loose stool (max 16 mg/ day for 5 days). *NB: can mask serious GI conditions.*

LORATADINE
Non-sedating antihistamine: see Cetirizine.

Dose: 10 mg od. Non-proprietary or as Clarityn.

LORAZEPAM
Benzodiazepine, short-acting.

Use: sedation[1] (esp acute behavioural disturbance/Ψ disorders, e.g. acute psychosis), status epilepticus[2].

CI/Caution/SE/Interactions: see Diazepam.

Dose: 0.5–2 mg po/im/iv prn (bottom of this range if elderly/ respiratory disease/naive to benzodiazepines; top of range if young/ recent exposure to benzodiazepines; max 4 mg/day)[1]; 0.1 mg/kg ivi at 2 mg/min (max 4 mg repeated once after 10 mins if necessary)[2]. **NB:** ↓**dose in RF**.

> ☠ Beware respiratory depression: have O_2 (± resuscitation trolley) at hand, esp if respiratory disease or giving high doses im/iv ☠.

▼ LOSARTAN/COZAAR

Angiotensin II receptor antagonist: specifically blocks renin– angiotensin system ∴ does not inhibit bradykinin and ⇒ dry cough.
Use: HTN (*for advice on stepped HTN Mx see p. 235*), Px of type 2 DM nephropathy (if ACE-i not tolerated*).
CI: P/B.
Caution: RAS, HCM, mitral/aortic stenosis, if taking drugs that ↑K^{+**}, **L/R/E**.
SE/Interactions: as captopril, but ↓dry cough (major reason for ACE-i intolerance*). As with ACE-i, can ⇒ ↑K^+(esp if taking ↑K^+ sparing diuretics/salt substitutes or if RF).
Dose: initially 25–50 mg od (↑ing to max 100 mg od). **NB:** ↓**dose in LF or RF**.

> ☠ **Beware if on other drugs that ↑K^+, e.g. amiloride, spironolactone, triamterene, ACE-i and ciclosporin. Don't give with oral K^+ supplements (inc dietary salt substitutes) ☠.

LOSEC see Omeprazole; PPI (ulcer-healing drug).

LUGOL'S SOLUTION

Oral I_2 solution (containing iodine and K^+ iodide).
Use: ↑T_4 if severe ('thyroid storm') or pre-operatively.
CI: B.
Caution: not for long-term Rx, **P**.
SE: hypersensitivity.
Dose: 0.1–0.3 ml tds (of solution containing 130 mg iodine/ml).

LYMECYCLINE

Tetracycline, broad-spectrum antibiotic (see Tetracycline).
Use: acne vulgaris, rosacea.
CI/Caution/SE/Interactions: as tetracycline.
Dose: 408 mg od for $\geq$8 wks (can $\uparrow$to bd for other indications).

MADOPAR see Co-beneldopa; L-dopa for Parkinson's.

MAGNESIUM SULPHATE (iv)

Mg^{2+} replacement.
Use: life-threatening asthma[1] (unlicensed indication), serious arrhythmias[2] (esp if torsades or if $\downarrow$K+; often caused by $\downarrow Mg^{2+}$), MI[3] (equivocal evidence of $\downarrow$mortality), eclampsia/pre-eclampsia[4] ($\downarrow$s seizures), symptomatic $\downarrow Mg^{2+}$ [5] (mostly 2° to GI loss).
Caution: monitor BP, respiratory rate and urine output, **L/R**.
SE: flushing, $\downarrow$BP, GI upset, thirst, $\downarrow$reflexes, weakness, confusion/drowsiness. Rarely arrhythmias, respiratory depression, coma.
Interactions: $\uparrow$risk of $\downarrow$BP with Ca^{2+} channel blockers.
Dose: 4–8 mmol ivi over 20 min[1]; 8 mmol iv over 10–15 min[2] (repeating once if required); 8 mmol ivi over 20 min then ivi of 65–72 mmol over 24 h[3]; 4 mg ivi over 5–10 min then ivi at 1 mg/h until 24 hr after the last seizure[4]; up to 160 mmol ivi/im according to need[5] (over up to 5 days). For iv injection, use concentrations of $\leq$20%; if using 50% solution dilute 1 part with $\geq$1.5 parts water for injection.

MANNITOL

Osmotic diuretic.
Use: cerebral oedema[1] (and glaucoma).
CI: pulmonary oedema, **H**.
SE: GI upset, fever/chills, oedema. Rarely seizures, HF.
Dose: 0.25–2 g/kg (2.5–20 ml/kg **10% solution**) as rapid ivi over 30–60 min[1].

MAXOLON see Metoclopramide; antiemetic (DA antagonist).

MEBEVERINE

Antispasmodic: direct action on GI muscle.

Use: GI smooth-muscle cramps (esp IBS, diverticulitis).

CI: ileus (paralytic).

Caution: porphyria, **P**.

SE: hypersensitivity/skin reactions.

Dose: 135–150 mg tds (20 min before food) or 200 mg bd of SR preparation (Colofac MR).

MEFENAMIC ACID/PONSTAN

Mild NSAID; non-selective COX inhibitor.

Use: musculoskeletal pain, dysmenorrhoea, menorrhagia.

CI/Caution/SE/Interactions: as ibuprofen, but also CI if IBD, caution if epilepsy or acute porphyria. Can ⇒ severe diarrhoea, skin reactions, stomatitis, paraesthesia, fatigue, haemolytic/aplastic ↓Hb, ↓Pt. No known interaction with baclofen or triazoles. Mild **W +**.

Dose: 500 mg tds.

MEFLOQUINE/LARIAM

Antimalarial; kills asexual forms of *Plasmodium*.

Use: malaria Px[1] (in areas of chloroquine-resistant falciparum spp) and rarely as Rx *if not taking the drug as Px*.

CI: hypersensitivity *to mefloquine or quinine*, Hx of neuro-Ψ disorders (inc depression, convulsions).

Caution: epilepsy, cardiac conduction disorders, **L/P/B**.

SE: GI upset, neuro-Ψ reactions (dizziness, ↓balance, headache, convulsions, sleep disorders, neuropathies, tremor, anxiety, depression, psychosis, hallucinations, panic attacks, agitation). Also cardiac fx (AV block, other conduction disorders, ↑ or ↓HR, ↑or ↓BP), hypersensitivity reactions.

Warn: can ↓driving/other skilled tasks and ⇒ neuro-Ψ reactions.

Interactions: ↑risk of seizures with quinine, chloroquine and hydroxychloroquine. ↓s fx of anticonvulsants (esp valproate and carbamazepine). ↑risk of arrhythmias with amiodarone, quinidine, moxifloxacin and pimozide. Avoid artemether/lumefantrine.

Dose: 250 mg once-wkly[1] (↓dose if Wt <45 kg)[SPC/BNF].

Need to start Px 2 1/2 wks before entering endemic area (to identify neuro-Ψ reactions; 75% of reactions occur by 3rd dose) and continue for 4 wks after leaving endemic area.

MEROPENEM
Carbapenem broad-spectrum antibiotic (β-lactam, but non-penicillin/non-cephalosporin).
Use: severe Gram +ve and –ve aerobic and anaerobic infections. Hospital acquired septicaemia.
Caution: β-lactam sensitivity (avoid if immediate hypersensitivity reaction) **L/R/P/B**.
SE: GI upset (N&V&D – inc AAC), ΔLFTs, headache, blood/skin disorders. Rarely seizures, SJS/TENS.
Monitor: LFTs.
Dose: 500 mg tds iv/ivi (↑to 1 g tds if severe infection or 2 g tds if meningitis or exacerbation of lower RTI in CF).
NB: ↑interval ± ↓dose if RF[SPC/BNF].

MESALAZINE
'New' aminosalicylate: as sulfasalazine, but with ↓sulphonamide SEs.
Use: UC (Rx/maintenance of remission).
CI: *hypersensitivity to any salicylates*, coagulopathies, **R** (caution only if mild), **L** (caution only if not severe).
Caution: **P/B/E**.
SE: GI upset, **blood disorders**, hypersensitivity (inc **lupus**), RF, headache.
Warn: report unexplained bleeding, bruising, fever, sore throat or malaise.
Monitor: U&E, FBC (stop drug if blood disorder suspected).
Interactions: fx ↓by lactulose. NSAIDs and azathioprine may ↑nephrotoxicity.
Dose: as Asacol (or Ipocol, Mezavant, Mesren, Pentasa and Salofalk). Preparations not interchangeable as delivery characteristics may vary.

MESNA

Binds to metabolite (acrolein) of thiol-containing chemotherapy agents (cyclophosphamide, ifosfamide), which are toxic to urothelium and can $\Rightarrow$ severe haemorrhagic cystitis. Give as Px before chemotherapy; see BNF for details.

METFORMIN

Oral antidiabetic (biguanide): $\Rightarrow$ ↑insulin sensitivity w/o affecting levels ($\Rightarrow$ ↓gluconeogenesis and ↓GI absorption of glucose and ↑peripheral use of glucose). Only active in presence of endogenous insulin (i.e. functional islet cells).

Use: type 2 DM: usually 1st-line if diet control unsuccessful (esp if obese, as $\Rightarrow$ less ↑Wt than sulphonylureas). Also used in PCOS (unlicensed; specialist use).

CI: DKA, ↑risk of lactic acidosis (e.g. RF, severe dehydration/infection/peripheral vascular disease, shock, major trauma, respiratory failure, alcohol dependence, **recent MI***, **general anaesthetic**** or iodine-containing radiology contrast media*), **L/R/P/B.**

SE: GI upset (esp initially or if ↑doses), taste disturbance. Rarely ↓vit B_{12} absorption, lactic acidosis[†] (stop drug).

Dose: Standard release tablets – initially 500 mg mane, ↑ing as required to max 2 g/day in divided doses. Modified release tablets – initially 500 mg daily, ↑ing as required to max 2 g daily in 1. *Take with meals.* NB: ↓dose in mild RF, avoid in severe RF.

> 🦂 *Both often coexist in coronary angiography: stop drug on day of procedure (giving insulin if necessary; see p. 204) and restart 48 h later, having checked that renal function has not deteriorated. Stop on day of surgery ahead of general anaesthetic** and restart when renal function normal 🦂.

METHADONE

Opioid agonist: ↓euphoria and long $t_{1/2}$ ($\Rightarrow$ ↓withdrawal symptoms) compared with other opioids.

Use: opioid dependence as aid to withdrawal.

CI/Caution/SE/Interactions: as morphine but levels ↓by ritonavir, but are ↑by voriconazole and cimetidine and ↑risk of

ventricular arrhythmias with atomoxetine and amisulpride. Can
↑QTc (caution if family history of sudden death).

Dose: *individual requirements vary widely according to level of
previous abuse*: sensible starting dose is 10–20 mg/day po, ↑ing by
10–20 mg every day until no signs or symptoms of withdrawal –
which usually stop at 60–120 mg/day. Then aim to wean off
gradually. Available as non-proprietary solutions (1 mg/ml) or as
Methadose (10 mg/ml or 20 mg/ml). Can give sc/im[SPC/BNF]. **NB:**
↓**dose if LF, RF or elderly.**

☠ Don't confuse solutions of different strengths ☠.

METHIONINE

Sulphur-containing amino acid: binds toxic metabolites of
paracetamol.

Use: paracetamol OD *<12 h post-ingestion* (ineffective after this)
and not vomiting, mostly when acetylcysteine ivi cannot be given
(e.g. outside hospital).

CI: metabolic acidosis.

Caution: schizophrenia (can worsen), **L**.

SE: N&V, irritability, drowsiness.

Interactions: can ↓fx of L-dopa.

Dose: 2.5 g po 4-hrly (for *4 doses only: total dose = 10 g*).

METHOTREXATE

Immunosuppressant, antimetabolite: dihydrofolate reductase
inhibitor (↓s nucleic acid synthesis).

Use: rheumatoid arthritis [1] (1st-line DMARD) and other
inflammatory joint and muscle disorders, **psoriasis** (if severe/
resistant), Ca (ALL, non-Hodgkin's lymphoma, choriocarcinoma,
various solid tumours), rarely in Crohn's disease.

CI: severe blood disorders, active infections, immunodeficiency,
R/L (if either significant, otherwise caution), **P** (females and
males must avoid conception for ≥3 months after stopping
treatment), **B**.

Caution: effusions (esp ascites and pleural effusions: drain before starting treatment as risk of ↑toxicity), ↑ rheumatoid nodules, blood disorders, UC, PU, ↓immunity, porphyria, **E**.

SE: mucositis/GI upset, myelosuppression, skin reactions. Rarely **pulmonary fibrosis/pneumonitis** (esp in RA), liver toxicity/ hepatic fibrosis (esp in psoriatics), neurotoxicity (inc necrotising demyelinating leukoencephalopathy), seizures, RF (esp tubular necrosis).

Monitor: U&Es, FBC, LFTs ± procollagen 3 protein (to monitor for hepatic fibrosis).

Interactions: NSAIDs (e.g. concomitant use in RA), **trimethoprim, co-trimoxazole,** corticosteroids (e.g concomitant use in RA), probenecid, nitrous oxide, pyrimethamine, clozapine, cisplatin, acitretin, ciclosporin all ⇒ ↑toxicity ± levels.

Warn: avoid over-the-counter NSAIDs*, report any clinical features of infection (esp sore throat).

Dose: Oral: start 7.5 mg once weekly (max oral weekly dose 20 mg)[1]. For other indications and routes see BNF/SPC. NB: ↓dose in RF. *Usually needs concomitant folic acid (range 5 mg once/wk–5 days/wk (omitted day of and day after, methotrexate)).*

☠ NB: dose is only once a week: potentially fatal if given daily ☠.

METHOTRIMEPRAZINE see Levomepromazine; DA antagonist.

METHYLDOPA

Centrally acting α₂ agonist.

Use: HTN; esp pregnancy-induced and 1° HTN during pregnancy. *For advice on HTN Mx see p. 235.*

CI: depression, phaeo, porphyria, **L** (if active liver disease).

Caution: Hx of depression/**L**, **R**.

SE: (minimal if dose <1 g/day) dry mouth, sedation, dizziness, weakness, headache, GI upset, postural ↓BP, ↓HR. Rarely **blood disorders, hepatotoxicity,** pancreatitis, Ψ disorders, Parkinsonism, lupus-like syndrome, false +ve direct Coombs' test.

Monitor: FBC, LFTs.

Interactions: ↑s neurotoxicity of lithium. Hypotensive fx ↑d by antidepressants, anaesthetics and salbutamol ivi. ☠ **Avoid with, or within 2 wks of, MAOIs** ☠.
Dose: initially 250 mg bd/tds (125 mg bd in elderly), ↑ing gradually at intervals ≥2 days (max 2 g/day in elderly) to max of 3 g/day. **NB:** ↓dose in RF.

METHYLPREDNISOLONE
Glucocorticoid (mild mineralocorticoid activity).
Use: acute flares of inflammatory diseases[1] (esp rheumatoid arthritis, MS), cerebral oedema, Rx of graft rejection.
CI/Caution/SE/Interactions: see Steroids section (p. 217).
Dose: acutely, 10–500 mg ivi[1]; up to 1g ivi od for up to 3 days[2]. Also available po and as im depot[BNF].

METOCLOPRAMIDE/MAXOLON
Antiemetic: D₂ antagonist: acts on central chemoreceptor trigger zone and directly stimulates GI tract (⇒ ↑motility).
Use: N&V, esp GI (gastroduodenal, biliary, hepatic) or opiate-/chemotherapy-induced.
CI: GI obstruction/perforation/haemorrhage (inc 3–4 days post-GI surgery), phaeo, **B**.
Caution: epilepsy, porphyria, **L/R/P/E**.
SE: extrapyramidal fx (see p. 278 – esp in elderly and young females: reversible if drug stopped w/in 24 h or with procyclidine), **drowsiness**, restlessness (akathisia), GI upset, behavioural/mood Δs, ↑prolactin. Rarely skin reactions, neuroleptic malignant syndrome.
Interactions: ↑s fx of NSAIDs and ciclosporin levels. ↑s risk of extrapyramidal fx of antipsychotics, SSRIs and TCAs.
Dose: 10 mg tds po/im/iv. **NB:** ↓dose if RF, LF, 15–19 yrs old or weight <60 kg.

METOLAZONE
Potent thiazide-like diuretic: as bendroflumethiazide, plus has additive diuretic fx with loop diuretics.
Use: oedema[1], HTN[2] (for advice on stepped HTN Mx see p. 235).

CI/Caution/SE/Interactions: see Bendroflumethiazide.
Monitor: e'lytes (esp $Na^+/K^+/Ca^{2+}$) closely.
Dose: 5–10 mg od po (mane), ↑ing if needed to max of 80 mg/day (rarely >20 mg/day[1]); initially 5 mg od, then on alternate days for maintenance[2].

METOPROLOL

β-Blocker, cardioselective ($β_1 > β_2$), short-acting.
Use: HTN[1] (*for advice on stepped HTN Mx see p. 235*), angina[2], arrhythmias[3], migraine Px[4], ↑T_4 (adjunct)[5].
CI/Caution/SE/Interactions: see Propranolol.
Dose: 50–100 mg bd po[1,4]; 50–100 mg bd/tds po[2,3]; 50 mg qds po[5]. MR od preparation (Lopresor SR) available. Can give 2–5 mg iv[SPC/BNF] repeating to max 10–15 mg. See p. 226 for use in AMI/ACS. NB: ↓**dose in LF**.

METRONIDAZOLE/FLAGYL

Antibiotic, 'cidal': binds DNA of anaerobic (and microaerophilic) bacteria/protozoa.
Use: anaerobic and protozoal infections, abdominal sepsis (esp *Bacteroides*), aspiration pneumonia, *C. difficile* (AAC), *H. pylori* eradication, *Giardia/Entamoeba* infections, Px during GI surgery. Also dental/gynaecological infections, bacterial vaginosis (*Gardnerella*), PID.
Caution: avoid with alcohol: drug metabolised to acetaldehyde and other toxins ⇒ flushing, abdominal pain, ↓BP ('disulfiram-like' reaction), acute porphyria, **L/P/B**.
SE: GI upset (esp N&V), taste disturbed, skin reactions. Rarely, drowsiness, headache, dizziness, dark urine, hepatotoxicity, blood disorders, myalgia, arthralgia, seizures (transient), ataxia, **peripheral neuropathy** (if prolonged Rx).
Interactions: can ↑busulfan, lithium, ciclosporin and phenytoin levels, **W +**.
Dose: 500 mg tds ivi/400 mg tds po for severe infections. Lower doses can be given po or higher doses pr (1 g bd/tds) according to indication[SPC/BNF]. NB: ↓**dose in LF**.

MICONAZOLE

Imidazole antifungal (topical) but *systemic absorption can occur*.
Use: oral fungal infections (give po), cutaneous fungal infections (give topically).
CI: L. Oral gel – in infants: impaired swallowing reflex, and up to 5–6 months if born pre-term.
Caution: acute porphyria, P/B.
SE: GI upset. Rarely hypersensitivity, hepatotoxicity.
Interactions: as ketoconazole, but less commonly significant. **W +.**
Dose: po: oral gel (Daktarin) 5–10 ml qds (after food); 2.5 ml bd (4 months–2 yrs), 5 ml bd (2–6 yrs), 5 ml qds (6 yrs+) or buccal tablets (Loramyc) 50 mg od mane. NB: with oral gel treat for 48 h after lesions healed. top: apply 1–2 times/day.

MIDAZOLAM

Benzodiazepine, very short-acting.
Use: sedation for stressful/painful procedures[1] (esp if amnesia desirable) and for agitation/distress in palliative care[2].
CI/Caution/SE/Warn/Interactions: see Diazepam.
Dose: 1.0–7.5 mg iv[1]; initially 2 mg (0.5–1 mg if elderly) over 60 sec, then titrate up slowly until desired sedation achieved using 0.5–1.0-mg boluses over 30 sec (can also give im[SPC/BNF]); 2.5–5 mg sc prn[2] (or via sc pump). Also available as buccal liquid (with 2.5, 5 or 10 mg/ml, 'special order' preparations) – unlicensed use.
NB: ↓dose in RF or elderly.

> 💀 Beware respiratory depression: have flumazenil and O_2 (± resuscitation trolley) at hand, esp if respiratory disease or giving high doses im/iv 💀.

MINOCYCLINE

Tetracycline antibiotic: inhibits ribosomal (30S subunit) protein synthesis; broadest spectrum of tetracyclines.
Use: acne[1], rosacea.
CI/Caution/SE/Interactions: as tetracycline, but ↓bacterial resistance, although ↑risk of SLE and irreversible skin/body fluid

discoloration. Can also use (with caution) in RF. Check hepatic toxicity every 3 months – discontinue if develops.
Dose: 100 mg od po[1] (can ↑to bd for other indications). Use for ≥ 6 weeks in acne.

MINOXIDIL

Peripheral vasodilator (arterioles >> veins): also ⇒ ↑CO, ↑HR, fluid retention ∴ *always needs concurrent β-blocker and diuretic.*
Use: HTN (if severe/Rx-resistant); *for HTN Mx advice see p. 235.*
CI: phaeo.
Caution: IHD, acute porphyria, R/P/B.
SE: **hypertrichosis, coarsening of facial features** (reversible, but makes it less suitable for women), ↑Wt, peripheral oedema, pericardial effusions, angina (dt ↑HR). Rarely, GI upset, gynaecomastia/breast tenderness, renal impairment, skin reactions.
Dose: initially 2.5–5 mg/day in 1 or 2 divided doses, ↑ing by 5–10 mg at an interval of at least 3 days if needed up to usual max of 50 mg/day. **NB: ↓dose in elderly and dialysis patients.** Also used topically for male-pattern baldness.

MIRTAZAPINE/ZISPIN

Antidepressant: Noradrenaline And Specific Serotonin Agonist (NASSA); specifically stimulates $5HT_1$ receptors (antagonises $5HT_{2C}/5HT_3$), antagonises central presynaptic α_2 receptors.
Use: depression, esp in elderly* or if insomnia†.
CI/Caution/SE: as fluoxetine, but ⇒ ↓**sexual dysfunction**/GI upset, ↑**sedation**† (esp during titration) and ↑**appetite/Wt** (can be beneficial in elderly*). Rarely, blood disorders (inc agranulocytosis**), Δ LFTs, convulsions, myoclonus, oedema.
Warn: of initial sedation, to not stop suddenly (risk of withdrawal) and to report signs of infection** (esp sore throat, fever): stop drug and check FBC if concerned.
Interactions: avoid with other sedatives (inc alcohol), artemether/lumefantrine. ☠ **Never give with, or ≤2 wks after, MAOIs** ☠.
Dose: initially 15 mg nocte, ↑ing to 30 mg after 1–2 wks (max 45 mg/day). *Note lower doses more sedating than higher doses.*

MISOPROSTOL

Synthetic PGE_1 analogue: ↓s gastric acid secretion.

Use: Px/Rx of PU (esp NSAID-induced). Unlicensed uses: po or topically to cervix for induction of labour, to induce medical abortion and to ripen cervix for surgical abortion; also pr in postpartum haemorrhage.

CI: ☠ **pregnancy** ☠ (actual or planned; only give to women of childbearing age if high risk of PU and contraceptives prescribed), **P/B**.

Caution: cardiovascular/cerebrovascular disease (can ⇒ ↓BP), IBD.

SE: diarrhoea. Rarely, other GI upset, rash, light-headedness, menstrual Δs, vaginal bleeding.

Warn: women of child-bearing age of risks to pregnancy and need for adequate contraception when taking.

Dose: most often used with diclofenac as Arthrotec. Also available with naproxen as Napratec. Both these preparations contain 200 microgram misoprostol per tablet, i.e. total daily dose < the ideal 800 microgram.

MMF see Mycophenolate mofetil; immunosuppressant.

MOMETASONE (FUROATE) CREAM OR OINTMENT/ ELOCON

Potent topical corticosteroid.

Use: inflammatory skin conditions, esp eczema.

CI: untreated infection, rosacea, acne.

SE: skin atrophy, worsening of infections, acne.

Dose: apply thinly od top (use 'ointment' in dry skin conditions).

MONTELUKAST/SINGULAIR

Leukotriene receptor antagonist: ↓s Ag-induced bronchoconstriction.

Use: *non-acute* asthma, esp if large exercise-induced component or associated seasonal allergic rhinitis.

Caution: acute asthma, Churg–Strauss syndrome **P/B**.

SE: headache, GI upset, myalgia, dry mouth/thirst. Rarely **Churg–Strauss syndrome**: asthma (± rhin-/sinus-itis) with systemic vasculitis and ↑EØ*.

Monitor: FBC* and for development of vasculitic (purpuric/non-blanching) rash, peripheral neuropathy, ↑respiratory/cardiac symptoms: all signs of possible Churg–Strauss syndrome.
Dose: 10 mg nocte (↓doses if <15 years old$^{SPC/BNF}$).

MORPHGESIC SR Morphine (sulphate) SR (10, 30, 60 or 100 mg). Given bd. NB: ↓dose if LF, RF or elderly.

MORPHINE (SULPHATE)
Opiate analgesic.
Use: severe pain (inc post-op), AMI and acute LVF.
CI: acute respiratory depression, acute severe obstructive airways disease, ↑risk of paralytic ileus, delayed gastric emptying, biliary colic, acute alcoholism, ↑ICP/head injury (respiratory depression ⇒ CO_2 retention and cerebral vasodilation ⇒ ↑ICP), phaeo. **H** (if 2° to chronic lung disease).
Caution: ↓respiratory reserve, obstructive airways disease, ↓BP/shock, acute abdomen, biliary tract disorders (NB: biliary colic is CI), pancreatitis, bowel obstruction, IBD, ↑prostate/urethral stricture, arrhythmias, ↓T_4, adrenocorticoid insufficiency, MG, **L** (can ⇒ coma), **R/P/B/E**.
SE: N&V (and other GI disturbance) constipation* (can ⇒ ileus), respiratory depression, ↓BP (inc orthostatic. NB: rarely ⇒ ↑BP), ↓/↑HR, pulmonary oedema, oedema, bronchospasm, ↓cough reflex, sedation, urinary retention, RF, biliary tract spasm, ↑pancreatitis, ΔLFTs, hypothermia, muscle rigidity/fasciculation/myoclonus, ↑ICP, dry mouth, vertigo, syncope, headache, miosis, sensory disturbance, pruritis, anorexia, allodynia, mood Δ(↑ or ↓), delirium, hallucinations, restlessness, seizures (at ↑doses), rhabdomyolysis, amenorrhoea, ↓libido, dependence. Rarely, skin reactions.
Interactions: ☠ MAOIs (don't give within 2 wks of) ☠. Levels ↓by ritonavir. ↓s levels of ciprofloxacin. ↑sedative fx with antihistamines, baclofen, alcohol (also ⇒ ↓BP), TCAs, antipsychotics (also ↓BP), anxiolytics/hypnotics, barbiturates and

moclobemide (also ⇒ ↑CNS and ↑/↓BP). ↑s fx of sodium oxybate, gabapentin.

Dose: Acute pain: 5–20 mg sc/im 4-hrly; 2.5–15 mg iv up to 4-hrly (2 mg/min). NB: iv doses are generally 1/4–1/2 im doses. **AMI:** 5–10 mg iv (1–2 mg/min), repeated if necessary. **Acute LVF:** 1–2.5 mg iv (1 mg/min). **Chronic pain:** use po as Oramorph solution or as MST Continus, Morphgesic, MXL, Sevredol or Zomorph tablets; dose adjustment may be required when switching brands. Also available pr as suppositories of 10, 15, 20 and 30 mg giving 15–30 mg up to 4-hrly. *Unless short-term Rx, always consider laxative Px**. Can ↑doses and frequency with expert supervision. Always adjust dose to response. **NB: ↓dose if LF, RF or elderly.**

☠ If ↓BMI or elderly, titrate dose up slowly, monitor O₂ sats and have naloxone ± resuscitation trolley at hand ☠.

MST CONTINUS Oral morphine (sulphate), equivalent in efficacy to Oramorph but SR: dose every 12 hrs. Need to specify if *tablets* (5, 10, 15, 30, 60, 100 or 200 mg) or *suspension* (sachets of 20, 30, 60, 100 or 200 mg to be mixed with water).

MUPIROCIN/BACTROBAN

Topical antibiotic for bacterial infections (esp eradication of nasal MRSA carriage); available as nasal ointment, applied bd/tds.

Local MRSA eradication protocols often exist; if not, then a sensible regimen is to give for 5 days and then swab 2 days later, repeating regimen if culture still positive.

MXL CAPSULES Morphine (sulphate) capsules (30, 60, 90, 120, 150 or 200 mg), equivalent in efficacy to Oramorph but SR: dose od. NB: ↓dose if LF, RF or elderly.

MYCOPHENOLATE MOFETIL (MMF)

Immunosuppressant: ↓s B-/T-cell lymphocytes (and ↓s Ab production by B-cells).

Use: transplant rejection Px, autoimmune diseases, vasculitis.
CI: P/B

Caution: active serious GI diseases[†], E.

Monitor: FBC and LFTs (wkly for 1st 4 weeks, 2-wkly for 2 months, then monthly for 1st year).

Warn: patient to report unexplained bruises/bleeding/signs of infection. Avoid strong sunlight*.

SE: GI upset, blood disorders (esp ↓NØ, ↓Pt), weakness, tremor, taste Δ, headache, ↑cholesterol, ↑or ↓K⁺. Rarely GI ulceration/bleeding/perforation[†], hepatotoxicity, skin neoplasms*.

Interactions: Levels ↓by rifampicin.

Dose: Specialist use only[SPC/BNF].

N-ACETYLCYSTEINE see Acetylcysteine; paracetamol antidote.

NALOXONE

Opioid receptor antagonist for opiate reversal if OD or over-Rx.

Caution: cardiovascular disease, if taking cardiotoxic drugs, physical dependence on opioids, H.

Dose: 0.4–2 mg iv (or sc/im), much larger doses may be needed for certain opioids (e.g. tramadol), repeating after 2 min if no response (or ↑ing if severe poisoning). *NB: Short-acting*: may need repeating every 2–3 min (to total 10 mg) then review and consider ivi (10 mg made up to 50 ml with 5% dextrose; useful start rate is 60% of initial dose over 1 h, then adjusted to response).

NALTREXONE

Opioid antagonist: ↓s euphoria of opioids if dependence and ↓s craving and relapse rate in alcoholic withdrawal (opioids thought to mediate alcohol addiction; not licensed for this in UK yet).

Use: Opioid and alcohol withdrawal; start >1 wk after stopping*.

CI: if still taking opioids (can precipitate withdrawal*), L (inc acute hepatitis), severe R.

Caution: P/B.

SE: GI upset, hepatoxicity, sleep and Ψ disorders.

Monitor: LFTs.

Warn: patient that trying to overcome opiate blockade OD can ⇒ acute intoxication.

Dose: initial dose 25 mg od po, thereafter 50 mg od (or 350 mg per week split into 2 × 100 mg and 1 × 150 mg doses); specialist use only.

NB: also ↓s fx of opioid analgesics.

NAPROXEN

Moderate-strength NSAID; non-selective COX inhibitor.

Use: rheumatic disease[1]; acute musculoskeletal pain and dysmenorrhoea[2]; acute gout[3].

CI/Caution/SE/Interactions: as ibuprofen, but somewhat ↑SEs, notably, ↑risk PU/GI bleeds. Lowest thrombotic risk of any NSAID. Probenecid ⇒ ↑serum levels. No known interaction with baclofen or triazoles. Mild **W +**.

Dose: 500 mg–1 g daily in 1–2 divided doses[1]; 500 mg initially then 250 mg 6–8-hrly (max 1.25 g/day)[2]; 750 mg initially then 250 mg 8-hrly[3]. Also available with misoprostol as Px against PU (as Napratec). **NB: Avoid or ↓dose in RF & consider gastroprotective Rx.**

NARATRIPTAN/NARAMIG

$5HT_{1B/1D}$ agonist for acute migraine.

CI/Caution/SE/Interactions: see Sumatriptan. Not recommended if >65 yrs.

Dose: 2.5 mg po (can repeat after ≥4 h if responded then recurs). Max 5 mg/24 h (2.5 mg if LF or RF, avoid if severe).

NARCAN see Naloxone; opiate antidote.

NICORANDIL

K^+-channel activator (⇒ arterial dilation ⇒ ↓afterload) with nitrate component (⇒ venous dilation ⇒ ↓preload).

Use: angina Px/Rx (unresponsive to other Rx).

CI: ↓BP (esp cardiogenic shock), LVF with ↓filling pressures, **B**.

Caution: hypovolaemia, acute pulmonary oedema, ACS with LVF and ↓filling pressures, **P**.

L/R/H = Liver, Renal and Heart failure (full key see p. xv)

SE: headache (often only initially*), **flushing**, dizziness, weakness, N&V, ↓BP, ↑HR (dose-dependent). Rarely GI/perianal ulcers (consider stopping drug), myalgia, angioedema, hepatotoxicity.

Interactions: ☠ risk of ↓↓BP with silden-/tadal-/varden-afil ☠.

Dose: 5–30 mg bd (start low, esp if susceptible to headaches*).

NICOTINIC ACID/NIASPAN

Water-soluble B-complex vitamin; ↓s synthesis of cholesterol/TGs and ↑s HDL-cholesterol.

Use: dyslipidaemia (↑cholesterol, ↑TG, ↓HDL-cholesterol) *added to statin or if statin not tolerated*.

CI: active bleeding, active PU disease. **L**(if severe)/**B**.

Caution: ACS, gout, history of PU, ↑alcohol intake, DM. **R/P**.

SE: GI upset, dyspepsia, flushing, itch, rash, headache ↑HR, ↓BP, syncope, SOB, oedema, ↑uric acid, ↑INR, ↓Pt, ↓phosphate, DM, muscle disorders. Rarely rhabdomyolysis, anorexia.

Warn: avoid alcohol or hot drink around time of tablet (↑flushing and itch); false +ve urine G result. Flushing prostaglandin mediated; can be avoided if ↓ initial dose taken with meals, or if taking aspirin give 30 mins before nicotinic acid.

Monitor: BG, CK (if ↑risk myopathy) and LFTs (if mild-moderate LF).

Interactions: ↑risk of myopathy with statins.

Dose: 375 mg (MR tablets) od nocte after low fat snack; ↑dose weekly for 4 wks then monthly if needed. Maintenance dose 1–2 g od nocte.

NIFEDIPINE

Ca^{2+} channel blocker (dihydropyridine): dilates smooth muscle, esp arteries (inc coronaries). Reflex sympathetic drive ⇒ ↑HR and ↑contractility ∴ ⇒ ↓HF cf other Ca^{2+} channel blockers (e.g. verapamil, and to a lesser degree diltiazem), which ⇒ ↓HR + ↓contractility. Also diuretic fx.

Use: angina Px[1], HTN[2] (*for advice on stepped HTN Mx see p. 235*), Raynaud's[3].

CI: cardiogenic shock, clinically significant aortic stenosis, ACS (inc w/in 1 month of MI).

Caution: angina or LVF can worsen (consider stopping drug), ↓BP, DM, BPH, acute porphyria **L/R/H/P/B**.

SE: flushing, headache, ankle oedema, dizziness, ↓BP, palpitations, poly-/nocturia, rash/pruritus, GI upset, weakness, myalgia, arthralgia, gum hyperplasia, rhinitis. Rarely, PU, hepatotoxicity.

Interactions: metab by **P450**. ↑s fx of digoxin, theophylline and tacrolimus. ↓s fx of quinidine. Quinu-/dalfo-pristin, ritonavir and grapefruit juice ↑fx of nifedipine. Rifampicin, phenytoin and carbamazepine ↓fx of nifedipine. Risk of ↓↓BP with α-blockers, β-blockers or Mg^{2+} iv/im.

Dose: 5–20 mg tds po[3]; use long-acting preparations for HTN/ angina, as normal-release preparations ⇒ erratic BP control and reflex ↑HR, which can worsen IHD (e.g. Adalat LA or Retard and many others with differing fx and doses[SPC/BNF]). **NB: ↓dose if severe LF.**

NITROFURANTOIN

Antibiotic: only active in urine (no systemic antibacterial fx).

Use: UTIs (but not pyelonephritis).

CI: G6PD deficiency, acute porphyria, **R** (also ⇒ ↓activity of drug: it needs to be concentrated in urine), infants <3 yrs old, **P/B**.

Caution: DM, lung disease, ↓Hb, ↓vitamin B, ↓folate, electrolyte imbalance, susceptibility to peripheral neuropathy, **L/E**.

SE: GI upset, pulmonary reactions (inc effusions, fibrosis), peripheral neuropathy, hypersensitivity. Rarely, hepatotoxicity, cholestasis, pancreatitis, arthralgia, alopecia (transient), skin reactions (esp exfoliative dermatitis), blood disorders, BIH.

Dose: 50 mg qds po (↑to 100 mg if severe chronic recurrent infection); od nocte if for Px. *Take with food.* Not available iv or im.

NB: can ⇒ false-positive urine dipstick for glucose and discolour urine.

L/R/H = Liver, Renal and Heart failure (full key see p. xv)

NORADRENALINE (= NOREPINEPHRINE)

Vasoconstrictor sympathomimetic: stimulates α-receptors $\Rightarrow$ vasoconstriction.

Use: $\downarrow$BP (unresponsive to other Rx).

CI: $\uparrow$BP, **P**.

Caution: thrombosis (coronary/mesenteric/peripheral), Prinzmetal's angina, post-MI, $\uparrow T_4$, DM, $\downarrow O_2$, $\uparrow CO_2$, hypovolaemia (uncorrected), **E**.

SE: can $\downarrow$BF to vital organs (esp kidney). Also headache, $\downarrow$HR, arrhythmias, peripheral ischaemia. $\uparrow$BP if over-Rx.

Interactions: ☠ risk of arrhythmias with halothane and cyclopropane ☠. Risk of $\uparrow$BP with clonidine, MAOIs and TCAs.

Dose: 80 microgram/ml ivi at 0.16–0.33 ml/min (adjust according to response). (☠ NB: *doses given here are for noradrenaline* **acid tartrate**, *not* **base** ☠).

NORETHISTERONE

Progestogen (testosterone analogue).

Use: endometriosis[1], dysfunctional uterine bleeding and menorrhagia[2], dysmenorrhoea[3], postponement of menstruation[4].

CI: liver/genital/breast cancers (unless progestogens being used for these conditions), atherosclerosis, undiagnosed vaginal bleeding, acute porphyria, Hx of idiopathic jaundice, severe pruritis, pemphigoid during pregnancy.

Caution: risk of fluid retention, TE disease, DM, depression. **L/H/R**.

SE: $\uparrow$weight, nausea, headache, dizziness, insomnia, drowsiness, breast tenderness, acne, depression, Δ libido, skin reactions, hirsuitism & alopecia.

Dose: 5 mg bd-tds po for $\geqslant$4–6 months, commencing on day 5 of cycle (can $\uparrow$ to 10 mg bd-tds (max 25 mg / day) if spotting occurs, $\downarrow$ing when stops)[1]; 5 mg tds po for 10 days for Rx (for Px give 5 mg bd po from day 19–26 of cycle)[2]; 5 mg tds po from day 5–24 for 3–4 cycles[3]; 5 mg tds po starting 3 days prior to expected menstruation onset (bleeding will commence 2–3 days after stopping)[4].

NUROFEN see Ibuprofen; NB: 'over-the-counter' use can ⇒ poor response to HTN and HF Rx.

NYSTATIN

Polyene antifungal.

Use: *Candida* infections: topically for skin/mucous membranes (esp mouth/vagina); po for GI infections (not absorbed).

SE: GI upset (at ↑doses), skin reactions.

Dose: po suspension: 100,000 units qds, usually for 1 wk, for Rx *after food*.

OFLOXACIN 0.3% EYE DROPS/EXOCIN

Topical antibiotic; mostly used for corneal ulcers[1] (only start if corneal Gram stain/cultures taken and specialist not available).

Caution: P/B.

SE: local irritation. Rarely dizziness, headache, numbness, nausea.

Dose: 1 drop 2–4 hourly for 1st 2 days then qds (max 10 days)[1]. See SPC for other uses.

OLANZAPINE/ZYPREXA

'Atypical' antipsychotic: D_1, D_2, D_4 and $5HT_2$ (+ mild muscarinic) antagonist.

Use: schizophrenia[NICE], mania, bipolar Px, acute sedation.

CI: B. If giving im also acute MI/ACS, ↓↓BP/HR, SSS or recent heart surgery. See also Chlorpromazine.

Caution: drugs that ↑QTc, dementia, cardiovascular disease (esp if Hx of or ↑risk of CVA/TIA), DM*, ↑prostate, glaucoma (angle closure), Parkinson's, Hx of epilepsy, blood disorders, paralytic ileus. ↑s fx of alcohol, **L/R/H/P/E**.

SE: sedation, ↑Wt, ankle oedema, Δ LFTs, postural ↓BP (esp initially ∴ titrate up dose slowly). ↑**glucose*** (rarely ☠ DM/DKA ☠). Also extrapyramidal/anticholinergic fx (see p. 278; often transient) and rarely neuroleptic malignant syndrome and hepatotoxicity.

Monitor: BG* (± HbA_{1C}), LFTs, U&Es, FBC, prolactin, Wt, lipids (and CK if neuroleptic malignant syndrome suspected). If giving im closely monitor cardiorespiratory function for ≥4 h post-dose, esp if given other antipsychotic or benzodiazepine.

L/R/H = Liver, Renal and Heart failure (full key see p. xv)

Interactions: metab by **P450** ∴ many, but most importantly, levels ↓by carbamazepine and smoking. ↑risk of ↓NØ with valproate. Levels may be ↑by ciprofloxacin. ↑risk of CNS toxicity with sibutramine. ↑risk of arrhythmias with drugs that ↑QTc and atomoxetine. ↑risk of ↓BP with general anaesthetics. ↓s fx of anticonvulsants.

Dose: 5–20 mg po daily (preferably nocte to avoid daytime sedation). Available in 'melt' form if ↓compliance/swallowing (as Velotab). Available in quick-acting im form (▼) for acute sedation; give 5–10 mg (2.5–5 mg in elderly) repeating 2 h later if necessary to max total daily dose, inc po doses, of 20 mg (max 3 injections/day for 3 days).

NB: im doses not recommended with im/iv benzodiazepines (↑risk of respiratory depression) which should be given ≥1 h later; if benzodiazepines already given, use with caution and closely monitor cardiorespiratory function.

OLMESARTAN/OLMETEC

Angiotensin II antagonist: see Losartan.
Use: HTN; *for advice on stepped HTN Mx see p. 235.*
CI: biliary obstruction, **P/B**.
Caution/SE/Interactions: see Losartan.
Dose: initially 10 mg od, ↑ing to max 40 mg (20 mg in LF, RF or elderly).

OMEGA-3-ACID ETHYL ESTERS 90/OMACOR

Essential fatty acid combination: 1 g capsule = eicosapentaenoic acid 460 mg and decosahexaenoic acid 380 mg.
Use: Adjunct to diet in type IIb and III ↑TG[1] (with statin) or type IV. Added for 2° prevention w/in 3 months of acute MI[2].
CI : B.
Caution: bleeding disorders, anticoagulants, DM **L/P**.
SE: GI; rarer: taste disorder, dry nose, dizziness, hypersensitivity, hepatotoxicity, headache, rash, ↓BP, DM, ↑WBC.
Monitor: LFTs, INR.
Dose: Capsules: 2–4 g od[1]; 1 g od[2]. Take with food.

OMEPRAZOLE/LOSEC

PPI: inhibits H^+/K^+ ATPase of parietal cells $\Rightarrow$ ↓acid secretion.

Use: PU Rx/Px (esp if on NSAIDs), gastro-oesophageal reflux disease (if symptoms severe or complicated by haemorrhage/ulcers/stricture)[NICE]. Also used for *H. pylori* eradication and ZE syndrome.

Caution: can mask symptoms of gastric Ca, **L/P/B**.

SE: GI upset, headache, dizziness, arthralgia, weakness, skin reactions. Rarely, hepatotoxicity, blood disorders, hypersensitivity.

Interactions: ↓ (and ↑) P450 ∴ many, most importantly ↑s phenytoin, cilostazol, diazepam, raltegravir and digoxin levels. ↓s fx of ataza-/nelfi-/tipra-navir, mild **W +**.

Dose: 20 mg od po, ↑ing to 40 mg in severe/resistant cases and ↓ing to 10 mg od for maintenance if symptoms stable; 20 mg bd for *H. pylori* eradication regimens. If unable to take po (e.g. perioperatively, ↓GCS, on ITU), give 40 mg iv od either over 5 min or as ivi over 20–30 min. **NB: max dose 20 mg if LF.**

> NB: also specialist use iv for acute bleeds. Usually as 8 mg/h ivi for 72 h if endoscopic evidence of PU (prescribed as divided infusions, as drug is unstable). Contact pharmacy ± GI team for advice on indications and exact dosing regimens.

ONDANSETRON

Antiemetic: $5HT_3$ antagonist: acts on central and GI receptors.

Use: N&V, esp if resistant to other Rx or severe postoperative/chemotherapy-induced.

Caution: GI obstruction (inc subacute), ↑QTc*, **L** (unless mild), **P/B**.

SE: constipation (or diarrhoea), headache, sedation, fatigue, dizziness. Rarely seizures, chest pain, ↓BP, Δ LFTs, rash, hypersensitivity.

Interactions: metab by **P450**. Levels ↓by rifampicin, carbamazepine and phenytoin. ↓s fx of tramadol. Avoid with drugs that ↑QTc*.

Dose: 8 mg bd po; 16 mg od pr; 8 mg 2–8-hrly iv/im. Max 24 mg/day usually (8 mg/day if LF). Can also give as ivi at 1 mg/h for max of 24 h. Exact dose and route depends on indication[SPC/BNF].

ORAMORPH Oral morphine solution for severe pain, esp useful for prn or breakthrough pain.

Dose: Multiply sc/im morphine dose by 2 to obtain approx equivalent^Oramorph dose. NB: ↓**dose if LF or RF.**

Solution mostly commonly used is 10 mg/5 ml, but can be 100 mg/5 ml ∴ *specify strength if prescribing in ml (rather than mg).*

OTOSPORIN Ear drops for otitis externa (esp if bacterial infection suspected): contains antibacterials (neomycin, polymyxin B) and hydrocortisone 1%.

Dose: 3 drops tds/qds.

OXYBUTYNIN

Anticholinergic (selective M_3 antagonist); antispasmodic (↓s bladder muscle contractions).

Use: detrusor instability (also neurogenic bladder instability, nocturnal enuresis).

CI: bladder outflow or GI obstruction, urinary retention, severe UC/ toxic megacolon, glaucoma (narrow angle), MG, **B.**

Caution: ↑prostate, autonomic neuropathy, hiatus hernia (if reflux), ↑T_4, IHD, arrhythmias, porphyria, **L/R/H/P/E.**

SE: antimuscarinic fx (see p. 276), GI upset, palpitations/↑HR, skin reactions – mostly dose-related and reportedly less severe in MR preparations*.

Dose: initially 5 mg bd/tds po (2.5 mg bd if elderly) ↑ing if required to max of 5 mg qds (bd if elderly). Also available as MR tablet (Lyrinel XL* 5–20 mg od) and transdermal patch (Kentera 36 mg; releases 3.9 mg/day and lasts 3–4 days).

OXYCODONE (HYDROCHLORIDE)/OXYNORM

Opioid for moderate/severe pain (esp in palliative care.)

CI: as fentanyl, plus acute abdomen, delayed gastric emptying, chronic constipation, cor pulmonale, acute porphyria. **L**(if moderate/ severe)/**R** (if severe), **P/B.**

Caution: all other conditions where morphine is CI/cautioned.

SE/Interactions: as morphine, but does not interact with baclofen, gabapentin and ritonavir.
Dose: 4–6-hrly po/sc/iv or as sc infusion. NB: 2.5 mg sc/iv = 5 mg po = approx 10 mg morphine po. Available in MR form as OxyContin (12-hrly). Available with naloxone (works locally to ↓GI SEs) as ▼ Targinact (12-hrly). NB: ↓dose if LF, RF or elderly.

OXYTETRACYCLINE
Tetracycline antibiotic: inhibits ribosomal protein synthesis.
Use: acne vulgaris (and rosacea).
CI/Caution/SE/Interactions: as tetracycline, plus caution in porphyria.
Dose: 500 mg bd po (1 h before food or on empty stomach) for ≥16 wks.

PABRINEX
Parenteral (iv or im) vitamins that come as a pair of vials. Vial 1 contains B_1 (thiamine*), B_2 (riboflavin) and B_6 (pyridoxine). Vial 2 contains C (ascorbic acid), nicotinamide and glucose.
Use: Acute vitamin deficiencies (esp thiamine*).
Caution: Rarely ⇒ anaphylaxis (esp if given iv too quickly; should be given over ≥ 30 mins). *Ensure access to resuscitation facilities.*

*See p. 273 for Wernicke's encephalopathy Px/Rx in alcohol withdrawal.

(DISODIUM) PAMIDRONATE
Bisphosphonate: ↓s osteoclastic bone resorption.
Use: ↑Ca^{2+} (esp metastatic: also ↓s pain)[1], Paget's disease[2], myeloma.
CI: P/B.
Caution: Hx of thyroid surgery, cardiac disease, **L/R/H**.
SE: 'flu-like symptoms (inc fever, transient pyrexia), GI upset (inc haemorrhage), dizziness/somnolence (common post-dose*), ↑ (or ↓) BP, seizures, musculoskeletal pain, osteonecrosis of jaw

(esp in cancer patients; consider dental examination or preventative Rx – MHRA advice), e'lyte Δs ($\downarrow PO_4$, $\downarrow$or $\uparrow K^+$, $\uparrow Na^+$, $\downarrow Mg^{2+}$), RF, blood disorders.

Monitor: e'lytes (inc U&E before each dose), Ca^{2+}, PO_4^-, before starting biphosphonate consider dental check as risk of osteonecrosis of the jaw.

Warn: not to drive/operate machinery immediately after Rx*.

Dose: 15–90 mg ivi according to indication ($\pm Ca^{2+}$ levels[1]). **NB: if RF max rate of ivi 20 mg/h (unless for life-threatening $\uparrow Ca^{2+}$).** *Never given regularly for sustained periods.*

PANCURONIUM

Neuromuscular blocker; as vecuronium but $\uparrow$duration of action (60–120 mins).

Use: neuromuscular blockade for surgery[1] or during intensive care[2].

CI: anaesthetist not confident of airway maintenance.

Caution: hypersensitivity to other neuromuscular blockers (allergic cross-reactivity), neuromuscular disease (MG/Eaton-Lambert syndrome, old polio), $\uparrow$BP, fluid/e'lyte Δ (unpredictable response). **L** (slower onset, $\uparrow$dose requirement, $\uparrow$recovery time) / **R** ($\uparrow$ duration of block).

SE: $\uparrow$HR, $\uparrow$BP, myopathy.

Warn: Don't drive for 24h after full recovery. Injection painful.

Monitor: Cardiac, respiratory & motor function.

Interactions: fx $\uparrow$ by aminoglycosides, clindamycin and polymyxins. Only administer after full recovery from neuromuscular blockade from suxamethonium. Corticosteroids can $\uparrow$ risk of myopathy. Tricyclic antidepressants can $\Rightarrow$ arrhythmia.

Dose: initially 100 micrograms/kg then 20 micrograms/kg iv as required[1]; initially 100 micrograms/kg (optional) then 60 micrograms/kg iv every 60–90 mins[2]. **NB:** *if obese (weight 30% above ideal body weight (IBW; see p.296)) use IBW for dose calculation.*

☠ Specialist use only; respiration needs assistance / control until drug inactivated or antagonised and anaesthetic / sedative to prevent awareness. ☠

PANTOPRAZOLE

PPI; as omeprazole, but ↓interactions and can ⇒ ↑TGs.

Dose: 20–80 mg mane po (↓ing to 20 mg maintenance if symptoms allow). If unable to take po (e.g. perioperatively, ↓GCS, on ITU), can give 40 mg iv over ≥2 min (or as ivi) od. ↑doses if ZE syndrome[SPC/BNF]. NB: ↓dose if RF or LF.

PARACETAMOL

Antipyretic & mild analgesic. Unlike NSAIDs, *has no anti-inflammatory fx*.

Use: mild pain (or moderate/severe in combination with other Rx), pyrexia.

Caution: alcohol dependence, **L** (CI if severe liver disease), **R**.

SE: *all rare*: rash, blood disorders, hepatic (rarely renal) failure – esp if over-Rx/OD (for Mx, see p. 279).

Interactions: may **W** + if prolonged regular use.

Dose: 0.5–1 g po/pr; 1 g (or 15 mg/kg if <50 kg) iv. All doses 4–6 hourly, max 4 g/day. Max 3 g/day iv (▼) in LF, dehydration, chronic alcoholism or chronic malnutrition. Minimum iv dosing interval in RF: 6-hrly. (For children, see Calpol.)

PAROXETINE/SEROXAT

SSRI antidepressant; as fluoxetine, but ↓$t_{1/2}$*.

Use: depression[1], other Ψ disorders (social/generalised anxiety disorder[1], PTSD[1], panic disorder[2], OCD[3]).

CI/Caution/SE/Interactions: as fluoxetine, but ↓frequency of agitation/insomnia, although ↑frequency of **antimuscarinic fx** (see p. 276), **extrapyramidal fx** (see p. 278) and **withdrawal fx*** (see p. 277). Avoid if <18 yrs old as may ↑suicide risk & hostility[SPC]. Also does not ↑carbamazepine levels (but its levels are ↓by carbamazepine) but ↑s galantamine levels. Risk of CNS toxicity if given with tramadol. Avoid if patient enters manic stage. **P**.

Dose: initially 20 mg[1,3] (10 mg[2]) mane, ↑ing if required to max 50 mg[1] or 60 mg[2,3].

NB: ↓dose if RF, LF or elderly.

Stop slowly over at least a few weeks, as short $t_{1/2}$ $\Rightarrow$ ↑risk of withdrawal syndrome.

PARVOLEX see Acetylcysteine; antidote for paracetamol poisoning.

PENICILLAMINE
Chelates copper/lead $\Rightarrow$ ↑elimination (also acts as DMARD): slow onset of action (6–12 wks).
Use: Wilson's disease*, copper/lead poisoning, rarely for rheumatoid arthritis (also autoimmune hepatitis, cystinuria).
CI: SLE, **R** (unless mild when only caution).
Caution: penicillin allergy (can also be penicillamine allergic), taking other nephrotoxic drugs, **P**.
SE: RF (esp immune nephritis $\Rightarrow$ proteinuria*: stop drug if severe), **blood disorders** (↓Pt, ↓NØ, agranulocytosis, aplastic ↓Hb), **rashes** (inc SJS, pemphigus), **taste Δs, GI upset** (esp nausea, but ↓s if taken with food). Can ↑neurological symptoms in Wilson's. Rarely hepatotoxicity, pancreatitis, autoimmune phenomena: poly-/dermato-myositis, Goodpasture's syndrome, lupus-/myasthenia-like syndromes.
Warn: immediately report sore throat, fever, infection, non-specific illness, unexpected bleeding/bruising, purpura, mouth ulcers or rash.
Monitor: FBC, U&Es, urine dipstick ±24-h collection*.
Interactions: ↑risk of agranulocytosis with clozapine. Absorption ↓by antacids and $FeSO_4$. Can ↓levels of digoxin.
Dose: 125–2000 mg daily^{SPC/BNF} depending on indication.
NB: consider ↓dose if RF or elderly.

Can $\Rightarrow$ ↓pyridoxine which often needs supplementing. Consider stopping if fever, lymphadenopathy, ↓Pt/NØ, proteinuria or worsening neuro symptoms. Sensitivity occurs in 10%; can restart with prednisolone – get senior advice.

PENICILLIN G see Benzylpenicillin.

PENICILLIN V see Phenoxymethylpenicillin.

PENTASA see Mesalazine; aminosalicylate for UC, with ↓SEs.

PEPPERMINT OIL

Antispasmodic: direct relaxant of GI smooth muscle.
Use: GI muscle spasm, distension (esp IBS).
SE: perianal irritation, indigestion. Rarely rash or other allergy.
Dose: 1–2 capsules tds, before meals and with water.

PEPTAC Alginate raft-forming oral suspension for acid reflux.
Dose: 10–20 ml after meals and at bedtime (NB: 3 mmol Na^+/5 ml).

PERINDOPRIL/COVERSYL

ACE-i; see Captopril.
Use: HTN (*for advice on stepped HTN Mx see p. 235*), HF, Px of IHD.
CI/Caution/SE/Monitor/Interactions: as Captopril, plus can ⇒ mood/sleep Δs.
Dose: 2–8 mg od$^{SPC/BNF}$, starting at 2–4 mg od. **NB: consider ↓dose if RF, elderly, taking a diuretic, cardiac decompensation or volume depletion.**

PETHIDINE

Opioid; less potent than morphine but quicker action ⇒ ↑euphoria + ↑abuse/dependence potential ∴ not for chronic use e.g. in palliative care.
Use: moderate/severe pain, obstetric and peri-op analgesia.
CI: acute respiratory depression, risk of ileus, ↑ICP/head injury/ coma, phaeo.
Caution: any other condition where morphine CI/cautioned.
SE: as morphine, but ↓constipation. Toxic metabolites can accumulate.
Interactions: as morphine but ☠ ↑risk of hyperpyrexia/ CNS toxicity with **MAOIs** ☠. Ritonavir ⇒ ↓levels and ↑s toxic metabolites. May ↑serotonergic effects of duloxetine. No known interaction with gabapentin or baclofen.
Dose: 25–100 mg up to 4-hrly im/sc (can give 2-hrly post-op or 1–3-hrly in labour with max 400 mg/24 hrs); 25–50 mg up to 4-hrly

slow iv. Rarely used po: 50–150 mg up to 4-hrly. **NB: ↓dose if LF, RF or elderly.**

PHENOBARBITAL (= PHENOBARBITONE)

Barbiturate antiepileptic: potentiates GABA (inhibitory neurotransmitter), antagonises fx of glutamate (excitatory neurotransmitter).

Use: status epilepticus (SEs and interactions limit other uses).

Caution: respiratory depression, acute porphyria, **L/R/P/B/E.**

SE: hepatitis, cholestasis, respiratory depression, sedation, ↓BP, ↓HR, ataxia, skin reactions. Rarely, paradoxical excitement (esp in elderly), blood disorders.

Interactions: ↑ **P450** ∴ many, most importantly ↓s levels/ fx of aripiprazole, antivirals, carbamazepine, Ca^{2+} antagonists, chloramphenicol, corticosteroids, ciclosporin, eplerenone, mianserin, tacrolimus, telithromycin, posa-/vori-conazole and OCP. Anticonvulsant fx ↓by antipsychotics, TCAs and SSRIs. Avoid with St John's wort. ↑s fx of sodium oxybate. Caution with other sedative drugs (esp benzodiazepines), **W–.**

Dose: total of 10 mg/kg as ivi at 50–100 mg/min (max total 1 g).

PHENOXYMETHYLPENICILLIN (= PENICILLIN V)

As benzylpenicillin (penicillin G) but active orally: used for ENT/ skin infections (esp erysipelas), Px of rheumatic fever/*S. pneumoniae* infections (esp post-splenectomy).

Dose: 0.5–1.0 g qds po (take on empty stomach; ≥ 1 hr before food or ≥ 2 hrs after food).

PHENTOLAMINE

α-Blocker, short-acting.

Use: HTN 2° to phaeo (esp during surgery).

CI: ↓BP, IHD (inc Hx of MI).

Caution: PU/gastritis, asthma, **R/P/B/E.**

SE: ↓BP, ↑HR, dizziness, weakness, flushing, GI upset, nasal congestion. Rarely, coronary/cerebrovascular occlusion, arrhythmias.

Interactions: see Doxazosin.
Dose: 2–5 mg iv (repeat if necessary).

PHENYLEPHRINE EYE DROPS

Topical sympathomimetic for pupil dilation (commonly used in combination with cyclopentolate or tropicamide).
Caution: cardiovascular disease, ↑HR, ↑T_4, children **E**.
SE: blurred vision, local irritation, ↑BP, ↑HR, arrhythmias, coronary artery spasm.
Dose: 1 drop. 2.5% drops most common (10% available but ↑risk of ↑BP).

PHENYTOIN

Antiepileptic: blocks Na^+ channels (stabilises neuronal membranes).
Use: all forms of epilepsy[1] (except absence seizures) inc status epilepticus[2].
CI: *if giving iv* (do not apply if po); sinus ↓HR, Stokes–Adams syndrome, SAN block, 2nd-/3rd-degree HB, acute porphyria.
Caution: DM, porphyria ↓BP, **L/H/P** (⇒ cleft lip/palate, congenital heart disease), **B**.
SE (acute): *dose-dependent*: drowsiness (also confusion/dizziness), **cerebellar fx** (see p. 278), **rash** (common cause of intolerance and rarely ⇒ SJS/TEN), N&V, diplopia, dyskinesia (esp orofacial). *If iv, risk of ↓BP* (from propylene glycol diluent), **arrhythmias*** (esp ↑QRS), '**purple glove syndrome**' (hand damage distal to injection site), CNS/respiratory depression.
SE (chronic): gum hypertrophy, coarse facies, hirsutism, acne, ↓folate (⇒ megaloblastic ↓Hb), Dupuytren's, peripheral neuropathy, rickets, osteomalacia. Rarely, blood disorders, hepatotoxicity, suicidal thoughts/behaviour.
Monitor: FBC**, keep serum levels at 10–20 mg/l (narrow therapeutic index). ☠ If iv, closely monitor BP and ECG* (esp QRS) ☠.
Warn: report immediately any rash, mouth ulcers, sore throat, fever, bruising, bleeding.
Interactions: metab by and ↑s P450 ∴ many; most importantly ↓s fx of OCP, doxycycline, Ca^{2+} antagonists (esp nifedipine), imatinib,

lapatinib, ciclosporin, keto-/itra-/posa-conazole, indinavir, quinidine, theophyllines, eplerenone, telithromycin, aripiprazole, mianserin, mirtazapine, paroxetine, TCAs and corticosteroids. Fx ↓by rifampicin, rifabutin, theophyllines, mefloquine, pyrimethamine, sucralfate, antipsychotics, TCAs and St John's wort. Levels ↑by NSAIDs (esp azapropazone), fluoxetine, mi-/flu-/vori-conazole, diltiazem, disulfiram, trimethoprim, cimetidine, esomeprazole, amiodarone, metronidazole, chloramphenicol, clarithromycin, isoniazid, sulphonamides, sulfinpyrazone, topiramate (levels of which are ↓) and ethosuximide. Complex interactions with other antiepileptics[SPC/BNF]. **W−** (or rarely **W** +).

Dose: po [1]: 150–500 mg/day in 1–2 divided doses[SPC/BNF]. iv [2]: load with 18 mg/kg ivi at max rate of 25–50 mg/min, then maintenance iv doses of approximately 100 mg tds/qds, adjusting to weight, serum levels and clinical response. If available give iv as pro-drug *fosphenytoin* (NB: doses differ).

NB: ↓dose if LF.

☠ Stop drug if ↓WCC** is severe, worsening or symptomatic ☠.

PHOSPHATE ENEMA

Laxative enemas; ⇒ osmotic H_2O retention ⇒ ↑evacuation.

Use: severe constipation (unresponsive to other Rx).

CI: acute GI disorders.

Caution: if debilitated or neurological disorder, **E**.

SE: local irritation.

Dose: 1 prn.

PHYLLOCONTIN CONTINUS see Aminophylline (MR).

Dose: initially 1 tablet (225 mg) bd po, then ↑ to 2 tablets bd after 1 wk according to serum levels. (Forte tablets of 350 mg used if smoker/other cause of ↓$t_{1/2}$, e.g. interactions with other drugs; see Theophylline.) NB: ↓**dose if LF**.

PHYTOMENADIONE

Intravenous vit K_1 for warfarin overdose/poisoning; see p. 216.

Caution: give iv injections slowly. NB: not compatible with NaCl **P**.

PICOLAX see Bowel preparations.
Dose: 1 sachet at 8 am and 3 pm the day before GI surgery or Ix.

PIOGLITAZONE/ACTOS

Thiazolidinedione (glitazone) antidiabetic; ↓s peripheral insulin resistance (and, to lesser extent, hepatic gluconeogenesis).
Use: type 2 DM in combination with a sulphonylurea (if metformin not tolerated) *or* metformin (if risk of ↓glucose with sulphonylurea unacceptable) *or* sulphonylurea + metformin (if obese, metabolic syndrome or human insulin unacceptable due to lifestyle/personal issues)[NICE].
CI: ACS (inc Hx of), previous or active bladder cancer, **H** (inc Hx of), **L/P/B**
Caution: peri-operatively cardiovascular disease. Omit pioglitazone peri-operatively as insulin needed. **R.**
SE: oedema (esp if HTN/CCF), ↓Hb, ↑Wt, GI upset (esp diarrhoea), headache, hypoglycaemia (if also taking sulphonylureas), ↑risk of distal fractures, rarely **hepatotoxicity**.
Monitor: LFTs. ☠ *Discontinue if jaundice develops* ☠ and for signs of HF.
Interactions: levels ↓by rifampicin and ↑by gemfibrozil.
Dose: initially 15–30 mg od (max 45 mg od)

PIPERACILLIN

Ureidopenicillin: antipseudomonal.
Use: only available with tazobactam* (β-lactamase inhibitor) as Tazocin, reserved for severe infections.
CI/Caution/SE/Interactions: see Benzylpenicillin.
Dose: see Tazocin*.

PIRITON see Chlorphenamine; antihistamine for allergies.

PLAVIX see Clopidogrel; anti-Pt agent for Px of IHD (and CVA).

POTASSIUM TABLETS see Kay-cee-L (syrup 1 mmol/ml),
Sando-K (effervescent 12 mmol/tablet) and Slow-K (MR non-

effervescent 8 mmol/tablet, reserved for when syrup/effervescent preparations are inappropriate; avoid if ↓swallow).

PRAMIPEXOLE/MIRAPEXIN

Dopamine agonist (non-ergot derived); use in early Parkinson's ⇒ ↓motor complications (e.g. dyskinesias) but ↓motor performance cf L-dopa.

Use: Parkinson's[1], moderate-severe restless legs syndrome (RLS)[2].

CI: B.

Caution: psychotic disorders, severe cardiovascular disease **R/H/P**.

SE: GI upset, sleepiness (inc sudden onset sleep), ↓BP (inc postural, esp initially), Ψ disorders (esp psychosis and impulse control disorders e.g. gambling and ↑sexuality), amnesia, headache, oedema.

Warn: sleepiness and ↓BP may impair skilled tasks (inc driving). Avoid abrupt withdrawal.

Monitor: ophthalmological testing if visual Δs occur.

Dose: initially 88 microgram tds[1] (or 88 microgram nocte for RLS[2]) ↑ing if tolerated/required to max 1.1 mg tds[1] (or 540 microgram nocte[2]). **NB: doses given for BASE (not SALT) & ↓dose if RF.**

PRAVASTATIN/LIPOSTAT

HMG-CoA reductase inhibitor: 'statin'; ↓s cholesterol/LDL (and TG).

Use/CI/Caution/SE/Monitor: see Simvastatin.

Interactions: ↑risk of myositis (± ↑levels) with ☠ fibrates ☠, nicotinic acid, daptomycin, ciclosporin and ery-/clari-thromycin.

Dose: 10–40 mg nocte. NB: ↓dose if RF (10 mg if moderate to severe RF).

PREDNISOLONE

Glucocorticoid (and mild mineralocorticoid activity).

Use: anti-inflammatory (e.g. rheumatoid arthritis, IBD, asthma, eczema), immunosuppression (e.g. transplant rejection Px, acute leukaemias), glucocorticoid replacement (e.g. Addison's disease, hypopituitarism).

CI: systemic infections (w/o antibiotic cover).

Caution/SE/Interactions: see p. 217.

Warn: carry steroid card (and avoid close contact with people who have chickenpox/shingles if patient has never had chickenpox).

Dose: usually 2.5–15 mg od po for maintenance. In acute/initial stages, 20–60 mg od often needed (depends on cause and often physician preference), e.g. acute asthma (40–50 mg od), acute COPD (30 mg od), temporal arteritis (40–60 mg daily). Take with food ($\downarrow Na^+$, $\uparrow K^+$ diet recommended if on long-term Rx). For other causes, consult[SPC/BNF], pharmacy or local specialist relevant to the disease. Also available as once or twice weekly im injection.

> 💀 Warn patient not to stop tablets suddenly (*can* $\Rightarrow$ *Addisonian crisis*). Requirements may $\uparrow$ if intercurrent illness/surgery. Consider Ca/vit D supplements/bisphosphonate to $\downarrow$ risk of osteoporosis and PPI to $\downarrow$ risk of GI ulcer 💀.

PREGABALIN/LYRICA

Antiepileptic; GABA analogue.

Use: epilepsy (partial seizures w or w/o 2° generalisation), neuropathic pain, generalised anxiety disorder.

CI: B.

Caution: avoid abrupt withdrawal, **H** (if severe) **R/P/E.**

SE: neuro-Ψ disturbance; esp **somnolence/dizziness** ($\Rightarrow$ falls in elderly), confusion, visual Δ (esp blurred vision), mood $\uparrow$ or $\downarrow$ (and *possibly* suicidal ideation/behaviour[†]), $\downarrow$libido, sexual dysfunction and vertigo. Also GI upset, $\uparrow$appetite/Wt, oedema and dry mouth. Rarely HF (esp if elderly and/or CVS disease).

Warn: seek medical advice if $\uparrow$suicidality or mood $\downarrow$s[†]. Don't stop abruptly as can $\Rightarrow$ withdrawal fx* (insomnia, headache, N&D, 'flu-like symptoms, pain, sweating, dizziness, pain).

Dose: 50–600 mg/day po in 2–3 divided doses[SPC/BNF]. **NB: stop over ≥1wk* and ↓dose if RF.**

PROCHLORPERAZINE/STEMETIL

Antiemetic: DA antagonist (phenothiazine ∴ also antipsychotic, but now rarely used for this).

Use: N&V (inc labyrinthine disorders).

CI/Caution/SE/Monitor/Warn/Interactions: as chlorpromazine, but CI are relative and $\Rightarrow$ ↓sedation. NB: can $\Rightarrow$ **extrapyramidal fx** (esp if elderly/debilitated) inc restlessness (akathisia); see p. 278.

Dose: *po:* acutely 20 mg, then 10 mg 2 h later (5–10 mg bd/tds for Px and labyrinthine disorders); **im:** 12.5 mg, then po doses 6 h later; *pr:* 25 mg then po doses 6 h later (5 mg tds pr for migraine). Available as quick-dissolving 3-mg tablets to be placed under lip (Ⓑuccastem); give 1–2 bd. NB: ↓**dose if RF.**

PROCYCLIDINE

Antimuscarinic: ↓s cholinergic to dopaminergic ratio in extrapyramidal syndromes $\Rightarrow$ ↓tremor/rigidity. No fx on bradykinesia (or tardive dyskinesia; may even worsen).

Use: extrapyramidal symptoms (e.g. Parkinsonism), esp if drug-induced[1] (e.g. antipsychotics; see p. 278).

CI: urinary retention (if untreated), glaucoma* (angle-closure), GI obstruction, MG.

Caution: cardiovascular disease, ↑prostate, tardive dyskinesia, **L/R/H/P/B/E.**

SE: antimuscarinic fx (see p. 276), Ψ disturbances, euphoria (can be drug of abuse), glaucoma*.

Warn: can ↓ability at driving/skilled tasks.

Dose: 2.5 mg tds po prn[1] (↑if necessary to max of 10 mg tds); 5–10 mg im/iv if acute dystonia or oculogyric crisis.

NB: do not stop suddenly: can $\Rightarrow$ rebound muscarinic fx.

PROMETHAZINE

Sedating antihistamine.

Use: insomnia[1]. Also used iv/im for anaphylaxis and po for symptom relief in chronic allergies.

CI: CNS depression/coma, MAOI w/in 14 days.

Caution: urinary retention, ↑prostate, glaucoma, epilepsy, IHD, asthma, porphyria, pyloroduodenal obstruction, **R** (↓dose), **L** (avoid if severe)/**P/B/E.**

SE: antimuscarinic fx (see p. 276), **hangover sedation**, headache.
Warn: can ↓ability at driving/skilled tasks.
Interactions: ↑s fx of anticholinergics, TCAs and sedatives/hypnotics.
Dose: 25 mg nocte[1] (can ↑dose to 50 mg).

PROPOFOL

Anaesthetic (iv).
Use: induction or maintenance of anaesthesia. Also for sedation during intensive care (if >16 years old*) or diagnostic procedures.
CI: anaesthetist not confident of airway maintenance, ICU sedation in children <16*, peanut or soya allergy.
Caution: hypovolaemia, ↓BP, cardiovascular disease, respiratory impairment, epilepsy, ↑ICP, **L/R/P/B** (for 24h)/**E**
SE: local pain, headache, N&V in recovery, anaphylaxis, extraneous muscle movements, convulsions (inc delayed onset), ↓HR (occasionally profound- treat with IV antimuscarinic), ↓BP, flushing, transient apnoea, hyperventilation, coughing, hiccup during induction, 💀 **propofol infusion syndrome*** if <16 yrs old in sedation in intensive care- potentially fatal, metabolic acidosis, HF, rhabdomyolysis, hyperlipidaemia, hepatomegaly) 💀, 💀 **arrhythmia** (↑/↓HR, asystole) 💀.
Warn: injection painful (can ↓ by giving into large vein or with iv lidocaine); don't drive/operate machinery for ≥12h (or longer depending on age, and patient condition); avoid alcohol before and for at least 8 hrs after.
Monitor: Cardiac / respiratory function. Have resus equipment readily available.
Interactions: other CNS depressants ↑ sedation & cardiorespiratory depression. Suxamethonium (↑risk of myocardial depression & ↓HR), ↑ hypotensive fx with adrenergic neurone blockers, α-blockers, antipsychotics, verapamil.
Dose: age, weight and drug concentration dependent[BNF/SPC]; titrated to effect, except when using 'rapid sequence induction'.

L/R/H = Liver, Renal and Heart failure (full key see p. xv)

☠ Should only be administered by, or under direct supervision of, personnel experienced in its use, with adequate training in anaesthesia and airway management, and when resuscitation equipment is available. Can $\Rightarrow$ apnoea and $\downarrow$BP within one arm-brain circulation time. ☠

PROPRANOLOL

β-Blocker (non-selective): $\beta_1 \Rightarrow \downarrow$HR and $\downarrow$contractility, $\beta_2 \Rightarrow$ vasodilation (and bronchoconstriction and glucose release from liver). Also blocks fx of catecholamines, $\downarrow$s renin production, slows SAN/AVN conduction.

Use: HTN[1] (*for advice on stepped HTN Mx see p. 235*), IHD (angina Rx[2], MI Px[3]), portal HTN[4] (Px of variceal bleed; NB: *may worsen liver function*), essential tremor[5], Px of migraine[6], anxiety[7], $\uparrow$T (symptom relief[8], thyroid storm[9]), arrhythmias[8] (inc severe[9]).

CI: asthma/Hx of bronchospasm, peripheral arterial disease (if severe), Prinzmetal's angina, severe $\downarrow$HR or $\downarrow$BP, SSS, 2nd-/3rd-degree HB, cardiogenic shock, metabolic acidosis, phaeo (unless used specifically with α-blockers), **H** (if uncontrolled).

Caution: COPD, 1st-degree HB, DM*, MG, Hx of hypersensitivity (may $\uparrow$ to *all* allergens), **L/R/P/B**.

SE: $\downarrow$HR, $\downarrow$BP, HF, peripheral vasoconstriction ($\Rightarrow$ cold extremities, worsening of claudication/Raynaud's), **fatigue, depression, sleep disturbance** (inc nightmares), hyperglycaemia (and $\downarrow$**sympathetic response to hypoglycaemia***), GI upset. Rarely, conduction/blood disorders.

Interactions: ☠ verapamil and diltiazem $\Rightarrow$ risk of HB and $\downarrow$HR ☠. Risk of $\downarrow$BP and HF with nifedipine. Risk of $\downarrow$BP with α-blockers. $\uparrow$s risk of bupiva-/lido-caine toxicity. $\uparrow$s risk of AV block, myocardial depression and $\downarrow$HR with amiodarone, flecainide. Levels of both drugs can $\uparrow$with chlorpromazine. Risk of $\uparrow$BP with moxisylyte. Risk of $\uparrow$BP (and $\downarrow$HR) with dobutamine, adrenaline and noradrenaline. Risk of withdrawal $\uparrow$BP with clonidine (stop β-blocker before slowly $\downarrow$ing clonidine).

Dose: 80–160 mg bd po[1]; 40–120 mg bd po[2]; 40 mg qds for 2–3 days, then 80 mg bd po[3] (start 5–21 days post-MI); 40 mg bd po[4] (↑dose if necessary); 40 mg bd/tds po[5,6]; 40 mg od po[7] (↑dose to tds if necessary); 10–40 mg tds/qds[8]; 1 mg iv over 1 min[9] repeating every 2 min if required, to max total 10 mg (or 5 mg in anaesthesia).

> **NB: ↓po dose in LF and ↓initial dose in RF.** Withdraw slowly (esp in angina); if not can ⇒ rebound ↑of symptoms.

PROPYLTHIOURACIL

Thionamide antithyroid (peroxidase inhibitor): ↓s I⁻ ⇒ I₂ ↓s and ∴ ↓T_{3/4} production, as carbimazole does, but also ↓s peripheral T_4 to T_3 conversion. Possible immunosuppressant fx.

Use: ↑T_4 (2nd-line in the UK; if carbimazole not tolerated).

Caution: L/R, P/B (can cause fetal/neonatal goitre/↓T_4 ∴ use min dose and monitor neonatal development closely; 'block-and-replace' regimen ∴ not suitable as high doses used for this).

SE: blood disorders (esp ☠ **agranulocytosis** ☠ stop drug if occurs), **skin reactions** (esp urticaria, rarely cutaneous vasculitis/lupus), fever. Rarely **hepatotoxicity**, nephritis.

Warn: patient to report symptoms of infection (esp sore throat) or of liver disease (e.g. anorexia, N&V, jaundice, pruritis), & signs of LF (explain symptoms).

Monitor: FBC, LFTs, clotting.

Dose: 200–400 mg po in divided doses until euthyroid, then ↓ to maintenance dose of 50–150 mg od. **NB: ↓dose if LF or RF.**

PROSCAR see Finasteride; antiandrogen for BPH (and baldness).

PROTAMINE (SULPHATE)

Protein (basic) that binds heparin (acidic).

Use: reversal of heparin (or LMWH) following over-Rx/OD or after temporary anticoagulation for extracorporeal circuits (e.g. cardiopulmonary bypass, haemodialysis).

Caution: ↑risk of hypersensitivity reaction if: (1) vasectomy, (2) infertile man, (3) allergy to fish.

L/R/H = Liver, Renal and Heart failure (full key see p. xv)

SE: ↓BP, ↓HR, N&V, flushing, dyspnoea. Rarely pulmonary oedema, hypertension, **hypersensitivity reactions**.
Dose: 1 mg per 80–100 units of heparin to be reversed (max 50 mg) iv/ivi at rate ≤ 5 mg/min; exact regimen depends on whether reversing heparin or LMWH and whether given iv or sc[BNF/SPC].
NB: $t_{1/2}$ of iv heparin is short; ↓doses of protamine if giving to reverse iv heparin >15 min after last dose – see SPC.

Max total dose 50 mg: ☠ *high doses can* ⇒ *anticoagulant fx!* ☠

PROXYMETHACAINE
Topical anaesthetic (lasts 20 min).
Use: eye examination (if painful eye or checking IOP).
SE: corneal epithelial shedding.
Dose: 1 drop prn (not for prolonged treatment).

PROZAC see Fluoxetine; SSRI antidepressant.

PULMICORT see Budesonide; inh steroid for asthma. 50, 100, 200 or 400 microgram/puff. ▼ Aerosol (not other preparations).

PYRAZINAMIDE
Antibiotic: 'cidal' only against intracellular and dividing mycobacteria (e.g. TB). Good CSF penetration*.
Use: TB Rx (for initial phase, see p. 267), TB meningitis*.
CI: acute porphyria, **L** (if severe, otherwise caution).
Caution: DM, gout (avoid in acute attacks), **P**.
SE: **hepatotoxicity****, ↑**urate**, GI upset (inc N&V), dysuria, interstitial nephritis, **arthr-/my-algia**, sideroblastic ↓Hb, ↓Pt, rash (and photosensitivity).
Monitor: LFTs**.
Warn: patients and carers to stop drug and seek urgent medical attention if signs of LF (explain symptoms).
Dose: up to 2 g daily usually given as part of combination product (500 mg tablets of just pyrazinamide available, but unlicensed)– exact dose varies according to Wt and whether Rx is 'supervised' or not[SPC/BNF].

PYRIDOSTIGMINE

Anticholinesterase: inhibits cholinesterase at neuromuscular junction ⇒ ↑ACh ⇒ ↑neuromuscular transmission.

Use: myasthenia gravis.

CI: GI/urinary obstruction.

Caution: asthma, recent MI, ↓HR/BP, arrhythmias, vagotonia, ↑T, PU, epilepsy, Parkinsonism, **R/P/B/E**.

SE: cholinergic fx (see p. 276) – esp if xs Rx/OD, where ↓BP, bronchoconstriction and (confusingly) weakness can also occur (= cholinergic crisis*); ↑**secretions** (sweat/saliva/tears) and miosis are good clues** of xs ACh.

Interactions: fx ↓d by **aminoglycosides** (e.g. gentamicin), **polymixins**, clindamycin, lithium, quinidine, chloroquine, propranolol and procainamide. ↑s fx of suxamethonium.

Dose: 30–120 mg po up to qds (can ↑to max total 1.2 g/24 h; if possible give <450 mg/24 h to avoid receptor downregulation).
NB: ↓dose if RF.

> ☠ ↑ing weakness can be due to *cholinergic crisis** as well as MG exacerbation; if unsure which is responsible**, get senior help (esp if ↓respiratory function) before giving Rx, as the wrong choice can be fatal! ☠

QUETIAPINE/SEROQUEL

Atypical (2nd generation) antipsychotic.

Use: schizophrenia[1], mania[2], depression in bipolar disorder[3]. Off-licence use for psychosis/behavioural disorders (esp in dementias, but use of antipsychotics in dementia generally not recommended).

CI: B.

Caution: cardiovascular disease, Hx of epilepsy, drugs that ↑QTc, **L/R/E/P**.

SE/Interactions/Warn/Monitor: as olanzapine but therapeutic doses are initially sedating and ↓BP requiring ∴ start with ↓dose*. Also levels ↑by ery-/clari-thromycin.

Dose: *Needs titration** (*see SPC/BNF*): initially 25 mg bd ↑ing daily to max 750 mg/day[1]; initially 50 mg bd ↑ing daily to max

800 mg/day[2]; initially 50 mg od ↑ing daily to max 600 mg/day[3]. If RF, LF or elderly start at 25 mg od ↑ing less frequently. Available in MR form (▼ Seroquel XL); initially 300 mg od then 600 mg od the next day[2], then adjust to response (if giving for depression[3] or if RF, LF or elderly start at 50 mg od then ↑cautiously[SPC/BNF]).

QUININE
Antimalarial: kills bloodborne schizonts.

Use: malaria Rx[1] (esp falciparum), nocturnal leg cramps[2].

CI: optic neuritis, tinnitus, haemoglobinuria, MG.

Caution: cardiac disease (inc conduction dfx, AF, HB), G6PD deficiency, H/P/E.

SE: visual Δs (inc temporary blindness, esp in OD), tinnitus (and vertigo/deafness), GI upset, headache, rash/flushing, hypersensitivity, confusion, hypoglycaemia*. Rarely blood disorders, AKI, cardiovascular fx (can ⇒ severe ↓BP in OD).

Monitor: blood glucose*, ECG (if elderly) and e'lytes (if given iv).

Interactions: ↑s levels of flecainide and digoxin. ↑s risk of arrhythmias with pimozide, moxifloxacin and amiodarone. ↑risk of seizures with mefloquine. Avoid artemether/lumefantrine.

Dose: 200–300 mg nocte po as quinine *sulphate*[2]. For malaria Rx, see p. 267 (**NB:** ↓iv maintenance dose if RF).

RABEPRAZOLE/PARIET
PPI; as omeprazole, but ↓interactions[BNF/SPC].

Dose: 20 mg od (↓to 10 mg od for maintenance). Max 120 mg/day (depending on indication).

RAMIPRIL/TRITACE
ACE-i; see Captopril.

Use: HTN[1] (*for advice on stepped HTN Mx see p. 235*), HF[2], Px post-MI[3]. Also Px of cardiovascular disease (if age >55 years and at risk)[4].

CI/Caution/SE/Monitor/Interactions: as captopril.
Dose: initially 1.25 mg od ($\uparrow$ing slowly to max of 10 mg daily)[1,2]; initially 2.5 mg bd then $\uparrow$to 5.0 mg bd after 2 days[3] (start 3–10 days post-MI) then maintenance 2.5–5 mg bd; initially 2.5 mg od ($\uparrow$ing to 10 mg)[4].
NB: $\downarrow$dose if RF.

RANITIDINE/ZANTAC

H_2 antagonist $\Rightarrow$ $\downarrow$parietal cell H^+ secretion.
Use: PU (Px if on long-term high dose NSAIDs[1], chronic Rx[2], a cute Rx[3]), reflux oesophagitis.
Caution: acute porphyria, **L/R/P/B**. ☠ *May mask symptoms of gastric cancer* ☠.
SE: *all rare*: GI upset (esp diarrhoea), dizziness, confusion, fatigue, blurred vision, headache, Δ LFTs (rarely hepatitis), rash. Very rarely arrhythmias (esp if given iv), hypersensitivity, blood disorders.
Dose: initially 150 mg bd po (or 300 mg nocte)[1,2], $\uparrow$ing to 600 mg/day if necessary but try to $\downarrow$ to 150 mg nocte for maintenance; 50 mg tds/qds iv[3] (or im/ivi[SPC/BNF])
NB: $\downarrow$dose if RF.

REOPRO see Abciximab; antiplatelet agent for MI/ACS.

RETEPLASE (=r-PA).

Recombinant plasminogen activator: thrombolytic.
Use/CI/Caution/SE: see Alteplase and p. 231 but only for Rx of AMI (i.e. not approved for CVA/other use).
Dose: 10 units as slow iv injection over $\leqslant$2 min, repeating after 30 min.

Concurrent unfractionated iv heparin needed for 48 h; see p. 232.

RIFABUTIN

Rifamycin antibiotic; see Rifampicin.
Use: TB: Rx of pulmonary TB[1] and non-tuberculous mycobacterial disease[2]. Also Px of *Mycobacterium avium* [3] (if HIV with $\downarrow$CD4).

CI/Caution/SE/Warn/Monitor/Interactions: as rifampicin, plus levels ↑ by macrolides, triazoles, imidazoles and antivirals (⇒ ↑risk of uveitis; ↓rifabutin dose) and ↓s carbamazepine and phenytoin levels.
Dose: 150–450 mg od[1]; 450–600 mg od[2]; 300 mg od[3]. **NB:** ↓dose if severe LF or RF.

RIFAMPICIN

Rifamycin antibiotic: 'cidal' ⇒ ↓RNA synthesis.
Use: TB Rx, *N. meningitidis* (meningococcal)/*H. influenzae* (type b) meningitis Px. Rarely for *Legionella*/*Brucella*/*Staphylococcus* infections.
CI: jaundice, are concurrently receiving saquinavir/ritonavir therapy, hypersensitivity to rifamycins or excipients.
Caution: acute porphyria, **L/R/P/B**.
SE: hepatotoxicity, GI upset (inc AAC), headache, fever, 'flu-like symptoms (esp if intermittent use), orange/red body secretions*, SOB, blood disorders, skin reactions, shock, AKI.
Warn: of symptoms/signs of liver disease; report jaundice/persistent N&V/malaise immediately. Warn about secretions*.
Monitor: LFTs, FBC (and U&Es if dose >600 mg/day).
Interactions: ↑ **P450** ∴ many; most importantly ↓s fx of OCP**, lamotrigine, phenytoin, sulphonylureas, tolbutamide, mefloquine, gefi-/nilo-tinib, digoxin, keto-/flu-/itra-/.posa-/vori-conazole, antivirals, telithromycin, nevirapine, ciclosporin, siro-/tacro-limus, imatinib, corticosteroids, haloperidol, aripiprazole, disopyramide, mefloquine, bosentan, propafenone, eplerenone and Ca^{2+} antagonists. **W–**.
Dose: for TB Rx, see p. 267; for other indications see SPC/BNF. (NB: well absorbed po; give iv *only* if ↓swallow.) **NB:** ↓dose if LF or RF.

Other contraception** needed during Rx.

RIFATER Combination preparation of rifampicin, isoniazid and pyrazinamide for 1st 2 months of TB Rx (⇒ ↓bacterial load/ infectiousness until sensitivities known); see p. 267.

RISEDRONATE

Bisphosphonate: ↓s osteoclastic bone resorption.

Use: osteoporosis (Px[1]/Rx[2], esp if postmenopausal or steroid -induced), Paget's disease[3].

CI: ↓Ca^{2+}, **R** (if eGFR <30 ml/min), **P/B.**

Caution: delayed GI transit/emptying (esp oesophageal abnormalities). Correct Ca^{2+} and other bone/mineral metabolism Δ (e.g. vit D and PTH function) before Rx, dental procedures in patients at risk of osteonecrosis of the jaw (e.g. chemotherapy).

SE: GI upset, **bone/joint/muscle pain, headache, rash**. Rarely iritis, dry eyes/corneal lesions, oesophageal stricture/inflammation/ulcer*, osteonecrosis of the jaw and atypical femoral fractures.

Warn: of symptoms of oesophageal irritation and if develop to stop tablets/seek medical attention. Must swallow tablets whole with full glass of water on an empty stomach ≥30 min before, and stay upright until breakfast*. Need to report thigh, hip or groin pain.

Interactions: Ca^{2+}-containing products (inc milk) and antacids (⇒ ↓absorption) ∴ separate doses as much as possible from risedronate. Also avoid iron and mineral suplements.

Dose: 5 mg od[1,2] (or 1 × 35-mg tablet/week as Actonel Once a Week [2]); 30 mg daily for 2 months[3].

▼ RISPERIDONE/RISPERDAL

'Atypical' antipsychotic: similar to olanzapine (⇒↓extrapyramidal fx cf 'typical' antipsychotics, esp tardive dyskinesia).

Use: psychosis/schizophrenia (acute and chronic)[NICE], mania & short term Rx (<6 wks) of persistent aggression unresponsive to non-pharmacological Rx in Alzheimer's.

CI: phenylketonuria (only if Quicklet form used).

Caution/SE: similar to olanzapine but ⇒↓sedation, ↑hypotension (esp initially: ↑dose slowly* (retitrate if many doses missed), ↓hyperglycaemia, ↑extrapyramidal fx; if ↑stroke risk.

Interactions: levels may be ↓by carbamazepine and ↑by ritonavir, fluoxetine and paroxetine. ↑risk of CNS toxicity with sibutramine. ↑mortality rate in elderly if taking furosemide. ↑risk of arrhythmias with drugs that ↑QTc and atomoxetine. ↑risk of ↓BP with general anaesthetics. ↓s fx of anticonvulsants. Avoid paliperidone.

Dose: initially 2 mg od titrating up if necessary, generally to 4–6 mg od (if elderly initially 0.5 mg bd titrating up if required to max 2 mg bd po). Also available as liquid or quick dissolving 1, 2, 3, or 4 mg tablets ('Quicklets') and as long-acting im 2-wkly injections ('Consta' ▼) for ↑compliance.

NB: ↓dose if LF or RF.

RITUXIMAB/MABTHERA

Monoclonal Ab against B lymphocytes (CD20+).

Use: Various B cell non-Hodgkin's lymphoma[1] (many indications for Diffuse Large B cell Lymphoma and Follicular Lymphoma[NICE]), RA[2] (in combination with methotrexate, in severe active cases with inadequate response to DMARDs, inc ≥1 TNF-α inhibitor[NICE]), SLE, vasculitis, CLL[NICE].

CI: active severe infections, hypersensivity to active substances or excipients, **B**.

Caution: IHD, if already on other cardiotoxic/cytotoxic drugs, with active or chronic infections (e.g. hepatitis B), **H** (avoid if severe and giving for RA)/**P**.

SE: ☠ infusion hypersensitivity/cytokine release syndrome* (mainly during 1st infusion: fever, chills, arrhythmias, ARDS and allergic reactions) ☠, tumour lysis syndrome, pancytopenia, ↓BP, ↑risk of PML, ↑infections.

Warn: withhold antihypertensive drugs 12 h prior to ivi. Remember to give patient alert card.

Monitor: BP, neurological function (PML), FBC.

Dose: seek expert advice and product literature for dose/rate[1], 1 g ivi initially and repeat once after 2 wks[2(see SPC/BNF)].

> ☠ Only give if full resuscitation facilities available. Interrupt ivi for severe reactions* and institute supportive care measures.

RIVASTIGMINE/EXELON

Acetylcholinesterase inhibitor that acts centrally (crosses BBB): replenishes ACh, which is ↓d in certain dementias.

Use: Alzheimer's disease[NICE] & Parkinson's disease dementia.
CI: L (if severe, otherwise caution), **B**.
Caution: conduction defects (esp SSS), PU susceptibility, Hx of COPD/asthma/seizures, bladder outflow obstruction, **R/P**.
SE: cholinergic fx (see p. 276), **GI upset** (esp nausea initially), **headache, dizziness,** behavioural/Ψreactions. Rarely GI haemorrhage, ↓HR, AV block, angina, seizures, rash.
Monitor: weight
Dose: 1.5 mg bd po initially (↑ing slowly to 3–6 mg bd: specialist review needed for clinical response and tolerance). Available as daily transdermal patch releasing 4.6 mg or 9.5 mg/24 h. Continue only if MMSE remains 10–20[NICE].

NB: If > several days doses missed retitration of dose required.

RIZATRIPTAN/MAXALT

$5HT_{1B/1D}$ agonist for acute migraine.
Use/CI/Caution/SE/Interactions: see Sumatriptan.
Dose: 10 mg po (can repeat after ⩾ 2 h if responded then recurs). Max 20 mg/24 h. **NB: give 5 mg doses if RF or LF (and avoid if either severe).**

ROCURONIUM

Aminosteroid neuromuscular blocker (see Vecuronium). Most rapid onset of the non-depolarising neuromuscular blockers (2 mins). Intermediate duration of action.
Use: neuromuscular blockade for surgery[1] or during intensive care[2].
CI: anaesthetist not confident of airway maintenance.
Caution: neuromuscular disease (MG, Eaton-Lambert, old polio), hypothermia, obesity, burns. **L/R/E**.
SE: ↑HR/BP (mild), prolonged paralysis and myopathy*.
Warn: Don't drive until 24h after full recovery. Injection painful.
Monitor: Cardiac, respiratory & motor function.
Interactions: fx ↑ by aminoglycosides, clindamycin and polymyxins. Only administer after full recovery from neuromuscular blockade of suxamethonium. Corticosteroids can ↑ myopathy risk*.

L/R/H = Liver, Renal and Heart failure (full key see p. xv)

Dose: initially 600 micrograms/kg iv then maintenance 150 micrograms/kg iv **or** initially 300–600 micrograms/kg/hr ivi adjusting to response[1]; initially 600 micrograms/kg iv (optional) then 300–600 micrograms/kg/hr ivi for 1st hr, then adjusting to response[2]. *NB: if obese (weight 30% above ideal body weight (IBW; see p.296)) use IBW for dose calculation.* ↓ Dose if elderly, LF or RF[SPC/BNF].

> 💀 Specialist use only. Needs respiratory assistance / control until drug inactivated or antagonised. Needs anaesthetic / sedative to prevent awareness. 💀

ROPINIROLE/REQUIP[1] or ADARTREL[2]

Dopamine agonist (non-ergot derived); use in early Parkinson's⇒ ↓motor complications (e.g. dyskinesias) but ↓motor performance cf L-dopa. Also adjunctive use in Parkinson's with motor fluctuations.

Use: Parkinson's[1], moderate-severe restless legs syndrome (RLS)[2].

CI: P/B.

Caution: major psychotic disorders, severe cardiovascular disease L/R.

SE: GI upset, sleepiness (inc sudden onset sleep),↓BP (inc postural, esp initially), Ψ disorders (esp psychosis and impulse control disorders, e.g. gambling and ↑sexuality), confusion, leg oedema, paradoxical worsening of restless legs syndrome symptoms or early morning rebound (may need to withdraw or reduce dose).

Warn: sleepiness and↓BP may impair skilled tasks (inc driving). Avoid abrupt withdrawal.

Dose: initially 250 microgram tds[1] (or 250 microgram nocte for RLS[2]) ↑ing if tolerated/required to max 8 mg tds[1] (or 4 mg nocte for RLS[2]). Available in MR preparation (Requip XL) 2–24 mg od[1].

ROSUVASTATIN/CRESTOR

HMG-Co A reductase inhibitor; 'statin' to ↓cholesterol (and TG).

Use/CI/Caution/SE: as simvastatin, but safe in porphyria, can ⇒ DM and proteinuria (and rarely haematuria). Avoid if severe RF.

Interactions: ↑risk of myositis with ☠ **fibrates** and **ciclosporin** ☠, **daptomycin**, **protease inhibitors**, **fusidic** and **nicotinic acid**. Levels ↓ by antacids. Mild **W +**.

Dose: initially 5–10 mg od. If necessary ↑ to 20 mg after ≥4 wks (if not of Asian origin or risk factors for myopathy/rhabdomyolysis, can ↑ to 40 mg after further 4 wks). **NB:↓dose if RF, Asian origin or other ↑risk factor for myopathy.**

(r)tPA (Recombinant) tissue-type plasminogen activator; see Alteplase.

SALBUTAMOL

β_2 Agonist, short-acting: dilates bronchial smooth muscle (and endometrium). Also inhibits mast-cell mediator release.

Use: chronic[1] and acute[2] asthma. Rarely↑K^+(give nebs prn), premature labour (iv).

Caution: cardiovascular disease (esp arrhythmias*, susceptibility to ↑QTc, HTN), DM (can ⇒ DKA, esp if iv ∴ monitor CBGs),↑T_4, **P/B**.

SE: *neurological* : fine tremor, headache, nervousness, behavioural/sleep Δs (esp in children); *CVS*:↑**HR**, palpitations/arrhythmias (esp if iv), ↑QTc*; *other* : ↓K^+, muscle cramps, lactic acidosis. Rarely hypersensitivity, **paradoxical bronchospasm**. Prolonged Rx ⇒ small↑risk of glaucoma.

Monitor: K^+ and glucose (esp if ↑ or iv doses).

Interactions: iv salbutamol ⇒ ↑risk of ↓↓BP with methyldopa.

Dose: 100–200 microgram (aerosol) or 200–400 microgram (powder) inh prn up to qds[1]; 2.5–5 mg qds 4-hrly neb[2]. If life-threatening (see p. 242), can ↑nebs up to every 15 min or give as ivi (initially 5 microgram/min, then up to 20 microgram/min according to response).

SALMETEROL/SEREVENT

Bronchodilator: long-acting β_2 agonist(LABA).

Use: 1st choice add-on for asthma Rx (on top of short-acting β_2 agonist and inh steroids). *Not for acute Rx!*

Caution/SE/Monitor: as salbutamol.

Dose: 50–100 microgram bd inh.

SALOFALK see Mesalazine; 'new' aminosalicylate for UC (↓SEs).

SANDOCAL Calcium supplement; available in '400' (400 mg calcium = 10 mmol Ca^{2+}) or '1000' (1 g calcium = 25 mmol Ca^{2+}) effervescent tablets.

SANDO-K
Effervescent oral KCl (12 mmol K^+/tablet).
Use: ↓K^+.
CI: $K^+ > 5.0$ mmol/l, **R** (if severe, otherwise caution).
Caution: GI ulcer/stricture, hiatus hernia, taking other drugs that ↑K^+ and cardiac disease.
SE: N&V, GI ulceration, flatulence.
Dose: according to serum K^+: start with 2–4 tablets/day if diet normal. Take with food. **NB:** ↓**dose in RF/elderly** (↑ if established ↓K^+).

SENNA/SENOKOT
Stimulant laxative; takes 8–12 h to work.
Use: constipation.
CI: GI obstruction.
Caution: **P** (try bulk forming or osmotic laxative 1st).
SE: GI cramps. If chronic use atonic non-functioning colon, ↓K^+.
Dose: 2 tablets nocte (can ↑ to 4 tablets nocte). Available as syrup.

SEPTRIN see Co-trimoxazole (sulfamethoxazole +trimethoprim).

SERC see Betahistine; histamine analogue for vestibular disorders.

SERETIDE Combination asthma or COPD inhaler with possible synergistic action: long-acting β_2 agonist (LABA) salmeterol 50 microgram (Accuhaler) or 25 microgram (Evohaler) + fluticasone (steroid) in varying quantities (50, 100, 125, 250 or 500 microgram/puff). Note different devices have different licensed indications.

SEROXAT see Paroxetine; SSRI antidepressant.

SERTRALINE/LUSTRAL

SSRI antidepressant; also increases dopamine levels; see Fluoxetine.

Use: depression[1] (also PTSD in women, OCD, social anxiety disorder & panic disorder). Relatively good safety record in pregnancy and breast-feeding.

CI/Caution/SE/Warn/Interactions: as fluoxetine, but↓incidence of agitation/insomnia, doesn't↑↑carbamazepine/phenytoin levels, but does ↑pimozide levels.

Dose: initially 50 mg od,↑ing in 50 mg increments over several weeks to max daily dose 200 mg (if>100 mg/day, must be divided into at least 2 doses)[1]. **NB:↓dose if LF.**

SEVELAMER HYDROCHLORIDE

PO_4^- binding agent; contains no Al/Ca^{2+} ∴ no risk of↑ing Al/Ca^{2+} (which can occur with other drugs, esp if on dialysis). Also ↓s cholesterol.

Use: ↑PO_4 (if on dialysis).

CI: GI obstruction.

Caution: GI disorders, P/B.

SE: GI upset.

Interactions: can↓ plasma levels of ciprofloxacin and immunosuppressants used in renal transplant patients.

Dose: initially 800–1600 mg tds po, then adjust to response[SPC/BNF].

SEVREDOL Morphine (sulphate) tablets (10, 20 or 50 mg).
Dose: see Oramorph.

SILDENAFIL/VIAGRA or REVATIO (▼)

Phosphodiesterase type-5 inhibitor: ↑s local fx of NO (⇒ ↑smooth-muscle relaxation ∴ ↑blood flow into corpus cavernosum).

Use: erectile dysfunction[1], pulmonary artery hypertension[2] (and digital ulceration under specialist supervision).

CI: recent CVA/MI/ACS,↓BP (systolic <90 mmHg), hereditary degenerative retinal disorders, Hx of non-arteritic anterior ischaemic optic neuropathy and conditions where vasodilation/sexual activity inadvisable. **L/H** (if either severe).

Caution: cardiovascular disease, LV outflow obstruction, bleeding disorders (inc active PU), anatomical deformation of penis, predisposition to prolonged erection (e.g. multiple myeloma/leukaemias/sickle cell disease), **R/P/B**.

SE: headache, flushing, GI upset, dizziness, visual disturbances, nasal congestion, hypersensitivity reactions. Rarely, serious cardiovascular events, priapism and painful red eyes.

Interactions: ☠ *Nitrates (e.g.GTN/ISMN/ISDN) and nicorandil can ↓↓BP ∴ never give together* ☠. Antivirals (esp rito-/ataza-/indi-navir) ↑its levels. ↑s hypotensive fx of α-blockers; avoid concomitant use. Levels ↑by keto-/itra-conazole

Dose: initially 50 mg approx 1 h before sexual activity[1], adjusting to response (1 dose per 24 h, max 100 mg per dose); 20 mg tds[2].
NB: ↓dose if RF or LF.

SIMVASTATIN/ZOCOR

HMG-CoA reductase inhibitor ('statin'): ⇒ ↓cholesterol(↓s synthesis), ↓LDL (↑s uptake), mildly ↓s TG.

Use: ↑cholesterol, Px of atherosclerotic disease: IHD (inc 1° prevention), CVA, PVD.

CI: acute porphyria, **L** (inc active liver disease or ΔLFTs), **P** (contraception required during, and for 1 month after, Rx), **B**.

Caution: ↓T_4, alcohol abuse, Hx of liver disease, **R** (if severe).

SE: hepatitis and myositis* (both rare but important), headache, GI upset, rash. Rarely pancreatitis, hypersensitivity.

Monitor: LFTs (and CK if symptoms develop*).

Interactions: ↑risk of myositis (± ↑levels) with ☠ fibrates ☠, clari-/ery-/teli-thromycin, itra-/keto-/mi-/posa-conazole, ciclosporin, protease inhibitors, nicotinic acid, fusidic acid, colchicine, danazol, amiodarone, verapamil, diltiazem, amlodipine, ranolazine and grapefruit juice. Mild **W +**.

Dose: 10–80 mg nocte (usually start at 10–20 mg[SPC/BNF]) ↑ing at intervals ≥ 4 wks.↓max dose if significant drug interactions[SPC/BNF].
NB:↓dose if RF or other ↑risk factor for myositis*.

☠ Myositis* can rarely ⇒**rhabdomyolysis**; ↑risk if ↓T₄, RF or taking drugs that ↑levels/risk of myositis (see above) ☠.

SINEMET see Co-careldopa; L-dopa for Parkinson's.

SLOW-K
Slow-release (non-effervescent) oral KCl (8 mmolK⁺/tablet).
Use: ↓K⁺ where liquid/effervescent tablets inappropriate.
CI/Caution/SE: as Sando-K, plus caution if ↓swallow.
Dose: according to serum K⁺: average 3–6 tablets/day. **NB:** ↓**dose if RF** (and caution if taking other drugs that ↑K⁺).

SODIUM BICARBONATE iv
Alkalinising agent.
Use: TCA overdose with ECG Δs; cardiac arrest* (only if due to ↑K⁺ or TCAs), rarely for severe metabolic acidosis due to xs bicarbonate loss.
SE: paradoxical intracellular acidosis, negative inotrope,↓s O₂ delivery (O₂ saturation curve shift to left), ↓K⁺, ↑Na⁺, ↑serum osmolality.
Dose: iv: available in 1.26%, 4.2% and 8.4% solutions; in cardiac arrest* give 50 mmol (50 ml of 8.4% solution) repeating if necessary. **NB:** *specialist use only* – strongly consider getting senior help before giving.

☠ Inflammatory if extravasates when given iv (⇒ tissue necrosis) ☠.

SODIUM VALPROATE see Valproate; antiepileptic.

SOTALOL
β-Blocker (non-selective); class II (+III) antiarrhythmic.
Use: Px of SVT (esp of paroxysmal AF), Rx of VT (if life-threatening/symptomatic, esp non-sustained or spontaneous sustained dt IHD or cardiomyopathy).
CI: as propranolol, plus ↑QT syndromes, torsades de pointes, **R** (if severe, otherwise caution).

Caution: as propranolol, plus electrolyte Δs ($\Rightarrow$ $\uparrow$risk of arrhythmias, esp if $\downarrow K^+$/$\downarrow Mg^{2+}$; $\therefore$ beware if severe diarrhoea).

SE: as propranolol, plus arrhythmias (can $\Rightarrow$ $\uparrow QT$ $\pm$ **torsades de pointes***, esp in females).

Interactions: as propranolol (NB: ☠ *Verapamil and diltiazem* $\Rightarrow$*risk of $\downarrow$HR and HB* ☠) plus disopyramide, quinidine, procainamide, amiodarone, moxifloxacin, mizolastine, dolasetron, ivabradine, TCAs and antipsychotics $\Rightarrow$ $\uparrow$**risk arrhythmias***.

Dose: 40–160 mg bd po ($\uparrow$if life-threatening to max 640 mg/day); 20–120 mg iv over 10 min (repeat 6-hrly if necessary). **NB:** $\downarrow$**dose if RF.**

Give under specialist supervision and with ECG monitoring.

SPIRIVA see Tiotropium; new inhaled muscarinic antagonist.
▼ Respimat (non HandiHaler).

SPIRONOLACTONE

K^+-sparing diuretic: aldosterone antagonist at distal tubule (also potentiates loop and thiazide diuretics).

Use: ascites (esp 2° to cirrhosis or malignancy), oedema, HF (adjunct to ACE-i and/or another diuretic), nephrotic syndrome, 1° aldosteronism.

CI: $\uparrow K^+$, $\downarrow Na^+$, Addison's, **P/B.**

Caution: porphyria, **L/R/E.**

SE: $\uparrow K^+$, **gynaecomastia**, GI upset (inc N&V), impotence, $\downarrow$BP,$\uparrow Na^+$, rash, confusion, headache, hepatotoxicity, blood disorders.

Monitor: U&E.

Interactions: $\uparrow$s digoxin and lithium levels. $\uparrow$s risk of RF with NSAIDs (which also antagonise its diuretic fx).

Dose: 100–400 mg/day po (25 mg od if for HF).

☠ Beware if on other drugs that $\uparrow K^+$, e.g. amiloride, triamterene, ACE-i, angiotensin II antagonists and ciclosporin. Do not give with oral K^+ supplements inc dietary salt substitutes ☠.

STEMETIL see Prochlorperazine; DA antagonist antiemetic.

STREPTOKINASE

Thrombolytic agent: ↑s plasminogen conversion to plasmin ⇒↑fibrin breakdown.

Use: AMI, TE of arteries (inc PE, central retinal artery) or veins (DVT, central retinal vein).

CI/Caution/SE: see p. 230.

Dose: AMI: 1.5 million units ivi over 60 min; **other indications:** 250,000 units ivi over 30 min, then 100,000 units ivi every hour for up to 12–72 h (see SPC).

STREPTOMYCIN

Aminoglycoside antibiotic.

Use: TB (if isoniazid resistance established before Rx); see p. 267.

CI/Caution/SE/Interactions: see Gentamicin.

STRONTIUM RANELATE/PROTELOS

↑s bone formation and ↓s bone resorption.

Use: postmenopausal osteoporosis[NICE] if bisphosphonates CI/not tolerated & aged >75 with previous fracture.

CI: VTE (inc Hx of), temporary or prolonged immobilisation, phenylketonuria (contains aspartame), **P/B.**

Caution: ↑risk of VTE, Δs urinary and plasma Ca^{2+} measurements. **R** (avoid if severe).

SE: severe allergic reactions* GI upset.

Warn: to report any skin rash* and immediately stop drug.

Interactions: absorption ↓ by concomitant ingestion of Ca^{2+} (e.g. milk) and Mg^{2+}. ↓s absorption of quinolones and tetracycline.

Dose: 2 g (1 sachet in water) po od at bedtime[SPC/BNF]. *Avoid food/milk 2 h before and after taking.*

☠ **Rash* can be early DRESS syndrome: D**rug **R**ash, **E**osinophilia and **S**ystemic **S**ymptoms (e.g. fever); lymphadenopathy and ↑WCC also seen early. Can⇒ LF, RF or respiratory failure ± death ☠.

SULFASALAZINE

Aminosalicylate: combination of the immune modulator 5-aminosalicylic acid (5-ASA) and the antibacterial sulfapyridine (a sulphonamide).

Use: rheumatoid arthritis[1]. Also UC[2] (inc maintenance of remission) and active Crohn's disease[2], but not 1st-line, as newer drugs (e.g. mesalazine) have ↓sulphonamide SEs; still used if well-controlled with this drug and with no SEs or if joint manifestations.
CI: sulphonamide or salicylate hypersensitivity, **R** (caution if mild).
Caution: slow acetylators, Hx of any allergy, porphyria, G6PD deficiency, **L/P** (give only under specialist care)/**B**.
SE: GI upset (esp ↓appetite/Wt), **hepatotoxicity**, **blood disorders**, **hypersensitivity** (inc severe skin reactions like Stevens–Johnson syndrome), seizures, lupus.
Monitor: LFTs, U&Es, FBC.
Warn: to report signs of blood disorders
Dose: 500 mg/day ↑ing to max 3 g/day[1]; 1–2 g qds po for acute attacks[2], ↓ing to maintenance of 500 mg qds – can also give 0.5–1.0 g pr bd after motion (as supps) ± po Rx.

SUMATRIPTAN/IMIGRAN

$5HT_{1B/1D}$ agonist.
Use: migraine (acute). Also cluster headache (sc route & unlicenced use intranasally).
CI: IHD, coronary vasospasm (inc Prinzmetal's), PVD, HTN (moderate, severe or uncontrolled). Hx of MI, CVA or TIA.
Caution: predisposition to IHD (e.g. cardiac disease), **L/H/P/B/E**.
SE: sensory Δs (tingling, heat, pressure/tightness), dizziness, flushing, fatigue, N&V, seizures, visual Δs and drowsiness.
Interactions: ↑risk of CNS toxicity with SSRIs, MAOIs, moclobemide and St John's wort. ↑risk of vasospasm with ergotamine and methysergide.
Dose: 50 mg po (can repeat after ≥2 h if responded then recurs and can ↑doses, **if no LF**, to 100 mg if required). Max 300 mg/24 h. Available sc or intranasally[BNF/SPC].

NB: frequent use may ⇒ medication overuse headache.

SUXAMETHONIUM

Depolarising neuromuscular blocker. Nicotinic ACh antagonist at neuromuscular junction.

Use: Muscle relaxation in general anaesthesia (short duration)

CI: anaesthetist not confident of airway maintenance, FHx of malignant hyperthermia, ↑K^+, major trauma, severe burns, neurological disease with acute major muscle wasting, prolonged immobilisation (↑K^+ risk), Hx or FHx congenital myotonic disease, Duchenne muscular dystrophy, ↓ plasma-cholinesterase activity (inc severe LF), conscious patient.

Caution: action irreversible (cf non-depolarising agents- see page 185), recovery is spontaneous (assisted ventilation must continue until muscle function restored), MG and Eaton-Lambert syndrome (resistant to action), cardiac / respiratory / neuromuscular disease, ↑IOP, severe sepsis (↑K^+ risk). **L/P/B** (resume once mother recovered from neuromuscular block)

SE: ↑ gastric pressure, ↑K^+, post-op muscle pain, myoglobinuria, myoglobinaemia, ↑IOP, flushing, rash, arrhythmias, cardiac arrest, bronchospasm, apnoea, prolonged respiratory depression. Painful fasciculations prior to neuromuscular block ∴ give after induction.

Monitor: cardiac and respiratory function.

Interactions: anticholinesterases (e.g. neostigmine) ↑ neuromuscular block. fx ↑ by aminoglycosides, clindamycin, vancymicin & polymixins. Myocardial depression and ↓HR risk with propofol. Can't be mixed with any other agent in same syringe.

Dose: IV: 1-1.5mg/kg; IM: up to 2.5mg/kg (max 150mg)

☠ Specialist use only; requires respiration assistance / control until drug inactivated or antagonised and anaesthetic / sedative to prevent awareness. ☠

SYMBICORT Combination asthma inhaler: each puff contains *x* microgram budesonide (steroid) + *y* microgram formoterol (long-acting β_2 agonist) in the following '*x/y*' strengths; '100/6', '200/6' and '400/12'.

SYNACTHEN SYNthetic ACTH (adreno cortico trophic hormone), also called tetracosactide.

Use: Dx of Addison's disease: in 'short' syncathen test will find ↓plasma cortisol 0, 30 and 60 min after 250 microgram iv/im dose.
CI: allergic disorders (esp asthma). NB: can ⇒ anaphylaxis.

TACROLIMUS (= FK 506)

Immunosuppressant (calcineurin inhibitor): ↓s IL-2-mediated LØ proliferation.
Use: Px of transplant rejection (esp renal). Also used topically as 0.1% or 0.03% ointment in moderate-severe atopic eczema unresponsive to conventional therapy (specialist use).
CI: macrolide hypersensitivity, immunodeficiency, **P** (exclude before starting), **B**.
Caution/SE: as ciclosporin, but ⇒ ↑neuro-/nephro-toxicity (although ⇒ ↓hypertrichosis/hirsutism); also **diabetogenic** and rarely ⇒cardiomyopathy (monitor ECG for hypertrophic Δs).
Interactions: metab by **P450** ∴ many, but most importantly: ↑s levels of 💀 ciclosporin 💀. Levels ↑ by clari-/ery-/teli-thromycin, quinu-/dalfo-pristin, chloramphenicol, antifungals, ataza-/rito-/nelfi-/saqui-navir, nifedipine, diltiazem and grapefruit juice. Levels ↓ by rifampicin, phenobarbital, phenytoin and St John's wort. Nephrotoxicity↑ by NSAIDs, aminoglycosides and amphotericin. Avoid with other drugs that ↑K+.
Dose: specialist use^SPC/BNF. **NB: may require ↓dose if LF**.

> 💀 Interactions important: ↑levels ⇒ toxicity; ↓levels may ⇒ rejection.
> Available in immediate release & modified release preparations with
> different dosing; Adoport, Capexion, Modigraf, Prograf, Tacni &
> Vivadex (bd) and Advagraf (MR od preparation) ∴ mustn't confuse 💀.

TADALAFIL/CIALIS/ADCIRCA (▼)

Phosphodiesterase type-5 inhibitor; see Sildenafil.
CI/Use/Caution/SE/Interactions: as sildenafil plus CI in moderate HF and uncontrolled HTN/arrhythmias.
Dose (*for erectile dysfunction*): initially 10 mg ≥30 min before sexual activity, adjusting to response (1 dose per 24 h, max 20 mg per dose, unless RF or LF when max 10 mg).

TAMOXIFEN

Oestrogen receptor antagonist.

Use: oestrogen receptor-positive Ca breast[1] (as adjuvant Rx: ⇒ ↑survival, delays metastasis), anovulatory infertility[2].

CI: P ** (exclude pregnancy before starting Rx).

Caution: ↑risk of TE* (if taking cytotoxics), porphyria, **B**.

SE: hot flushes, GI upset, menstrual/endometrial Δs (☠ inc Ca: if Δ vaginal bleeding/discharge or pelvic pain/pressure ⇒ urgent Ix ☠). Also fluid retention, exac of bony metastases pain. Many other gynaecological/blood/skin/metabolic Δs (esp lipids, LFTs).

Warn: of symptoms of endometrial cancer and TE* (and to report calf pain/sudden SOB). If appropriate, advise non-hormonal contraception**.

Interactions: W +.

Dose: 20 mg od po[1]; for anovulatory infertility[2] see SPC/BNF.

TAMSULOSIN/FLOMAXTRA XL

α-Blocker ⇒ internal urethral sphincter relaxation (∴⇒ ↑bladder outflow) and systemic vasodilation.

Use: BPH.

CI/Caution/SE/Interactions: as doxazosin plus **L** (if severe).

Dose: 400 microgram mane (after food).

TAZOCIN Combination of piperacillin (antipseudomonal penicillin) + tazobactam (β-lactamase inhibitor).

Use: severe infections/sepsis (mostly in ITU setting or if resistant to other antibiotics).

CI/Caution/SE/Interactions: as benzylpenicillin.

Dose: 2.25–4.5 g tds/qds iv. NB: ↓to **bd/tds** if RF.

TEGRETOL see Carbamazepine; antiepileptic.

TEICOPLANIN

Glycopeptide antibiotic.

Use: serious Gram-positive infections (mostly reserved for MRSA).

Caution: vancomycin sensitivity, **R/P/B/E**.

SE: GI upset, hypersensitivity/skin reactions, blood disorders, nephrotoxicity, ototoxicity (but less than vancomycin), ΔLFTs, local reactions at injection site.

Monitor: U&Es, LFTs, FBC, auditory function (esp if chronic Rx or on other oto-/nephro-toxic drugs, e.g. gentamicin, amphotericin B, ciclosporin, cisplatin and furosemide). Drug levels may be monitored in some situations – consult local guidelines/experts.

Dose: if weight < 70 kg, initially 400 mg iv/ivi every 12 hrs for 3 doses, then 400 mg od (subsequent doses can be given im). If weight >70 kg, initially 6 mg/kg iv/ivi every 12 hrs for 3 doses, then 6 mg/kg od. **NB: ↑dose if sepsis, septic arthritis, osteomyelitis, severe burns or endocarditis and ↓dose if RF; see SPC/BNF.**

▼ TELMISARTAN/MICARDIS

Angiotensin II antagonist; see Losartan.

Use: HTN; *for advice on stepped HTN Mx see p. 235.*

CI: biliary obstruction, **L** (if severe, otherwise caution), **P/B.**

Caution/SE/Interactions: as Losartan, plus ↑s digoxin levels.

Dose: 20–80 mg od (usually 40 mg od). **NB: ↓dose if LF or RF.**

TEMAZEPAM

Benzodiazepine, short-acting.

Use: insomnia.

CI/Caution/SE/Interactions: see Diazepam.

Dose: 10 mg nocte (can ↑dose if tolerant to benzodiazepines, but beware respiratory depression). *Dependency common:* max 4-wk Rx. **NB: ↓dose if LF, severe RF or elderly.**

TENECTEPLASE (= TNK-tPA)/METALYSE

Recombinant thrombolytic; advantageous as given as single bolus.

Use: Acute myocardial infarction (i.e. not approved for CVA/ other use).

CI/Caution/SE: see p. 231, plus **B.**

Dose: iv bolus over 10 sec according to weight: ≥90 kg, 50 mg; 80–89 kg, 45 mg; 70–79 kg, 40 mg; 60–69 kg, 35 mg; <60 kg, 30 mg.

Concurrent unfractionated iv heparin or enoxaparin is needed for 24–48 h; see p. 209.

TERAZOSIN/HYTRIN

α-Blocker ⇒ internal urethral sphincter relaxation (∴⇒ ↑bladder outflow) and systemic vasodilation.

Use: BPH[1] (and rarely HTN[2]).

Caution: Hx of micturition syncope or postural ↓BP, **P/B/E**.

SE/Interactions: see Doxazosin. '1st-dose collapse' common.

Dose: initially 1 mg nocte, ↑ing as necessary to max 10 mg/day[1] (or 20 mg/day[2]).

TERBINAFINE/LAMISIL

Antifungal: oral[1,2] or topical cream[3].

Use: ringworm[1] (*Tinea* spp) dermatophyte nail infections[2], fungal skin infections[3]. NB: ineffective in yeast infections.

Caution: psoriasis (may worsen), autoimmune disease (risk of lupus-like syndrome), **L/R** (neither apply if giving topically), **P/B**.

SE: headache, GI upset, mild rash, joint/muscle pains. Rarely neuro-Ψ disturbances, blood disorders, hepatic dysfunction, serious skin reactions (stop drug if progressive rash).

Dose: 250 mg od po for 2–6 wks[1] or 6 wks–3 months[2]; 1–2 topical applications/day for 1–2 wks[3].

TERBUTALINE/BRICANYL

Inhaled β[2] agonist similar to salbutamol.

Dose: 500 microgram od–qds inh (powder or aerosol); 5–10 mg up to qds neb. Can also give po/sc/im/iv[SPC/BNF].

TETRACYCLINE

Tetracycline broad-spectrum antibiotic: inhibits ribosomal (30S subunit) protein synthesis.

Use: acne vulgaris[1] (or rosacea), genital/tropical infections (NB: doxycycline often preferred).

CI: age <12 years (**stains/deforms teeth**), acute porphyria, **R/P/B**.

Caution: may worsen MG or SLE, **L**.

SE: GI upset (rarely AAC), oesophageal irritation, headache, dysphagia. Rarely hepatotoxicity, blood disorders, photosensitivity, hypersensitivity, visual Δs (rarely 2° to BIH; stop drug if suspected).

Interactions: ↓absorption with milk (do not drink 1 h before or 2 h after drug), antacids and Fe/Al/Ca/Mg/Zn salts. ↓s fx of OCP (small risk). ↑risk of BIH with retinoids. Mild **W +**.

Dose: 500 mg bd po[1], otherwise 250–500 mg tds/qds po. **NB: max 1 g/24 h in LF.**

NB: swallow tablets whole with plenty of fluid while sitting or standing and take >30 min before food.

THEOPHYLLINE

Methylxanthine bronchodilator. *Theories of action*: (1) ↑s intracellular cAMP; (2) adenosine antagonist; (3) ↓s diaphragm fatigue. NB: additive fx with β_2 agonists (but with ↑risk of SEs, esp ↓K^+).

Use: severe asthma/COPD: acute (iv as aminophylline; see p. 243) or chronic (po).

CI: hypersensitivity to any 'xanthine' (e.g. aminophylline/ theophylline), acute porphyria.

Caution: cardiac disease (risk of arrhythmias*), epilepsy, ↑T_4, PU, HTN, fever, porphyria, acute febrile illness, **L/P/B/E**.

SE: (tachy)**arrhythmias***, seizures (esp if given rapidly iv), **GI upset** (esp **nausea**), CNS stimulation (restlessness, insomnia), headache, ↓K^+.

Monitor: K^+, serum levels (4–6 h post dose) as narrow therapeutic window (10–20 mg/l = 55–110 micromol/l) but toxic fx can occur even in this range.

Interactions: metab by **P450** ($\Rightarrow$ very variable $t_{1/2}$): **levels ↑d in** HF/LF*/viral infections/elderly, and if taking **fluvoxamine/ cimetidine/ciprofloxacin/norfloxacin/macrolides (ery-/clari-thromycin)/propranolol/'flu vaccines/fluconazole/ketoconazole/ OCP/Ca^{2+} channel blockers. Levels ↓d in** smokers/chronic alcohol abuse, and if taking phenytoin/carbamazepine/phenobarbital/ rifampicin/ritonavir/St John's wort. ↑risk of convulsions with quinolones.

Dose: MR preparations preferred (↓SEs) and doses vary with brand[SPC/BNF]; range 200–500 mg bd. *Available iv as aminophylline.* **NB: ↓dose if LF***. Note: dose adjustment may be necessary if smoking started or stopped during chronic treatment.

THIAMINE (= vitamin B1).

Use: replacement for nutritional deficiencies (esp in alcoholism).

Dose: 100 mg bd/tds po in severe deficiency (25 mg od if mild/chronic).

> For iv preparations, see Pabrinex and p. 272 for Mx of acute alcohol withdrawal.

THYROXINE (= LEVOTHYROXINE).

Synthetic T_4 (NB: thyroxine often now called 'levothyroxine').

Use: $\downarrow T_4$ Rx (for maintenance); **NB:** acutely, e.g. myxoedema coma, liothyronine (T_3) often needed – see p. 257.

CI: $\uparrow T_4$.

Caution: panhypopituitarism/other predisposition to adrenal insufficiency (*corticosteroids needed 1st*), chronic $\downarrow T_4$, cardiovascular disorders (esp HTN/IHD; can worsen)*, DI, DM**, **P/B/E**.

SE: features of $\uparrow T_4$ (should be minimal unless xs Rx): D&V, tremors, restlessness, headache, flushing, sweating, heat intolerance, angina, arrhythmias, palpitations, $\uparrow$HR, muscle cramps/weakness, $\downarrow$Wt. Also osteoporosis (esp if xs dose given; use min dose necessary).

Interactions: can Δ digoxin and antidiabetic** requirements, $\uparrow$fx of TCAs and $\downarrow$levels of propranolol. **W +**.

Monitor: baseline ECG to help distinguish Δs due to ischaemia or $\downarrow T_4$.

Dose: 25–200 microgram mane (titrate up slowly, esp if >50 yrs old/$\downarrow\downarrow T_4$/HTN/IHD*).

TIMOLOL EYE DROPS/TIMOPTOL

β-Blocker eye drops; $\downarrow$aqueous humour production.

Use: glaucoma (2nd line), ocular HTN (1st line); not useful if on systemic β-blocker.

CI: asthma, $\downarrow$HR, HB, **H** (if uncontrolled).

Caution/SE/Interactions: as propranolol* plus can ⇒ local irritation.

Dose: 1 drop bd (0.25% or 0.5%). Also available in long-acting od preparations TIMOPTOL LA (0.25 and 0.5%) and NYOGEL /

TIOPEX (0.1%). Timolol 0.5% also available in combination with other classes of glaucoma medications; carbonic anhydrase inhibitors (dorzolamide Cosopt, brinzolamide ▼ Azarga), PG analogues (latanoprost Xalacom, travoprost Duotrav, bimatoprost Ganfort) α-agonists (brimonidine Combigan).

☠ Systemic absorption possible despite topical application* ☠.

TINZAPARIN/INNOHEP

Low-molecular-weight heparin (LMWH).

Use: DVT/PE Rx[1] and Px[2] (inc pre-operative). Not licensed for MI/unstable angina (unlike other LMWHs).

CI/Caution/SE/Monitor/Interactions: as heparin, plus CI if breast feeding (**B**) and caution in asthma (⇒ ↑hypersensitivity reactions).

Dose: (all sc) 175 units/kg od[1]; 50 units/kg or 4500 units od[2] (3500 units od if low risk).

Consider monitoring anti-Xa (3–4 h post dose) ± dose adjustment if RF (i.e. creatinine >150), severe LF, pregnancy, Wt >100 kg or <45 kg; see p. 209.

TIOTROPIUM/SPIRIVA

Long-acting inh muscarinic antagonist for COPD/(unlicenced for asthma) similar to ipratropium, but only for chronic use and caution in RF.

SE: dry mouth, urinary retention, glaucoma.

Dose: 18 microgram dry powder inhaler or 5 microgram by soft mist inhaler (▼ Respimat) od inh.

TIROFIBAN/AGGRASTAT

Antiplatelet agent: glycoprotein IIb/IIIa receptor inhibitor – stops binding of fibrinogen and inhibits platelet aggregation.

Use: Px of MI in unstable angina/NSTEMI (*if last episode of chest pain w/in 12 h*), esp if high risk and awaiting PCI[NICE] (see p. 233).

CI: abnormal bleeding or CVA w/in 30 days, haemorrhagic diathesis, Hx of haemorrhagic CVA, intracranial disease (neoplasm/aneurysm/AVM), severe HTN, ↓Pt, ↑INR/PT, **B**.

Caution: ↑risk of bleeding (e.g. drugs, recent bleeding/trauma/procedures; see^{SPC/BNF}), **L** (avoid if severe), **H** (if severe), **R/P**.
SE: bleeding, nausea, fever, ↓Pt (reversible).
Monitor: FBC (baseline, 2–6 h after giving, then at least daily).
Dose: 400 *nanograms*/kg/min for 30 min, then 100 *nanograms*/kg/min for ≥48 h (continue for 12–24 h post-PCI), for max of 108 h. Needs concurrent heparin. **NB: ↓dose if RF**.

Specialist use only: get senior advice or contact on-call cardiology.

TOLBUTAMIDE
Oral antidiabetic (short-acting sulphonylurea).
Use/CI/Caution/SE/Interactions: as gliclazide. Can also ⇒ headache and tinnitus. fx ↑ by azapropazone.
Dose: 0.5–2.0 g daily in divided doses, with food. **NB: ↓dose if RF or LF**.

TOLTERODINE/DETRUSITOL
Antimuscarinic, antispasmodic.
Use: detrusor instability; urinary incontinence/frequency/urgency.
CI/Caution/SE: as oxybutynin (SEs mostly antimuscarinic fx; see p. 276) plus caution if Hx of, or taking drugs that, ↑QTc, **P/B**.
Interactions: ↑risk of ventricular arrhythmias with amiodarone, disopyramide, flecainide and sotalol.
Dose: 1–2 mg bd po. **NB: ↓dose if RF or LF**. (MR preparation available as 4 mg od po; not suitable if RF or LF.)

tPA (= tissue-type plasminogen activator) see Alteplase.

TRAMADOL
Opioid. Also ↓s pain by ↑ing 5HT/noradrenergic transmission.
Use: moderate/severe pain (esp musculoskeletal).
CI/Caution: as codeine, but also CI in uncontrolled epilepsy, **P/B**. Not suitable as substitute in opioid-dependent patients.
SE: as morphine, but ↓respiratory depression, ↓constipation, ↓addiction. ↑confusion (esp in elderly) compared to codeine.
Interactions: as codeine; also ↑risk convulsions with SSRIs/TCAs/antipsychotics, ↑risk serotonin syndrome with SSRIs. Carbamazepine and ondansetron ↓ its fx. **W +**.

L/R/H = Liver, Renal and Heart failure (full key see p. xv)

Dose: 50–100 mg up to 4-hrly po/im/iv, max 400 mg/day. Post-op: initially 100 mg im/iv, then 50 mg every 10–20 min prn (max total dose of 250 mg in 1st hr), then 50–100 mg 4–6-hrly (max 600 mg/ day). **NB: ↓dose if RF, LF or elderly.**

TRANDOLAPRIL/GOPTEN

ACE-i for HTN (*for advice on stepped HTN Mx see p. 235*), HF and LVF post-MI.

CI/Caution/SE/Monitor/Interactions: see Captopril.

Dose: initially 0.5 mg od, ↑ing at intervals of 2–4 wks if required to max 4 mg od (max 2 mg if RF). ↓doses if given with diuretic. If for LVF post-MI, start ≥3 days after MI.

TRANEXAMIC ACID

Antifibrinolytic: inhibits activation of plasminogen to plasmin.

Use: bleeding: acute bleeds[1] (esp 2° to anticoagulants, thrombolytic/ anti-Pt agents, epistaxis, haemophilia), menorrhagia[2], hereditary angioedema[3].

CI: TE disease, Hx of convulsions, **R** (if severe, otherwise caution).

Caution: gross haematuria (can clot and obstruct ureters), DIC, **P**.

SE: GI upset, colour vision Δs (stop drug), TE.

Dose: 15–25 mg/kg bd/tds po (if severe, 0.5–1 g tds iv)[1]; 1 g tds po for 4 days (max 4 g/day)[2]; 1–1.5 g bd/tds po[3]. **NB: ↓dose if RF.**

TRAVOPROST EYE DROPS/TRAVATAN

Topical PG analogue for glaucoma; see Latanoprost.

Use/CI/Caution/SE: see Latanoprost.

Dose: 1 drop od, preferably in the evening.

TRIAMTERENE

K$^+$-sparing diuretic (weak); see Amiloride.

Use/CI/Caution/SE: as amiloride, but ⇒ less ↓BP ∴ not used for HTN (unless used with other drugs), plus **L** (avoid if severe).

Warn: urine may go blue.

Interactions: ↑s lithium and phenobarbital levels. NSAIDs ↑risk of RF and ↑K$^+$.

Dose: almost exclusively used with stronger K$^+$-wasting diuretics in combination preparations (e.g. co-triamterzide). For use alone, initially give 150–250 mg daily, ↓ing to alternate days after 1wk.

> ☠ Beware if on other drugs that ↑K$^+$, e.g. amiloride, spironolactone, ACE-i, angiotensin II antagonists and ciclosporin. Do not give with oral K$^+$ tablets or dietary salt substitutes ☠.

TRI-IODOTHYRONINE
See Liothyronine; synthetic T$_3$ mostly used in myxoedema coma.

TRIMETHOPRIM
Antifolate antibiotic: inhibits dihydrofolate reductase.
Use: UTIs (rarely other infections).
CI: blood disorders (esp megaloblastic ↓Hb).
Caution: ↓folate (or predisposition to), porphyria, R/P/B/E.
SE: see Co-trimoxazole (Septrin), but much less frequent and severe (esp BM suppression, skin reactions). Also **GI upset**, rash, rarely other hypersensitivity.
Warn: those on long-term Rx to look for signs of blood disorder and to report fever, sore throat, rash, mouth ulcers, bruising or bleeding.
Interactions: ↑s phenytoin levels. ↑s risk of arrhythmias with amiodarone, antifolate fx with pyrimethamine and toxicity with ciclosporin, azathioprine, mercaptopurine and methotrexate. **W +**.
Dose: 200 mg bd po (100 mg nocte for chronic infections or as Px if at risk; NB: risk of ↓folate if long-term Rx). **NB: ↓dose if RF**.

TROPICAMIDE EYE DROPS
Antimuscarinic: mydriatic (lasts approx 4 hrs), weak cycloplegic.
Use: dilated retinal examination. See also 'Dilating eye drops'.
CI: untreated acute angle closure glaucoma.
Caution: ↑IOP* (inc predisposition to), inflamed eye (↑risk of systemic absorption).
SE: transient stinging & blurred vision & ↓accommodation. Rarely precipitation of acute angle closure glaucoma (↑risk if >60 yrs, long sighted, family history).

Warn: unable to drive until can read car number plate at 20 metres (approx 4 hrs).
Dose: 1 drop 1.0% solution 15–20 min before examination. 0.5% in children <1 yr old. NB: Rare cause of acute angle closure glaucoma* (esp if >60 yrs or hypermetropic).

TURBOHALER Inh delivery device for asthma drugs.

(SODIUM) VALPROATE

Antiepileptic and mood stabiliser: potentiates and ↑s GABA levels.
Use: epilepsy[1], mania (and off-licence for other Ψ disorders).
CI: acute porphyria, personal or family Hx of severe liver dysfunction, **L** (inc active liver disease).
Caution: SLE, ↑bleeding risk*, **R**, **P** (⇒ neural-tube/craniofacial dfx, Px folate), **B**.
SE: sedation, cerebellar fx (see p. 278; esp tremor, ataxia), headache, GI upset, ↑Wt, SOA, alopecia, skin reactions, ↓cognitive/motor function, Ψ disorders, encephalopathy (2° to ↑ammonia). Rarely but seriously **hepatotoxicity, blood disorders** (esp ↓Pt*), **pancreatitis** (mostly in 1st 6 months of Rx).
Warn: of clinical features of pancreatitis and liver/blood disorders. Inform women of childbearing age of teratogenicity/need for contraception.
Monitor: LFTs, FBC ± serum levels *pre-dose* (therapeutic range 50–100 mg/l; useful for checking compliance but ↓use for efficacy).
Interactions: fx ↓d by antimalarials (esp mefloquine), antidepressants (inc St John's wort), antipsychotics and some antiepileptics[SPC/BNF]. Levels ↑by cimetidine & carbopenems. ↑s fx of aspirin and primidone. ↑risk of ↓NØ with olanzapine. Mild **W** +.
Dose: initially 300 mg bd, ↑ing to max of 2.5 g/day[1]. NB: ↓dose if RF. Can give false-positive urine dipstick for ketones.

▼ VALSARTAN/DIOVAN

Angiotensin II antagonist; see Losartan.
Use: HTN[1] (*for advice on stepped HTN Mx see p. 235*), MI with LV failure/dysfunction[2], heart failure[3].

CI: biliary obstruction, cirrhosis, **L** (if severe)/**P/B**.

Caution/SE/Interactions: see Losartan (inc warning r/e drugs that ↑K[+]).

Dose: initially 80 mg od[1] (**NB: give 40 mg if** ⩾**75 yrs old, LF, RF or** ↓**intravascular volume**) or 20 mg bd[2,3], ↑ing if necessary to max 320 mg od[1]/160 mg bd[2] or 40 mg bd[3].

VANCOMYCIN

Glycopeptide antibiotic. Poor po absorption (unless bowel inflammation*), but still effective against *C. difficile*** as acts 'topically' in GI tract.

Use: serious Gram-positive infections[1] (inc endocarditis Px and systemic MRSA), AAC[2] (give po)**.

Caution: Hx of deafness, IBD* (only if given po), avoid rapid infusions (risk of anaphylaxis), **R/P/B/E**.

SE: nephrotoxicity, ototoxicity (stop if tinnitus develops), **blood disorders, rash, hypersensitivity** (inc anaphylaxis, severe skin reactions), nausea, fever, phlebitis/irritation at injection site.

Monitor: serum levels: keep predose trough levels 10–15 mg/l; start monitoring after 3rd dose (1st dose if RF); NB: higher trough recommended in osteomyelitis, endocarditis. Also monitor U&Es, FBC, urinalysis (and auditory function if elderly/RF).

Interactions: ↑nephrotoxicity with ciclosporin. ↑ototoxicity with loop diuretics. ↑s fx of suxamethonium.

Dose: 1–1.5 g bd ivi at 10 mg/min[1]; 125 mg qds po[2]. **NB:** ↓dose if RF or elderly.

NB: if ivi given too quickly ⇒ ↑risk of anaphylactoid reactions (e.g. ↓BP, respiratory symptoms, skin reactions).

VARDENAFIL/LEVITRA

Phosphodiesterase type-5 inhibitor; see Sildenafil.

Use/CI/Caution/SE/Interactions: as sildenafil plus CI in hereditary degenerative retinal disorders, caution if susceptible to (or taking drugs that) ↑QTc, and levels ↑by grapefruit juice.

L/R/H = Liver, Renal and Heart failure (full key see p. xv)

Dose: initially 10 mg approx 25–60 min before sexual activity, adjusting to response (1 dose per 24 h, max 20 mg per dose). **NB: halve dose if LF, RF, elderly or taking α-blocker.**

VECURONIUM (BROMIDE)

Aminosteriod non-depolarising neuromuscular blocker. Intermediate duration of action (30–40 mins). Competitively inhibits ACh receptor at neuromuscular junction. Reversible with anticholinesterases.
Use: neuromuscular blockade for surgery.
CI: anaesthetist not confident of airway maintenance.
Caution: hypersensitivity to other neuromuscular blockers (allergic cross-reactivity), MG and hypothermia prolong activity (use lower doses), fluid/e'lyte Δ (unpredictable response), burns (resistance can develop), cardiovascular disease (↓rate of administration); obesity (↑duration of action), **L** / **R**.
SE: ↓ or ↑ HR. Rarely acute myopathy*.
Monitor: Cardiac, respiratory and motor function.
Interactions: fx ↑by aminoglycosides, clindamycin & polymyxins. Corticosteroids can ↑ myopathy[1].
Dose: initially 80–100 micrograms/kg iv; then maintenance *either* 20–30 micrograms/kg iv (max. 100 micrograms/kg in caesarian section) *or* 0.8–1.4 micrograms/kg/min ivi, adjusting to response. *NB: if obese (weight 30% above ideal body weight (IBW; see p.296)) use IBW for dose calculation.*

> ☠ Specialist use only; respiration needs assistance / control until drug inactivated or antagonised and anaesthetic / sedative to prevent awareness. ☠

VENLAFAXINE/EFEXOR

Serotonin and Noradrenaline Reuptake Inhibitor (SNRI): antidepressant with ↓sedative/antimuscarinic fx cf TCAs. ↑danger in OD/heart disease than other antidepressants.
Use: depression[1], generalised anxiety disorder.
CI: very high risk of serious cardiac ventricular arrhythmia (e.g. significant LV dysfunction, NYHA class III/IV), uncontrolled HTN, **P.**

Caution: Hx of mania, seizures or glaucoma, **L/R** (avoid if either severe) **H/B**.

SE: GI upset, ↑BP (dose-related; monitor BP if dose >200 mg/day), **withdrawal fx** (see p. 277; common even if dose only a few hours late), **rash** (consider stopping drug, as can be 1st sign of severe reaction*), insomnia/agitation, dry mouth, sexual dysfunction, ↑weight, drowsiness, dizziness, SIADH and ↑QTc.

Warn: report rashes* and can ↓driving/skilled task ability. Don't stop suddenly.

Monitor: BP if heart disease ± ECG.

Interactions: ☠ *Never give with, or ≤2 wks after, MAOIs* ☠. ↑s risk of bleeding with aspirin/NSAIDs and CNS toxicity with selegiline/sibutramine. Avoid artemether/lumefantrine. ↑s levels of clozapine. Mild **W +**.

Dose: 37.5–187.5 mg bd po[1]; start low and ↑dose if required. Efexor XL MR od preparation available (max 225 mg od). *NB: halve dose if moderate LF (PT 14–18 s) or RF (GFR 10–30 ml/min).*

VENTOLIN see Salbutamol; β-agonist bronchodilator.

VERAPAMIL

Ca^{2+} channel blocker (rate-limiting type): fx on heart (⇒ ↓HR, ↓contractility*) > vasculature (dilates peripheral/coronary arteries); i.e. reverse of the dihydropyridine type (e.g. nifedipine). Only Ca^{2+} channel blocker with useful antiarrhythmic properties (class IV).

Use: HTN[1] *(for advice on stepped HTN Mx see p. 235)*, angina[2], narrow complex tachyarrhythmias (SVTs, esp instead of adenosine if asthma)[3].

CI: ↓BP, ↓HR (<50 bpm), 2nd-/3rd-degree HB, ↓LV function, SAN block, SSS, AF or atrial flutter 2° to WPW, acute porphyria. **H** * (inc Hx of).

Caution: AMI, 1st degree HB, **L/P/B**.

SE: constipation (rarely other GI upset), HF, ↓BP (dose-dependent), HB, headache, dizziness, fatigue, ankle oedema, hypersensitivity, skin reactions.

Interactions: ↑risk of AV block and HF with ☠ β-blockers ☠ disopyramide, flecainide, dronedarone and amiodarone. ↑s hypotensive fx of antihypertensives (esp α-blockers) and anaesthetics. ↑s levels/fx of digoxin, theophyllines, carbamazepine, quinidine, ivabradine, dabigatran and ciclosporin. Levels/fx ↓by rifampicin, barbiturates and primidone. ↑risk of myopathy with simvastatin. Sirolimus ↑s levels of both drugs. Levels may be ↑by clari-/ery-thromycin and ritonavir. Risk of VF with ☠ iv dantrolene ☠.

Warn: fx ↑d by grapefruit juice (avoid).

Dose: 80–160 mg tds po[1]; 80–120 mg tds po[2]; 40–120 mg tds po[3]; 5–10 mg iv (over 2 min (3 min in elderly) with ECG monitoring), followed by additional 5 mg iv if necessary after 5–10 min[3]. MR (od/bd) preparations available[BNF]. **NB:** ↓oral dose in LF.

VIAGRA see Sildenafil; phosphodiesterase inhibitor.

VITAMIN K see Phytomenadione.

VOLTAROL see Diclofenac; moderate-strength NSAID.

WARFARIN

Oral anticoagulant: blocks synthesis of vitamin-K-dependent factors (II, VII, IX, X) and proteins C and S.

Use: Rx/Px of TE; see p. 212.

CI: severe HTN, PU, severe bleeding, haemorrhagic CVA, **P**.

Caution: recent surgery, bacterial endocarditis, 48 hrs post-partum, **L/R** (avoid if creatinine clearance <10 ml/min)/**B**.

SE: haemorrhage, rash, fever, diarrhoea. Rarely other GI upset, 'purple-toe syndrome', skin necrosis, hepatotoxicity, hypersensitivity.

Warn: fx are ↑d by alcohol and cranberry juice (avoid).

Dose: see p. 214.

> ☠ NB: **W +** and **W–** denote significant interactions throughout this book: take particular care with antibiotics and drugs that affect cytochrome **P450** (see p. 279) ☠.

XALATAN see ▼ Latanoprost; topical PG analogue for glaucoma.

ZALEPLON

'Non-benzodiazepine' hypnotic; see Zopiclone.

Use/CI/Caution/SE/Interactions: see Zopiclone.
Dose: 10 mg nocte (5 mg if elderly). **NB: halve dose if LF (avoid if severe), severe RF or elderly.**

ZANTAC see Ranitidine; H antagonist.

ZESTRIL see Lisinopril; ACE-i.

ZIDOVUDINE (AZT)

Antiviral (nucleoside analogue): reverse-transcriptase inhibitor.
Use: HIV Rx (and Px, esp of vertical transmission).
CI: severe ↓NØ or ↓Hb (caution if other blood disorders), acute porphyria, **B.**
Caution: ↓B12, ↑risk of lactic acidosis, **L/R/P/E.**
SE: blood disorders (esp ↓Hb or ↓WCC; monitor FBC), **GI upset, headache, fever,** taste Δs, sleep disorders. Rarely hepatic/pancreatic dysfunction, myopathy, seizures, other neurological/Ψ disorders.
Interactions: levels ↑ by fluconazole. fx ↓ by ritonavir. ↑myelosuppression with ganciclovir. ↑risk of ↓Hb with ribavirin. ↓s fx of stavudine and tipranavir.
Dose: see SPC/BNF.

ZIRTEK see Cetirizine; non-sedating antihistamine for allergies.

ZOLEDRONIC ACID/ZOMETA

Bisphosphonate: ↓s osteoclastic bone resorption.
Use: Px of bone damage[1] in advanced bone malignancy, damage or Rx of ↑Ca^{2+} in malignancy[2], Rx of Paget's disease of bone[3], Rx of osteoporosis (postmenopausal or in men)[4].
CI: P/B.
Caution: cardiac disease, dehydration*, ↓Ca^{2+}/PO_4^{2-}/Mg^{2+}. **L** (if severe)/**R/H.**
SE: 'flu-like syndrome, fever, bone pain, fatigue, N&V. Also arthr-/my-algia, ↓Ca^{2+}/PO_4^{2-}/Mg^{2+}, pruritus/rash, headache, conjunctivitis, RF, hypersensitivity, blood disorders (esp ↓Hb) and **osteonecrosis** (esp of jaw; consider dental examination or preventive Rx before starting drug).

Monitor: Ca^{2+}, PO_4^{2-}, Mg^{2+}, U&E. Ensure patient adequately hydrated predose* and advise good dental hygiene.
Dose: 4 mg ivi every 3–4 weeks[1]; 4 mg ivi as single dose[2]. Also available as once yearly preparation (▼ Aclasta) 5 mg ivi over ≥ 15 mins[3,4]. NB: ↓dose in RF.

ZOLMITRIPTAN/ZOMIG

$5HT_{1B/1D}$ agonist for acute migraine.
Use/CI/Caution/SE/Interactions: as sumatriptan plus CI in WPW or arrhythmias assoc with accessory cardiac conduction p'way.
Dose: 2.5 mg po (can repeat after ≥ 2 h if responded then recurs and can ↑doses to 5 mg if required). Max 10 mg/24 h (5 mg/24 h if moderate-severe LF). Available intranasally[BNF/SPC].

ZOLPIDEM

'Non-benzodiazepine' hypnotic; see Zopiclone.
Use/CI/Caution/SE/Interactions: as Zopiclone but CI in psychotic illness, **P.**
Dose: 10 mg nocte. NB: halve dose if LF (avoid if severe), severe RF or elderly.

ZOMORPH Morphine sulphate capsules (10, 30, 60, 100 or 200 mg), equivalent in efficacy to Oramorph but SR: 12-hrly doses.

ZOPICLONE

Short-acting hypnotic (cyclopyrrolone): potentiates GABA pathways via same receptors as benzodiazepines (although isn't a benzodiazepine!): can also ⇒ dependence* and tolerance.
Use: insomnia (not long-term*).
CI: respiratory failure, sleep apnoea (severe), marked neuromuscular respiratory weakness (inc unstable MG), **L** (if severe**), **B.**
Caution: Ψ disorders, Hx of drug abuse*, muscle weakness, MG, **R/P/E.**
SE: *all rare*: GI upset, taste Δs, behavioural/Ψ disturbances (inc psychosis, aggression), hypersensitivity.

Interactions: Levels ↑by ritonavir, erythromycin and other enzyme inhibitors. Levels ↓ by rifampicin. Sedation ↑'d by other sedative medications and alcohol.

Dose: 7.5 mg nocte, ↑ing to 15 mg if necessary. **NB: halve dose if LF (avoid if severe**)**, severe RF or elderly.

ZOTON see Lansoprazole; PPI.

ZYBAN see Bupropion; adjunct to smoking cessation.

Drug selection

Analgesia in the ED	178
Antiemetics in the ED	179
Local anaesthesia	181
Procedural sedation and analgesia	182
Rapid sequence induction	184
Drug infusion guideline	186

ANALGESIA IN THE ED

Patients commonly present with pain to the emergency department (ED). All require prompt treatment whilst the underlying cause(s) are addressed.

Physical and psychological approaches such as splinting, elevation, ice or heat, with reassurance and explanation are as important (and usually much quicker) than relying on pharmacological agents.

When opiate analgesia is indicated for severe acute pain, give this iv titrated to effect.

GENERAL RULES

- Look for/treat the underlying cause(s) and reassess cause at each step.

- All opioids can ⇒ constipation, respiratory depression and ↓GCS (esp if elderly or RF – even low doses). Can also ⇒ coma if LF.

- All NSAIDs can ⇒ PU (related to strength of drug and length of Rx. Consider PPI or changing to COX2 inhibitor^{NICE}) Can also ⇒ AKI if fluid depleted (∴rehydrate 1st or avoid).

Step 4
- Strong opioid:
  iv if acute (e.g. morphine)
  po if chronic (e.g. **oramorph**)

Step 3
- High dose weak opioid e.g.:
  – dihydrocodeine 30 mg qds
  – tramadol 50–100 mg qds (also has 5HT fx: ↓SEs for same analgesia)

Step 2
- Compound prep. of paracetamol with low dose weak opioid (e.g. cocodamol or codydramol) or weak opioid alone (e.g. dihydrocodeine)

Step 1
- **Simple analgesia:** paracetamol 1 g qds usually 1st-line as few SEs.

  NSAIDs 2nd-line; 1st line if predominant inflammatory component, e.g.:
  – ibuprofen 200–400 mg tds po for mild pain.
  – diclofenac (**Voltarol**) 50 mg tds im/po or 75 mg SR bd im/po or 100 mg pr (max 150 mg/day) for moderate pain.
- **Consider specialist analgesia** according to cause, e.g. buscopan for colic, colchicine for gout, antacids for reflux, GTN for angina. For neuropathic pain try amitriptyline, gabapentin or pregabalin.

Figure 2.1 Analgesia ladder. (Stepwise approach based on WHO pain relief ladder for cancer pain.)

- Regular Rx ↓s recurrences *but always review to check whether still needed.*
- If pain ↓s, 'step down' (see Figure 2.1) and ensure adequate prn analgesia in case ↑s again.
- Pain has many adverse medical fx and is rarely refractory unless incorrectly/under-treated.
- Pain out of proportion to that expected may indicate an unrecognised serious underlying cause such as compartment syndrome, vascular compromise, necrotising fasciitis etc.
- If pain persists, get senior or specialist help (e.g. anaesthetist or pain team).

ANTIEMETICS IN THE ED

Commonly used 1st-line/narrow-spectrum antiemetics. See Figure 2.2.

Causes of nausea/vomiting:

- *GI:* surgical (obstruction, peritonism, pancreatitis, biliary colic) and gen medical (oesophagitis, gastritis, PU).
- *Neurological:* migraine, ↑ICP (esp tumour), meningo-encephalitis, Menière's, labyrinthitis.
- *Metabolic:* ↑Ca^{2+} (also ↓Na^+, ↑K^+), DKA, AKI, Addison's.
- *Infection:* gastroenteritis, UTI (often presenting symptom in elderly), respiratory infection (coughing).
- *Drugs:* esp opiates, chemotherapy/cytotoxics, antibiotics (esp erythromycin, metronidazole). Also dopamine agonists, antidepressants (esp fluoxetine), theophyllines, colchicine, $FeSO_4$ and acutely amiodarone/digoxin.
- *Poisoning:* paracetamol; aspirin; agents above
- *Other:* pregnancy, MI (esp inferior, often with atypical pain if DM/elderly).

General rules

- Look for/treat reversible causes (see p. 179).
- Reassess causes at each step.
- Start iv/im/sc switching to po when able.
- Don't stop Rx unless cause removed.

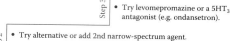
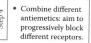

Step 4
- Combine different antiemetics: aim to progressively block different receptors.

Step 3
- Try levomepromazine or a 5HT$_3$ antagonist (e.g. ondansetron).

Step 2
- Try alternative or add 2nd narrow-spectrum agent.
- Consider dexamethasone if cause is brain tumour (or other cause of ICP) or chemotherapy.

Step 1
- Start narrow-spectrum (1st line) drug: choose most appropriate agent from the table below.

Figure 2.2 Antiemetic ladder – (designed for cancer patients;) step 4 is rarely needed in the ED.

Class	Example	Good for	Beware
Butyrophenone (D$_2$ antagonist)	**Haloperidol** 0.5–1.5 mg sc/po	Opiates, general anaesthetic, postoperative, chemo-/radio-therapy (if mild), 1st choice in LF	⇒ ↑ prolactin, extrapyramidal fx, ↓s seizure threshold, ↓BP
Phenothiazine (D$_2$ antagonist)	**Levomepromazine** 6.25–25 mg od or bd po/sc/iv	Broad spectrum: useful when cause unclear/ multifactorial	⇒ sedation, ↓BP ↓s seizure threshold
Benzamine (D$_2$ antagonist)	**Metoclopramide** 10 mg tds po/sc/ im/iv (Maxolon)	(GI causes ↑s GI motility[a]), migraine, drugs (esp opiates)	⇒ ↑ prolactin, extrapyramidal fx, 🚫 CI if GI obstruction 🚫 [a]

Benzamine (D_2 antagonist)	**Domperidone** 10–20 mg tds po or 30–60 mg bd pr *(not iv or im)*	Parkinson's disease[b], morning-after pill, chemotherapy	$\Rightarrow \uparrow$ prolactin, but minimal sedation and extrapyramidal fx[b], QT-prologation
Antihistamines	**Cyclizine** 50 mg tds po/sc/im/iv	GI obstruction[a]/ postoperative N&V, vestibular/ labyrinthine disorders. Antiemetic of choice in LF	$\Rightarrow$ Antimuscarinic fx (esp sedation). Avoid in IHD($\downarrow$s beneficial cardiodynamic fx of opiates)
$5HT_3$ antagonists	**Ondansetron** 4–8 mg bd po/ im/iv (16 mg od pr) **Granisetron Tropisetron**	Severe/resistant cases (esp chemo-/radio-therapy)	Minimal side effects: headache, constipation, dizziness

[a] Prokinetic fx of metoclopramide by anticholinergic drugs (see p. 276), esp cyclizine if also used in this setting.

[b] Extrapyramidal fx possible with all D2 antagonists (see p. 278) but less so with domperidone.

LOCAL ANAESTHESIA

Used for wound exploration and repair; painful procedures such as chest drain placement, LP and large cannula insertion or ABG puncture; local blocks such as ring block or femoral nerve block, and regional blocks such as Bier's.

SAFE USAGE
- Exclude allergy (ask), local infection (look), bleeding disorder (if nerve block planned).
- Know maximum safe doses (see Table 2.1).

Table 2.1 Maximum recommended safe dose and duration of action of common local anaesthetics

Drug	Dose (mg/kg)[a]	Duration (hr)
Lignocaine	3	0.5–1
Lignocaine with adrenaline	7	2–5
Bupivacaine	2	2–4
Prilocaine	6	0.5–1.5

[a] A 1% solution contains 10 mg/mL

- Lay patient down and aspirate for blood prior to local anaesthetic infiltration (avoids inadvertent systemic delivery).
- Recognise features of systemic toxicity and call for senior help (see Table 2.2).

PROCEDURAL SEDATION AND ANALGESIA

Must *only* be performed when two doctors are available, in a suitable monitored resuscitation area, on a carefully selected patient, with experienced (ideally credentialed) staff and full documentation including informed consent.

GENERAL PRINCIPLES

- Consider for brief painful procedure such as fracture manipulation, dislocation reduction, cardioversion or abscess drainage.
- Patients should ideally be fasted, haemodynamically stable, and without pre-existing cardiorespiratory impairment.
- Capnography is recommended as well as pulse oximetry (essential).
- Agent(s) chosen are given at minimum dose to achieve adequate sedation and analgesia for the particular procedure (see Table 2.3).
- Make certain patient is fully recovered after a period of observation before discharging home. Certain criteria must be fulfilled before they are ready to go (see Table 2.4).

Table 2.2 Features of systemic local anaesthetic toxicity (in order of increasing plasma levels)

Circumoral tingling

Dizziness

Tinnitus

Visual disturbance

Muscular twitching

Confusion

Convulsions

Coma

Apnoea

Cardiovascular collapse (highest plasma levels)

Table 2.3 IV procedural sedation drug doses for 70 kg adult. Reduce doses in the elderly, or with small muscle bulk

Drug	Initial IV bolus	Subsequent titrated IV boluses	Maximum cumulative dose
Morphine	2.5 mg	2.5 mg	10–15 mg
Fentanyl	25–50 microgram	25 microgram	150–200 microgram
Midazolam	2 mg	1 mg	10 mg
Diazepam	5 mg	2.5 mg	10 mg
Propofol	40–50 mg	20 mg	150 mg
Ketamine	20–30 mg	10–20 mg	120 mg
Etomidate	5–7 mg	2 mg	20 mg

Table 2.4 Criteria for discharge following procedural sedation in adults

Alert and oriented, or has returned to pre-procedure state

Ambulates safely, or has returned to pre-procedure state

Comfortable and has discharge analgesia arranged

Discharged into care of a responsible adult

No driving or similar for a minimum of 8 hours

Avoid alcohol or other CNS depressants for 12–24 hours

Warn about the potential for post-procedure pain, unsteadiness or dizziness. Seek medical attention if significant or disabling

RAPID SEQUENCE INDUCTION

Rapid sequence induction (RSI) is the simultaneous administration of sedation and a short-acting muscle relaxant in predetermined doses to enable laryngoscopy and placement of an endotracheal tube (ETT).

It is *only* performed by doctors trained in the technique including how to manage the difficult airway, in a suitable monitored resuscitation area, with experienced (ideally credentialed) staff, on a patient at risk of aspiration (full stomach, or critically ill or injured) to create, maintain and/or protect the airway, plus to facilitate ventilation.

GENERAL PRINCIPLES

- Drugs given fall into three groups: premedication agents (discretionary); induction agents to rapidly achieve anaesthesia; and muscle relaxants including rapid onset/short acting to place the ETT (suxamethonium or rocuronium) and then long acting for maintaining paralysis (see Table 2.5).
- Maintenance of oxygenation is paramount, including a period of pre-oxgenation, then throughout the procedure, and in any failed intubation drill including for the difficult airway.
- Confirm ETT placement using end-tidal CO_2 monitoring to avoid missing inadvertent oesophageal intubation.

Table 2.5 Drugs for rapid sequence induction (RSI) intubation

Drug	Dose	Action	Onset (min)	Duration (min)
Premedication agents				
Atropine	0.02 mg/kg	Vagal blockade	1	30
Lidocaine	1.5 mg/kg	Decreases ICP	1	30
Fentanyl	1.5 microgram/kg	Analgesic	2	30
Morphine	0.15 mg/kg	Analgesic	4	120
Midazolam	0.05 mg/kg	Anxiolytic	2	30
Vecuronium	0.01 mg/kg	Defasciculation	2	10
Induction agents				
Thiopentone	1–5 mg/kg	Rapid-onset sedation (+ decreases ICP)	0.5	10
Propofol	1–2 mg/kg	Sedation	1	10
Fentanyl	10–20 microgram/kg	Sedation, analgesic	1	20
Midazolam	0.05–0.1 mg/kg	Rapid-onset sedation	2	10
Diazepam	0.1 mg/kg	Rapid-onset sedation	2	20
Ketamine	1 mg/kg	Dissociative state	2	20
Muscle relaxants				
Suxamethonium	1.5 mg/kg	Depolarizing MR[a]	0.5	5
Rocuronium	1.0 mg/kg	Non-depolarizing MR[a]	1	30
Vecuronium	0.2 mg/kg	Non-depolarizing MR	2	40

(Continued)

Table 2.5 (Continued) Drugs for rapid sequence induction (RSI) intubation

Drug	Dose	Action	Onset (min)	Duration (min)
Atracurium	0.5 mg/kg	Non-depolarizing MR	3	30
Pancuronium	0.1 mg/kg	Non-depolarizing MR	3	40

ICP, intracranial pressure; MR, muscle relaxant.

a Short acting.

DRUG INFUSION GUIDELINE

Drug infusions are common in critical care areas where monitoring and close supervision are standard. Each hospital/area will have their preferred dilutions and delivery systems.

SAFE USAGE
- Checking and re-checking drug doses added is essential, as is reviewing the clinical effects for improvement or complications.
- See Table 2.6 for drug and dose calculations in adults based on body weight of 70–80 kg.

Table 2.6 Critical care area drug infusion guideline

Drug	Loading dose	Paediatric infusion range (< 30 kg)	Dilution Infusion pump (IP)	Syringe driver	Concentration	Adult dose (70–80 kg) Dose per hour	Volume per hour
Adrenaline (epinephrine)	According to condition 1–100 micrograms/kg	0.05–1.0 micrograms/kg/min	6 mg in 100 mL DS	3 mg in 50 mL DS	60 micrograms/mL	2–20 micrograms/min	2–20 mL/h
Aminophylline [b]*Standard*	5.0 mg/kg in 100 mL DS over 20 min by IP	0.5–0.9 mg/kg/h	1000 mg in 500 mL DS 500 mg in	—	2 mg/mL	0.5–0.9 mg/kg/h	17.5–30 mL/h
[a]*Transport*	5.0 mg/kg in 100 mL DS over 20 min by IP	0.5–0.9 mg/kg/h	100 mL DS	250 mg in 50 mL DS	5 mg/mL	0.5–0.9 mg/kg/h	7–13 mL/h
Amiodarone [b]*Standard*	2–5 mg/kg in 100 mL DW over 30 min by IP	5–15 micrograms/kg/min	600 mg in 500 mL DW glass bottle. Discard at 12 h	—	1.2 mg/mL	20–60 mg/h (max. 15 mg/kg/24h)	17–52 mL/h
[a]*Transport*	2–5 mg/kg in 100 mL DW over 30 min by IP	5–15 micrograms/kg/min	300 mg in 100 mL DW	150 mg in 50 mL DW	3 mg/mL	20–60 mg/h (max. 15 mg/kg/24h)	7.5–22 mL/h

(Continued)

Table 2.6 (Continued) Critical care area drug infusion guideline

Drug	Loading dose	Paediatric infusion range (< 30 kg)	Dilution		Concentration	Adult dose (70–80 kg)	
			Infusion pump (IP)	Syringe driver		Dose per hour	Volume per hour
Clonazepam	1.0–2.0 mg	5–10 micrograms/kg/h	10 mg in 100 mL DS	5 mg in 50 mL DS	0.1 mg/mL	0.35–0.7 mg/h	3.5–7.0 mL/h
Dobutamine	—	2–30 micrograms/kg/min	250 mg in 100 mL DS	125 mg in 50 mL DS	2.5 mg/mL	2–30 micrograms/kg/min	2–30 mL/h
Dopamine	—	Renal: 0.5–2.5 micrograms/kg/min Inotrope: 5–20 micrograms/kg/min	200 mg in 100 mL DS	100 mg in 50 mL DS	2 mg/mL	Renal: 0.5–2.5 micrograms/kg/min Inotrope: 5–20 micrograms/kg/min	Renal: 1–5 mL/h Inotrope: 10–40 mL/h
Fentanyl	1–5 micrograms/kg	1–10 micrograms/kg/h	1000 micrograms in 100 mL DS	500 micrograms in 50 mL DS	10 micrograms/mL	50–200 micrograms/h	5–20 mL/h
Glyceryl trinitrate (GTN) [b] Standard	—	1–10 micrograms/kg/min	200 mg in 500 mL DW. Use glass bottle/low-absorption set	—	400 micrograms/mL	0.4–8 mg/h	1–20 mL/h

[a]Transport	—	1–10 micrograms/kg/min	50 mg in 100 mL DW	25 mg in 50 mL DW	500 micrograms/mL	0.5–10 mg/h	1–20 mL/h
Insulin (short-acting)	2–20 units	0.03–0.3 units/kg/h	100 units in 100 mL NS	50 units in 50 mL NS	1 unit/mL	2–20 units/h	2–20 mL/h
Isoprenaline							
Low dose	50–100 micrograms increments	0.5–7.5 micrograms/min	1 mg in 100 mL DS	0.5 mg in 50 mL DS	10 micrograms/mL	0.5–7.5 micrograms/min	2–30 mL/h
High dose	—	0.05–1.0 micrograms/kg/min	6 mg in 100 mL DS	3 mg in 50 mL DS	60 micrograms/mL	2–20 micrograms/min	2–20 mL/h
Ketamine	IV: 1–2 mg/kg IM: 5–10 mg/kg	5–20 micrograms/kg/min	1000 mg in 100 mL DS	500 mg in 50 mL DS	10 mg/mL	0.3–1.2 mg/kg/h	2–10 mL/h
Lignocaine (lidocaine)							
[b]*Standard*	1–2 mg/kg	15–50 micrograms/kg/min	Pre-mixed: 2 g in 500 mL DW	Pre-mixed: 2 g 500 mL DW	4 mg/mL	*8 mg/min **4 mg/min ***2 mg/min	*120 mL/h for 20 min **60 mL/h for 60 min ***30 mL/h for 24 h
[a]*Transport*	1–2 mg/kg	15–50 micrograms/kg/min	2 g in 100 mL DW	1 g in 50 mL DW	20 mg/mL 50 mL DW	*8 mg/min **4 mg/min ***2 mg/min	*24 mL/h for 20 min **12 mL/h for 60 min ***6 mL/h for 24 h

(Continued)

Table 2.6 (Continued) Critical care area drug infusion guideline

Drug	Loading dose	Paediatric infusion range (< 30 kg)	Dilution Infusion pump (IP)	Syringe driver	Concentration	Adult dose (70–80 kg) Dose per hour	Volume per hour
Magnesium sulphate *49.3% solution in 5 mL = 10 mmol = 2.47 g*	0.15–0.3 mmol/kg = 10–20 mmol (adult) Dilute in 50 mL DS Infuse: 2 min (VT) to 20 min (pre-eclampsia)	0.05–0.1 mmol/ kg/h	40 mmol in 100 mL DS	20 mmol in 50 mL DS	0.4 mmol/mL or 0.1 g/mL	2–8 mmol/h 0.5–2.0 g/h	5–20 mL/h
Methyl prednisolone *Spinal injury*	30 mg/kg over 30 min by IP	5.4 mg/kg/h	4 g in 100 mL. Reconstitute in water BP Dilute in DS	2 g in 50 mL. Reconstitute in water BP Dilute in DS	40 mg/mL	5.4 mg/kg/h for 23 h	10 mL/h (70 kg)
Midazolam	0.05–0.1 mg/ kg in 1–2.5 mg increments	10–100 micro-grams/kg/h	50 mg in 100 mL DS	25 mg in 50 mL DS	0.5 mg/mL	2.5–10 mg/h	5–20 mL/h
Morphine	2.5–15 mg in 2.5 mg increments	10–50 micro-grams/kg/h	100 mg in 100 mL DS	50 mg in 50 mL DS	1 mg/mL	2–10 mg/h	2–10 mL/h

Drug							
Naloxone	0.4–2.0 mg (max. 10 mg)	10 micrograms/kg/h	4 mg in 100 mL DS	2 mg in 50 mL DS	40 micrograms/mL	0.5–1.0 mg/h	12.5–25 mL/h
Nimodipine	—	6–30 micrograms/kg/h	10 mg in 50 mL dispensed	10 mg in 50 mL dispensed	0.2 mg/mL	0.4–2.0 mg/h. Titrate to maintain MAP	Start 2 mL/h Increase 2 mL/h every hour to max. of 10 mL/h
Noradrenaline (norepinephrine)	—	0.05–1.0 micrograms/kg/min	6 mg in 100 mL DS	3 mg in 50 mL DS	60 micrograms/mL	2–20 micrograms/min	2–20 mL/h
Octreotide	50–200 micrograms	3–5 micrograms/kg/h	1000 micrograms in 100 mL DS	500 micrograms in 50 mL DS	10 micrograms/mL	25–100 micrograms/h	2.5–10 mL/h
Phenobarbitone (phenobarbital)	15–25 mg/kg in 100 mL DS over 20–30 min (max. 50 mg/min) by IP	—	—	—	—	—	—
Phenytoin	15–18 mg/kg in 100 mL NS over 20–30 min (max. 50 mg/min) by IP	—	—	—	—	—	—

(Continued)

Table 2.6 (Continued) Critical care area drug infusion guideline

Drug	Loading dose	Paediatric infusion range (< 30 kg)	Dilution Infusion pump (IP)	Dilution Syringe driver	Concentration	Adult dose (70–80 kg) Dose per hour	Adult dose (70–80 kg) Volume per hour
Procainamide	10 mg/kg (max. 1000 mg) in 100 mL DW over 30 min by IP	20–80 micro-grams/kg/min	1000 mg in 100 mL DW	500 mg in 50 mg DW	10 mg/mL	2–6 mg/min	12–36 mL/h
Propofol	Sedation: 0.5–1.0 mg/kg Induction: 2–3 mg/kg	1–10 mg/kg/h	—	500 mg in 50 mL (dispensed as 20-mL and 50-mL amps, both with 10 mg/mL)	10 mg/mL	Sedation 1–2 mg/kg/h Anaesthesia 5–10 mg/kg/h	Sedation 7–15 mL/h Anaesthesia 35–70 mL/h
rt-PA (alteplase)	15-mg bolus (15 ml)	—	100 mg in 100 ml water BP	—	1 mg/ml	(a) 15-mg bolus (b) 0.75 mg/kg (max 50 mg) over 30 min (c) 0.5 mg/kg (max 35 mg) over 60 min	

r-PA (reteplase)	10-U bolus in 2 min. After 30 min, second 10-U bolus in 2 min	—	2 vials/ prefilled syringes/ reconstitution devices and needles		
Salbutamol (asthma)	5–10 micrograms/kg in 100 ml DS over 10 min	1.0–5.0 micrograms/kg/min	6 mg in 100 ml DS	60 micrograms/ml	5–50 micrograms/min	5–50 ml/h
Salbutamol (obstetric)	5–10 micrograms/kg in 100 ml DS over 10 min	0.2–1.0 micrograms/kg/min	6 mg in 100 ml DS	60 micrograms/ml	10–50 micrograms/ min	10–50 ml/h
Sodium nitroprusside	—	0.05–10 micrograms/kg/min	100 mg in 500 mL DW in glass bottle Protect from light Discard at 24 h	Min 200 micrograms/mL Max 800 micrograms/ min	0.05–10 micrograms/ kg/min (max. 1.5 mg/kg/24h)	1–210 mL/h 500 mL/24h
Streptokinase *AMI*	1.5 million units in 100 mL NS over 45 min by IP	—	—	15 000 units/ mL	2.5 mL/min	150 mL/h

(Continued)

Table 2.6 (Continued) Critical care area drug infusion guideline

Drug	Loading dose	Paediatric infusion range (< 30 kg)	Dilution Infusion pump (IP)	Syringe driver	Concentration	Adult dose (70–80 kg) Dose per hour	Volume per hour
PE, DVT, etc.	250 000 units in 100 mL NS over 30 min by IP	1500–2000 units/kg/h	500 000 units in 100 mL NS	—	5000 units/mL	100 000 units/h	20 mL/h
Thiopentone (thiopental)	3–6 mg/kg (0.5 mg/kg in shock)	1–5 mg/kg/h	2500 mg in 100 mL water BP Protect from light	1250 mg in 50 mL water BP Protect from light	25 mg/mL	75–350 mg/h	3–15 mL/h
Vecuronium	0.1 mg/kg	0.05–0.1 mg/kg/h	100 mg in 100 mL. Reconstitute in water BP Dilute in DS	50 mg in 50 mL. Reconstitute in water BP Dilute in DS	1.0 mg/mL	4–8 mg/h	4–8 mL/h

AMI, acute myocardial infarct; DS, dextrose saline, or any isotonic crystalloid; DVT, deep vein thrombosis; DW, 5% dextrose in water; IM, intramuscular; IP, infusion pump; IV, intravenous; MAP, mean arterial pressure; NS, normal saline; PE, pulmonary embolus; VT, ventricular tachycardia; water BP, water for injection.

[a] Standard: use in Emergency department.

[b] Transport: use for retrievals/interhospital transfers.

Reproduced by kind permission of Associate Professor CT Myers, Director and Head, Department of Emergency Medicine, The Prince Charles Hospital, Brisbane.

How to prescribe

Intravenous fluids	196
Insulin	204
Anticoagulants	209
Steroids	217
Sedation in the ED	219
Controlled drugs	221

INTRAVENOUS FLUIDS

The same degree of care should be taken when 'prescribing' intravenous fluids in the emergency department (ED) on the fluid order form, as when writing up drugs on the medication chart.

See Table 3.1 for the composition of the iv fluids most commonly used in the ED.

CRYSTALLOIDS

Isotonic: used for replacement and or maintenance regimens:

- *Normal (0.9%) saline*: 1 litre contains 154 mmol Na^+. Use as replacement and maintenance fluid in all situations, unless local protocol dictates otherwise. Caution in $\uparrow Na^+$ and liver dysfunction.
- *Hartmann's solution:* compound sodium lactate, used instead of normal saline (note 1 litre contains 5 mmol K^+). Avoid if RF.
- *Glucose* saline:* 1 litre contains mixture of NaCl (30 mmol Na^+) and glucose (4% = 222 mmol). Although considered useful as contains correct proportions of constituents (excluding KCl, which can be added to each bag) for 'average' daily requirements (see below), it will soon lead to hyponatraemia longer term (days), and does not account for individual patient needs. Also used as ivi in insulin sliding scales (see p. 205).
- *5% glucose*:* 1 litre contains 278 mmol (=50 g) glucose, which is rapidly taken up by cells and included only to make the fluid isotonic (calories are minimal, at 200 kcal). Used as method of giving pure H_2O and as ivi with insulin sliding scales (see p. 205).

NB: commonest cause of $\downarrow Na^+$ in hospital is overuse of glucose saline or 5% glucose as fluid replacement (often post-op).

Table 3.1 Composition of commonly used fluids

	Na (mmol/L)	Cl (mmol/L)	K (mmol/L)	Ca (mmol/L)	Mg (mmol/L)	Other constituents (/L)	Osmolarity mOsm/L (osmolality mOsm/kg)	pH
CRYSTALLOIDS								
0.9% sodium chloride (*normal saline*)	154	154	–	–	–	–	308 (300)	4.0–7.0
0.45% sodium chloride (*half normal saline*)	77	77	–	–	–	–	154 (150)	4.0–7.0
Hartmann's solution (*compound sodium lactate*)	131	111	5	2	–	29 mmol lactate	280 (274)	5.0–7.0
Modified Hartmann's	131	135	29.5	2	–	29 mmol lactate	329 (324)	
Ringer's lactate	130	109	4	3	–	28 mmol lactate	272	
5% dextrose	–	–	–	–	–	50 g dextrose	278 (252)	3.5–6.5

(Continued)

Table 3.1 (Continued) Composition of commonly used fluids

	Na (mmol/L)	Cl (mmol/L)	K (mmol/L)	Ca (mmol/L)	Mg (mmol/L)	Other constituents (/L)	Osmolarity mOsm/L (osmolality mOsm/kg)	pH
						Composition of commonly used intravenous fluids		
10% dextrose	–	–	–	–	–	100 g dextrose	556 (505)	3.5–6.5
50% dextrose	–	–	–	–	–	500 g dextrose	2778 (2525)	3.5–6.5
3.3% dextrose, 0.3% sodium chloride (3 and a 1/3)	51	51	–	–	–	33 g dextrose	286 (284)	3.5–6.5
4% dextrose, 0.18% sodium chloride (4 and a 1/5)	30	30	–	–	–	40 g dextrose	284 (282)	3.5–6.5
8.4% sodium bicarbonate	1000	–	–	–	–	1000 mmol HCO$_3^-$	–	–

Plasma-Lyte	140	98	5	–	1.5	27 mmol acetate 23 mmol gluconate	294 (294)	4.0–6.5
Plasma-Lyte–Replacement and Glucose 5%	140	98	5	–	1.5	27 mmol acetate 23 mmol gluconate 50 g dextrose	547 (573)	4.0–6.0
Plasma-Lyte Maintenance and 5% Glucose	40	40	13	–	1.5	16 mmol acetate 50 g dextrose	363 (389)	
COLLOIDS								
Gelofusine	154	120	–	–	–	40 g succinylated gelatin	274	7.4+/-0.3
Albumin 4%	140	128	<2	–	–	40 g albumin 6.4 mmol octanoate		

(Continued)

Table 3.1 (Continued) Composition of commonly used fluids

					Composition of commonly used intravenous fluids		
	Na (mmol/L)	Cl (mmol/L)	K (mmol/L)	Ca (mmol/L)	Mg (mmol/L)	Other constituents (/L)	Osmolarity mOsm/L (osmolality mOsm/kg)	pH
Haemaccel	145	145	5.1	6.25	–	35 g Polygeline	301 (293)	7.3+/−0.3
Dextran 40 in 0.9% Saline	150	150	–	–	–	Dextran 40 g	(325)	6.0
Dextran 40 in 5% Dextrose	–	–	–	–	–	Dextran 40 g dextrose 50 g	(349)	5.0
Dextran 70 in 0.9% Saline	150	150	–	–	–	Dextran 70 g	(306)	6.0
Dextran 70 in 5% Dextrose	–	–	–	–	–	Dextran 70 g dextrose 50 g	(325)	4.5

Non-isotonic: only for specialist/emergency situations by those experienced in their use:

- *Hypertonic (5%) saline*: 1 litre contains 856 mmol Na$^+$; given for severe symptomatic hyponatraemia, i.e. with seizures.
  ☠ Seek specialist help first ☠.
- *Hypotonic (0.45%) saline*: for severe ↑Na$^+$ (e.g. HHS).
- *10% and 20% glucose**: for mild/moderate hypoglycaemia.
- *50% glucose**: for severe hypoglycaemia (see p. 251), or if insulin being used to lower K$^+$ (see p. 269).
- *Sodium bicarbonate (1.26% or move rarely 1.4%)*: useful replacement for 0.9% saline if ↓pH or ↑K$^+$ which often coexist. Not isotonic so caution re: salt load and accompanying fluid retention. ☠ Seek specialist help from nephrologists/others accustomed to its use ☠.

*NB: glucose = dextrose. Low-strength glucose solutions used to be called dextrose solutions; this is now being phased out.

COLLOIDS
Plasma expanders and substitutes helpful to ↑/maintain plasma oncotic pressure.

- Gelofusine: succinylated gelatin used in resuscitation of shock (non-cardiogenic). NB: electrolyte content is often overlooked: 1 litre Gelofusine has 154 mmol Na$^+$.
- *Albumin*: prepared from whole blood and containing soluble proteins and electrolytes, but no clotting factors etc. May be fluid of choice in sepsis.
- HAEMACCEL: bovine-derived polygeline (derivative of gelatin), may cause anaphylaxis.

DAILY FLUID AND ELECTROLYTE REQUIREMENTS (STANDARD)
Standard daily fluid and electrolyte requirement: For a 70 kg adult male is approx 30–40 ml/kg H$_2$O (3 litres); 1.5–2.0 mmol/kg Na$^+$ (100–150 mmol Na$^+$); and 0.5–1.0 mmol/kg K$^+$ (40–70 mmol K$^+$).

When no expected oral intake (↓GCS, unsafe swallow, post-CVA, preoperative, etc), this may be provided as follows:

Date	Infusion Fluid	Volume	Additives If Any Drug and Dose	Rate of Admin	Dura-tion	Dr's Signature	Time Start-ed	Time Com-pleted	Set Up by Sig-nature	Batch No.
08/01	5% Glucose	1 litre	20 mmol KCl		8h	TN				
08/01	Normal saline	1 litre			8h	TN				
08/01	5% Glucose	1 litre	20 mmol KCl		8h	TN				

Figure 3.1 Drug chart showing how to write up intravenous fluids.

This '1 sour (0.9% saline), 2 sweet (5% glucose)' regimen may be used in fit pre-operative patients. Otherwise, if there are abnormal losses such as fever, vomiting, diarrhoea etc, use normal (0.9%) saline unless liver failure (see below) or if Na^+ outside normal range (↓ or ↑).

Always get senior help if unsure, as incorrectly prescribed fluids can be as dangerous as any other incorrectly used drug.

Individual fluid and electrolyte requirements may differ substantially according to:

- Body habitus, age, residual oral intake, if on multiple iv drugs (which are sometimes given with significant amounts of fluid).
- Insensible losses (normally about 1 litre/day). ↑skin losses if fever or burns. ↑lung losses in hyperventilation or inhalation burns.
- GI losses (normally about 0.2 litre/day). Any vomiting (↑Cl^- content) or diarrhoea (↑K^+ content) must be taken into account as well as less obvious causes, e.g. ileus, fistulae.
- Fluid compartment shifts, esp vasodilation with distributive shock if sepsis/anaphylaxis.

K^+ CONSIDERATIONS

Do not give at >10 mmol/h iv unless K^+ dangerously low, when it can be given quicker (see p. 270).

Post-op surgical patients often need less K^+ in 1st 24 h, as K^+ is released by cell necrosis (∴ proportional to extent of surgery).

HANDY HINTS

- Check the following before prescribing any iv fluid:
  - *Clinical markers of hydration:* temperature, skin turgor, mucous membranes, JVP, peripheral oedema, pulmonary oedema (basal crackles). Easy to overlook, yet simple and useful signs!
  - *Recent input and output:* if at all concerned, ask nurses to commence a strict fluid balance chart. Consider also starting a daily weight chart.
  - Recent U&Es, esp K^+. Can use VBG to get an urgent result, before lab bloods are available.
- In general, encourage oral fluids (often overlooked in the ED): homeostasis (if normal) is safer, less expensive and less consuming of doctor/nurse time than iv fluids. Beware of shock, fever, vomiting, diarrhoea or ileus (iv fluid will be needed); ↓swallow; fluid overload (esp if HF or RF); ↓GCS; or if homeostasis disorders (esp SIADH).
- Take extreme care if major organ failure:
  - *Heart failure*: heart can quickly become 'overloaded' and ⇒ acute LVF. Even if not currently in HF, beware if predisposed (e.g. Hx of HF or IHD).
  - Renal failure: unless pre-renal cause (e.g. hypovolaemia), do not give more fluid than residual renal function can deal with. Seek help from senior doctor if at all concerned; good fluid Mx greatly influences outcomes in this group. Use saline unless specialist advice taken.
  - Liver failure: often preferable to use 5% glucose. Serum Na^+ may be ↓d, but total body Na^+ is often ↑d. Additional saline will end up in the wrong compartment (e.g. peritoneal fluid ∴↑ing ascites) but may be essential to ensure renal perfusion (RF often coexists).
- If in doubt, give 'fluid challenges': small volumes (normally 200–500 ml) of fluid over short periods of time, to see whether

clinical response to BP, urine output or left ventricular function is beneficial or detrimental before committing to longer-term fluid strategy.

> It can be difficult to elicit all this information under time pressure. The trick is to know when to take extreme care. Be particularly careful if you do not know the patient, i.e. a handover, and be wary when asked to 'just write up another bag' without reviewing the patient. You may be asked to prescribe fluids when no longer necessary or even when they may be harmful. To save time for those on ward call (and to ↑ the chances of your patient getting appropriate fluids), leave clear instructions with the nurses and on the drug chart for as long as can be sensibly predicted (esp over weekends/long holidays).

INSULIN

See page 252 for DKA and HHS management.

TYPES
Many types of insulin exist, with differences in the timing of action onset **O**, peak **P** and duration **D**.

Acute use, e.g. sliding scales (see below), acute control:

- **Soluble** (aka normal/neutral) can be given iv (and sc as other types), e.g. Actrapid, Humulin S:
  - **iv: O/P** immediate, **D** 0.5 h.
  - **sc: O** 0.5–1 h, **P** 2–4 h, **D** 6–8 h.

Maintenance use, i.e. normal control (sc only):

- **Aspart** (NovoRapid), **lispro** (Humalog) or **glulisine** (▼ Apidra): recombinant human analogues. Rapid onset ⇒ ↑eating flexibility (can give immediately before meals; other types of sc insulin must be given 30 min before), ↓duration ⇒ fewer hypos (esp before meals). **O** 0.25 h, **P** 1–3 h, **D** 2–5 h. + usually given with intermediate- or long-acting insulin ('basal/bolus' regime).

- **Isophane**: intermediate-acting e.g. Humulin I, Insulatard or Insuman Basal, mostly given bd.
- **Glargine**: long-acting recombinant insulin with delayed and prolonged absorption from sc injection site ⇒ constant, more 'physiological' basal supply; mostly given od but can be split into bd dosing (e.g. Lantus).
- **Detemir**: long-acting analogue. Binds to albumin and has different action from that of glargine but similar advantages. Give od or bd (e.g. Levemir).

Biphasic insulins: contain mixtures of intermediate- or long-acting insulin (e.g. isophane) with short-acting soluble insulin (e.g. aspart or lispro); e.g. Humalog Mix 25, Humulin M3, Insuman Comb 15, Insuman Comb 25, Novomix 30. Usually given bd (sometimes od).

   Short-acting insulins: can also be given by continuous sc infusion, using a portable pump, which gives basal insulin with patient-activated boluses.

SLIDING SCALE INSULIN

= Variable rate insulin ivi. Aim is for optimal blood glucose control in diabetics if (i) NBM/preoperative, (ii) MI*/ACS*, (iii) severe concurrent illness (e.g. sepsis), (iv) recovery after DKA/HHS.

   See page 252 for DKA where a fixed rate ivi is recommended rather than sliding scale (not universal, so follow local protocols).

How to write an insulin sliding scale on a fluid chart

Date/ Time	Infusion Fluid	Volume	Additives If Any Drug and Dose	Rate of Admin	Dura-tion	Dr's Signature	Time Start-ed	Time Com-pleted	Set Up by Sig-nature	Batch No.
08/01	Normal saline	50 ml	ACTRAPID 50 units	As below		TN				
08/01	Glucose saline	1 litre								
		CBG (= BM)	INSULIN ivi (ml/h)							
		0–4	0.5(+ call Dr if CBG < 2.5)							
		4.1–7	1							
		7.1–9	2							
		9.1–11	3							
		11.1–13	4							
		≥13.1	6							
Always run glucose saline (4% glucose + 0.18% saline) ivi at 125 ml per hour if CBG (BM) <15.										

Figure 3.2 Drug chart, showing slide scale.

This is one approach and ∴ suggested only as an *initial* regimen: requirements will vary widely between individuals and within an individual over time (esp with intercurrent illness, e.g. infection). Regular review and adjustment is essential – see below. Use your hospital's protocol where possible.

Important points
- Carefully consider need for starting a sliding scale, especially if patient eating/drinking normally and there is no other compelling indication.
- A poorly managed sliding scale ⇒ fluctuating glucose and ↑length of admission. prn insulin not recommended due to risk of hypoglycaemia.
- ☠ When prescribing any insulin, never abbreviate the word 'units' to 'U' (as 'U' can be mistaken for 'O' leading to ten-fold dosing error) ☠ .

- Check cannula patency before adjusting sliding scale (if not working could be why BG not improving/↓ing).
- Give 5% glucose or glucose saline (4% glucose with 0.18% saline, or 5% glucose with 0.45% saline and 0.15% KCl) ivi at 125 ml/h when CBG <15 mmol/l. If RF or mild HF give 5% glucose ivi at a slower rate. If severe HF give 10% glucose (preferably via central line) at 60–70 ml/h. KCl content should be adjusted according to individual needs.
- Discuss clearly with nursing staff the frequency of CBG measurement required. Sicker patients need CBGs every 1 h, ideally with regular (2–4 hrly) laboratory BG readings (to confirm accuracy). If not that sick and CBGs stable, check 2–4 hrly.
- Stop oral hypoglycaemics but remember to reintroduce them before ceasing sliding scale!

*NB: glucose = dextrose. Low-strength glucose solutions used to be called dextrose solutions; this is now being phased out.

Initial insulin dose and adjustments

Prescribe 50 units of soluble insulin (Actrapid or Humulin S) in 50 ml normal (0.9% NaCl) saline to run via a syringe driver according to one of the regimens (A, B, C, D) below.
  Prime the line by flushing with 5 ml of the solution before attaching to the patient (as the plastic tubing adsorbs insulin) ∴ remaining volume will be 45 ml.

1 Start with regimen A, unless known severe insulin resistance (i.e. normally takes ≥100 units sc insulin/day), in which case start with B.
2 If BG >10 (or >7 during acute MI, where target BG even lower) for 3 consecutive hourly tests and is ↑ing (or ↓ing by <25% in the past hour), step up to next sliding scale (i.e. if on A, step up to B; if on B, step up to C, etc).
3 If BG <3.5 mmol/l, step down to next scale (i.e. if on B, step down to A; if on C, step down to B, etc).

CBG(=BM)	Insulin ivi (units/h)			
	Regime A	Regime B	Regime C[b]	Regime D[b]
0.0–4.0[a]	0.5	0.5	0.5	0.5
4.1–7.0	1	2	3	4
7.1–9.0	2	4	6	8
9.1–11.0	3	6	9	12
11.1–13.0	4	8	12	16
>13.0	6	12	18	24

[a] Stop ivi for 15 min if severe hypoglycaemia (CBG <2.5 or symptoms) and give Rx as on
p. 251. Otherwise treat more gently with 5–10% glucose ivi and maintain insulin infusion
(esp if DKA).

[b] Rarely needed; used mostly for patients with severe insulin resistance (i.e. on more than 100
units insulin/day before admission).

(Reproduced with permission from Professor S Kumar, Dr A Rahim and Dr P Dyer,
Endocrinology Department, University of Warwick Medical School.)

Coming off a sliding scale

Once eating/drinking normally and CBGs normal/stable, consider
coming off sliding scale. This is rarely achieved within the ED (more
commonly occurs on the ward):

- Post-DKA, change back only if blood free of ketones and pH
  back to normal.
- Avoid hypos by continuing ivi until 1st sc dose starts to work
  (usually 10–30 min). Always change from iv to sc before a meal.

How to start sc regimen (always consult senior doctor if unsure):

1 Calculate daily requirements by doubling the number of units
  used in the past 12 h from the sliding scale. Note what fluids
  were given during this period.
2 Start qds sc regimen. If patient is well and CBGs stable, this step
  can be omitted (i.e. go straight to a bd regimen). Give 1/3 of
  total daily dose at 10 pm (as intermediate, e.g. isophane, or long
  acting, e.g. glargine or determir, insulin) and give remaining 2/3

(as short-acting soluble insulin) divided equally between pre-breakfast, pre-lunch and pre-evening meal doses.

3 Or start a bd sc regimen: give 60% of daily dose pre-breakfast and the remaining 40% pre-evening meal, both doses as biphasic 30/70 insulin (e.g. Humulin M3).

ANTICOAGULANTS

HEPARIN

Immediate and short-term Rx/Px of TE. Two main types: low-molecular-weight heparins (LMWHs) and unfractionated heparin. Also used in ACS (see p. 226).

LMWHs

Give sc. ↑convenience (↓monitoring, can give to outpatients). ↓incidence of HIT* and osteoporosis cf unfractionated heparin, so now preferred for most indications (esp MI/ACS, DVT/PE Rx and pre-cardioversion of AF). Types include:

- Enoxaparin (Clexane), dalteparin (Fragmin), and tinzaparin (Innohep) are the most common. Each hospital tends to use one in particular; ask staff which one they stock or call pharmacy.
- Prophylaxis does not need monitoring but do not use for >7–10 days if creatinine >150.

Monitoring of treatment with LMWH

Via peak anti-Xa assay: usually necessary only if renal impairment (i.e. creatinine >150), pregnancy or at extremes of Wt (i.e. <45 kg or >100 kg). Take sample 3–4 h post dose, which is therefore usually done on the wards.

HIT* = heparin-induced thrombocytopenia
Much more common with unfractionated heparin but can occur with all heparins. Watch for ↓ing platelet count. Get senior help if concerned. Discuss investigation and Mx with haematologist.

If HIT confirmed, stop heparin immediately – danaparoid (Orgaran) or lepirudin (Refludan) may be substituted.

UNFRACTIONATED HEPARIN

Given iv*: rapidly reversible (immediately if protamine given; see p. 212), which is useful if patient at ↑risk of bleeding, or following use of extracorporeal circuits such as haemodialysis or cardiopulmonary bypass.

- Is also used with recombinant fibrinolytics in AMI, but due to difficulty keeping in therapeutic range, LMWH increasingly preferred where possible – discuss with senior.
- *Can be given sc (only for Px), but now largely replaced by LMWH.

Starting iv unfractionated heparin

1 *Load with 5000** units as iv bolus*: prescribe on the 'once-only' section of the drug chart (give 10 000** units in severe PE).
2 Set up ivi at 15–25 units/kg/h: usually = 1000–2000 units/h. A sensible starting rate is 1500 units/h, which can be achieved by adding 25 000 units of heparin to 48 ml of normal saline to make 50 ml of solution (500 units/ml), then run at 3 ml/h via a syringe driver.
3 This can be written up as follows:

Date/ Time	Infusion Fluid	Volume	Additives if Any Drug and Dose	Rate of Admin	Dura-tion	Dr's Signature	Time Start-ed	Time Com-pleted	Set Up by Sig-nature	Batch No.
08/01	Normal saline	50 ml	HEPARIN 25,000 units			TN				
	run at 3 ml per hour as ivi									

Figure 3.3 Drug chart showing how to write up intravenous heparin infusion.

NB
Dosing for co-therapy with fibrinolytics (according to ESC guidelines) is slightly different; see p. 231.

Monitoring

Via APTT ratio (= Activated Partial Thromboplastin Time of patient plasma divided by that of control plasma). Results can (rarely) be given as patient's exact APTT: the normal range is 35–45 sec. You then need to calculate the ratio: take the middle of the normal range for your lab (e.g. 40 sec) for your calculations.

Target ratio is commonly 1.5–2.5, but this can vary: check your hospital's protocol and aim for the middle of range.

NB: there is no national (let alone international) consensus on methods of measuring APTT, so results are not yet standardised!

Don't take sample from drip arm (unless from site distal to ivi).

Although usually done on the inpatient ward, check APTT ratio after 6 h, then 6–10 h until stable, and then daily at a minimum, adjusting to the following regimen: (based on APTT *ratio* therapeutic range of 1.5–2.5).

APTT ratio	Action
<1.2	Give 5000-unit bolus iv and ↑ivi by 200–250 units/h
1.2–1.5	Give 2500-unit bolus iv and ↑ivi by 100–150 units/h
1.5–2.5	No change
2.5–3.0	↓ivi by 100–150 units/h
>3.0	Stop ivi for 1h then restart ivi, ↓ing by 200–250 units/h

Adjustments are safest made by writing a fresh ivi prescription at a different strength, but the same effect can also be achieved by calculating the appropriate rate change to the original prescription.

Variable rate of ivi: using fixed prescription of 25 000 units heparin in 50 ml saline:

Desired heparin ivi rate (units/h)	Rate of ivi (ml/h)	Desired heparin ivi rate (units/h)	Rate of ivi (ml/h)
1000	2.0	1500	3.0
1050	2.1	1550	3.1

Desired heparin ivi rate (units/h)	Rate of ivi (ml/h)	Desired heparin ivi rate (units/h)	Rate of ivi (ml/h)
1100	2.2	1600	3.2
1150	2.3	1650	3.3
1200	2.4	1700	3.4
1250	2.5	1750	3.5
1300	2.6	1800	3.6
1350	2.7	1850	3.7
1400	2.8	1900	3.8
1450	2.9	1950	3.9

Overtreatment/overdose (all heparins)

If significant bleeding, stop heparin and observe: iv heparin has short $t_{1/2}$ (30 min–2 h), so fx wear off quickly.

If bleeding continues or is life-threatening, consider iv protamine (1 mg per 80–100 units of heparin to be neutralised as ivi over 10 min. ↓doses if giving >15 min after heparin stopped). Seek expert help from haematology on-call if in any doubt!

NB: protamine is less effective against LMWH, and repeat administration may be required.

▼ FONDAPARINUX

New parenteral anticoagulant (synthetic pentasaccharide). Licensed for use in Rx of VTE and MI/ACS and Px of VTE in medical patients and patients undergoing orthopaedic or abdominal surgery. Monitoring is not necessary.

Also useful for Px of VTE for patients with history of HIT* or allergy to heparin. See BNF/SPC for dosing. NB: Caution if RF or LF.

WARFARIN

Patients are rarely started on warfarin whilst in the ED, but may present awaiting an INR (see below) and need that day's dose prescribed.

Basics

Oral anticoagulant for long-term Rx/Px of TE: loading (see below) usually takes several days and as it is initially prothrombotic, heparin (LMWH), which is effective immediately, is used as short-term cover until therapeutic levels are achieved.

Monitoring

Use INR = ratio of patient's PT (prothrombin time) to a control raised to the power of a variable dependent on exact reagents used in each lab.

A target INR is set at the start of Rx, according to indication (see below); variations of ±0.5 are acceptable.

BCSH guidelines for target INRs. Adapted with permission from *British Journal of Haematology* 2011; **154**(3): 311–24.

Indication	Target INR (± 0.5)
DVT/PE[a]	2.5
Thrombophilia (if symptomatic)[b]	2.5
Paroxysmal nocturnal haemoglobinuria (PNH)[c]	2.5
AF[d] (or other causes of cardiac emboli[e])	2.5
Bioprosthetic heart valves[f]	2.5
Mechanical heart valves[g]	3.5

[a] Treat for = 6 weeks if calf vein thrombosis, for = 3 months if provoked proximal (peroneal or above) DVT/PE, for = 6 months or lifelong if idiopathic venous TE or permanent risk factors. If recurrent DVT/PE whilst on therapeutic Rx, target INR = 3.5. Discuss all other than 1st presentation with anticoagulant service.

[b] Arterial thrombosis in antiphospholipid syndrome is exception with target INR 3.5.

[c] Paroxysmal nocturnal haemoglobinuria (PNH); only under guidance of consultant haematologist.

[d] Maintain INR >2.0 for 3 weeks before and 4 weeks after elective DC cardioversion.

[e] Dilated cardiomyopathy, mural thrombus post-MI or rheumatic value disease.

[f] Only for first 3–6 months post value insertion at discretion of each centre.

[g] New generation aortic values INR target 3.0.

Although not in the BCSH guidelines, a target INR of 2.5 is widely agreed for nephrotic syndrome (generally once albumin <20 g/l).

Starting warfarin Rx i.e. for acute thrombosis: (rarely done in the ED)

Check INR before 1st dose and every day for 4 days, then assess stability of INR and adjust accordingly. If on LMWH, do not stop until 2 days after therapeutic INR achieved.

For loading regimens, where possible use your hospital's own guidelines, since these often vary. Otherwise, it is sensible to use the BCSH guidelines:

Warfarin loading regimen. Adapted with permission of BMJ group from Fennerty A, et al. BMJ 1984; 288: 1268–1270.

Day 1		Day 2		Day 3		Day 4	
INR	Dose (mg)	INR	Dose (mg)	INR	Dose (mg)	INR	Dose[a] (mg)
<1.4	10	<1.8	10	<2.0	10	<1.4	>8
		1.8	1	2.0–2.1	5	1.4	8
		>1.8	0.5	2.2–2.3	4.5	1.5	7.5
				2.4–2.5	4	1.6–1.7	7
				2.6–2.7	3.5	1.8	6.5
				2.8–2.9	3	1.9	6
				3.0–3.1	2.5	2.0–2.1	5.5
				3.2–3.3	2	2.2–2.3	5
				3.4	1.5	2.4–2.6	4.5
				3.5	1	2.7–3.0	4
				3.6–4.0	0.5	3.1–3.5	3.5
				>4.0	0	3.6–4.0	3
						4.1–4.5	Miss 1 day then 2 mg
						>4.5	Miss 2 days then 1 mg

[a] Predicted maintenance dose.

Situations when dose (especially loading) may need review
↓**dose**: if age >80 yrs, LF, HF, post-op, poor nutrition, ↑baseline
INR or taking drugs that potentiate warfarin, so check for **W+**
symbols in this book (includes almost all antibiotics).
↑**dose**: if taking drugs that inhibit warfarin, so check for **W−**
symbols in this book.
Herbal remedies/non-prescription drugs: can have significant
interactions – always ask patients if taking any, as they may not
realise the importance (e.g. glucosamine can ↑INR). Check each
one with your hospital's drug information office for significance.
Alcohol and diet: can affect dosing, especially if intake varies –
the goalposts will move for an individual's therapeutic range.
It is a common misconception that BMI influences response.

Slow loading: give 3–5 mg for 5–7 days which achieves therapeutic
levels with less overshoot and may be preferable for outpatient
initiation in atrial fibrillation. (BCSH guidelines 3rd edition 2005
update www.bcshguidelines.com)

Interrupting warfarin

If interrupting warfarin (e.g. before operation/procedure), assess
thrombotic risk and use bridging anticoagulation with LMWH as
necessary; do not reload post-op as above, but restart at usual dose
+50% for 2 days, then return to usual dose *if no contraindications*
(e.g. bleeding/taking **W+** drugs).

Make small infrequent dose changes unless INR dangerously
high or low. 'Steering a supertanker' is a good analogy; there
is often significant delay between dose changes and their fx, so
don't fiddle!

Warfarin and pregnancy

Warfarin is contraindicated in early pregnancy (teratogenic during
weeks 6–12). Women of childbearing age must be counselled by a
specialist prior to planning pregnancy (inc informed to do pregnancy
test whenever a period is >2 days late).

Any woman who is pregnant and on warfarin must be converted immediately to LMWH under specialist guidance.

> **Overtreatment/overdose**
> *Seek expert help from senior doctor or haematology on-call* as xs vitamin K will make re-anticoagulation difficult. The fx can last for weeks ∴ ⇒ ↑risk of recurrence of condition that warfarin was started for.

Recommendations for Mx of excess warfarin (BCSH guidelines). Adapted with permission from *British Journal of Haematology* 2011; 154(3): 311–24.

INR	Action
3.0–6.0 if target 2.5 (4.0–6.0 if target 3.5)	↓dose or stop warfarin; restart when INR <5.0
6.0–8.0 and no/minor bleeding	Stop warfarin; restart when INR <5.0
>8.0 and no/minor bleeding	Stop warfarin; restart when INR <5.0 If other bleeding risks (e.g. age > 70 yrs, Hx of bleeding complications *or* liver disease) give phytomenadione (vit K$_1$) 0.5mg[a] iv or 5mg po
Major bleeding, e.g. ↓ing Hb or cardiodynamic instability	Stop warfarin Phytomenadione (vit K$_1$) 5 or 10 mg iv, repeating 24 h later if necessary Prothrombin complex concentrate 30–50 units/kg not exceeding 3000 units (if unavailable give FFP[b] 15ml/kg)

[a] Since publication of BCSH guidelines some advise larger doses of iv vit K, e.g. 2 mg

[b] Although not stated in BCSH guidelines, note that FFP is not fully effective in warfarin reversal.

DABIGATRAN

Dabigatran etexilate (▼ Pradaxa), an oral direct thrombin inhibitor, is a new oral anticoagulant licensed for once-daily administration for extended thromboprophylaxis after elective total knee or hip replacement[NICE].

Although it does not require monitoring of anticoagulant fx, and has fewer drug–food interactions than warfarin, it can pose a challenge in a patient with an acute problem such as an intracranial bleed, as it is not reversible (unlike warfarin).

NB: Caution if LF or RF. Note may also be associated with an increased risk of MI or ACS.

STEROIDS

CORTICOSTEROIDS

Commonly used systemic drugs include:

Drug	Equivalent dose	Main uses
Prednisolone	5 mg	Acute asthma/COPD, rheumatoid arthritis (po)
Methylprednisolone	4 mg	Acute flares rheumatoid arthritis/MS (iv)
Dexamethasone	750 microgram	↑ICP, CAH, Dx Cushing's (iv/po)
Hydrocortisone	20 mg	Acute asthma/COPD (iv)

Therapeutic effects

Glucocorticoid fx predominate; mineralocorticoid fx for all these are mild apart from hydrocortisone (has moderate fx) and dexamethasone (has minimal fx ∴ used when H_2O and Na^+ retention are particularly undesirable, e.g. ↑ICP).

Side effects: (i.e. Cushing's syndrome!)

- *Metabolic:* Na^+/fluid retention*, hyperlipoproteinaemia, leukocytosis, negative K^+/Ca^{2+}/nitrogen balance, generalised fluid/electrolyte abnormalities.
- *Endocrine:* hyperglycaemia/↓GTT (can ⇒ DM), adrenal suppression.
  - *Fat*: truncal obesity, moon face, interscapular ('buffalo hump') and suprascapular fat pads.

  — *Skin*: hirsutism, bruising/purpura, acne, striae, ↓healing, telangiectasia, thinning.
  — *Other*: impotence, menstrual irregularities/amenorrhoea, ↓growth (children), ↑appetite*.
- *GI*: pancreatitis, peptic/oesophageal ulcers: give PPI if on ↑doses.
- *Cardiac*: HTN, CCF, myocardial rupture post-MI, TE.
- *Musculoskeletal*: proximal myopathy, osteoporosis, fractures (can ⇒ avascular necrosis).
- *Neurological*: ↑epilepsy, ↑ICP/papilloedema (esp children on withdrawal of corticosteroids).
- *Ψ*: mood Δs (↑ or ↓), psychosis (esp at ↑doses), dependence.
- *Ocular*: cataracts, glaucoma, corneal/scleral thinning.
- *Infections*: ↑susceptibility, ↑rapidity (↑severity at presentation), TB reactivation, ↑risk of chickenpox/shingles/measles.

> **SEs are dose-dependent**
> If patient is on a high dose, make sure this is intentional: it is possible in fluctuating (e.g. inflammatory) illnesses for a patient to be left on high doses by mistake. Seek specialist advice if unsure.
> If on long term Rx consider giving Ca/vit D supplements/ bisphosphonate to ↓risk of osteoporosis, and PPI to ↓risk of GI ulceration.

> **Cautions**
> These can mostly be worked out from the SEs. Take care if patient already has any condition that is a potential SE. Systemic corticosteroids are CI in systemic infections (w/o antibiotic cover).
> NB: avoid live vaccines. If never had chickenpox, avoid exposure.

Interactions

Apply to all systemic Rx. fx can be ↓d by rifampicin, carbamazepine, phenytoin and phenobarbital. fx can be ↑d by erythromycin, ketoconazole, itraconazole and ciclosporin (whose own fx are ↑d by methylprednisolone).

↑risk of ↓K^+ with amphotericin and digoxin.

Withdrawal effects

Sudden withdrawal can precipitate acute adrenal insufficiency
(= Addisonian crisis; ☠ can be fatal ☠ see p. 256): ↓BP, ↑HR,
postural hypotension, weakness, myalgia, abdominal pain, vomiting,
↓Wt, confusion leading to coma, and characteristic e'lyte changes
with ↓BG, ↓Na^+, ↑K^+, ↑urea, ↑Ca. Note intercurrent infection/AMI/
trauma may also precipitate an Addisonian crisis.

∴ must withdraw corticosteroids slowly if patient has had >3 wks Rx
(or a shorter course w/in 1 year of stopping long-term Rx), other causes
of adrenal suppression, received high doses (>40 mg od prednisolone
or equivalent), or repeat doses in evening, or repeat course.

Thus intercurrent illness, trauma, surgery also need ↑doses to avoid
precipitating relative withdrawal.

Steroid Rx card should be carried by all patients on prolonged Rx.

MINERALOCORTICOIDS, e.g. fludrocortisone

Used for Addison's disease and acute adrenocortical deficiency (but
rarely needed for hypopituitarism).

Are also used for orthostatic/postural hypotension. Main SEs are
H_2O/Na^+ retention.

SEDATION IN THE ED

ACUTE SEDATION

Consider for the acutely agitated, disturbed or violent patient in the ED.

Note: procedural sedation and analgesia before a brief painful
procedure is described on page 182.

Important points

Delirium (acute confusional state)

- Delirium is the abrupt onset of clouding of consciousness
  that may fluctuate, disorientation in time and place, impaired
  memory, visual, olfactory or tactile hallucinations, and illusions.

There is restlessness, irritability, emotional lability and poor comprehension.

- Look for and treat hypoxia, drug intoxication or withdrawal (esp alcohol/opiates), sepsis including meningitis, cerebral event inc trauma, endocrine and metabolic causes (esp hypoglycaemia).

Violent or disturbed patient

- Most commonly the result of alcohol intoxication, or other recreational drugs such as cocaine, amphetamines or phencyclidine. Other causes inc mental illness such as mania or paranoid schizophrenia, as well as acute delirium as above (always check a CBG, and vital signs when able).
- A well-lit calm room and verbal reassurance may be all that is required. Call for senior help early. Follow with a 'show of force', with physical restraint as a last resort.
- Oral medications should be tried if possible, before parenteral.

There are two main choices – benzodiazepines and antipsychotics: ☺good for/reasons to choose; ☹bad for/reasons to not give.

Benzodiazepines

- ☺Alcohol withdrawal, anxiety.
- ☹Respiratory disease (⇒ respiratory depression; care if COPD/ asthma), elderly (⇒ falls and rarely paradoxical agitation/ aggression but can use with caution/↓ doses).
- *Lorazepam* 0.5–1 mg po/im/iv (maximum 4 mg/24 h). Shorter-acting than diazepam ∴ better if hepatic impairment.
- *Diazepam* 2–5 mg po/iv (if iv preferably as Diazemuls) or 10–20 mg pr. Can ↑doses$^{SPC/BNF}$ esp if tolerance/much previous exposure to benzodiazepines.
- *Midazolam* 1.0–7.5 mg iv: titrate up slowly, according to response. Wears off relatively quicker.

Antipsychotics

- ☺Taking benzodiazepines, elderly (use with caution, esp if ↑ risk of CVA), delirium (non-alcohol withdrawal), psychosis (e.g. hallucinations/delusions/schizophrenia).

- ☹ Antipsychotic-naive, alcohol withdrawal, cardiac disease, movement disorders (esp Parkinson's; de novo extrapyramidal fx are also common – see p. 278).
- *Haloperidol* 0.5–5 mg po (or im/iv if necessary). 1–2 mg is sensible starting dose for delirium in elderly. 5 mg is safe for acute psychosis in young adults. Maximum 18 mg im or 30 mg po in 24 h.
- If suspect *acute schizophrenia* use atypical antipsychotic as 1st-line[NICE], e.g. olanzapine 10 mg po ($\Rightarrow \downarrow$SEs) – now also available im.

CONTROLLED DRUGS

These drugs are rarely if ever prescribed to take home from the ED, except for severe acute pain or palliative care. NB: Chronic users of controlled drugs should *only* receive new supplies from authorised/licensed medical practitioners.

Note: special 'Prescription requirements' apply in the UK to 'schedule' 1, 2 or 3 drugs only, the most likely of which might be prescribed by a junior doctor are morphine, diamorphine, fentanyl, methadone, oxycodone (and less commonly buprenorphine or pethidine). The following must be written 'so as to be indelible, e.g. written by hand, typed or computer generated' (*NB: this is a recent change from previously having to be written by hand – only the signature now needs to be handwritten*):

- Date
- The patient's full name and address and, where appropriate, age
- Drug name plus its form* (and, where appropriate, strength)
- Dosing regimen (NB: the directions 'take one as directed' constitutes a dose but 'as directed' does not)
- Total amount of drug to be dispensed in words and figures (e.g. for morphine 5 mg qds for one week (5 mg×4 times a day×7 days = 140) write: '140 milligrams = one hundred and forty milligrams')
- Prescriber's address must be specified (should already be on prescription form, e.g. hospital address).

*Omitting the form (e.g. tablet/liquid/patch) is a common reason for an invalid prescription. It is often assumed to be obvious from the prescription (e.g. fentanyl as a patch or Oramorph as a liquid), but it still has to be written even if only one form exists.

These requirements *do not* apply to temazepam (despite being schedule 3), schedule 4 drugs (e.g. benzodiazepines) and schedule 5 drugs (such as codeine, dihydrocodeine/DF118 and tramadol). For full details on controlled drug guidance in the UK see www.dh.gov.uk/controlleddrugs.

Medical emergencies

Cardiopulmonary resuscitation (CPR) 225
Anaphylaxis 225
Acute coronary syndrome (ACS) 226
Acute LVF 234
Hypertension and accelerated
   hypertension 235
Atrial fibrillation 240
Acute severe asthma 242
Pneumonia 244
COPD exacerbation 247
Pulmonary embolism 248
Acute upper GI haemorrhage 249
Hypoglycaemia 251
DKA 252
HHS (HONK) 255
Addisonian crisis 256
Myxoedema coma/crisis 257
Thyrotoxic crisis/thyroid storm 257
Meningitis 258

Seizures   260
TIA and stroke   261
Severe sepsis or septic shock   264
Febrile neutropenia   265
Urinary tract infections   265
GI infections   266
TB pneumonia   267
Malaria   267
Electrolyte disturbances   269
Alcohol withdrawal   271
Acute poisoning   274

CARDIOPULMONARY RESUSCITATION (CPR)

See algorithms for adult BLS and adult ALS inside front cover.

CPR is required if a collapsed person is unconscious or unresponsive, not breathing, and has no pulse in a large artery such as the carotid or femoral. The following may also be seen: occasional/ineffectual (agonal) gasps, pallor or cyanosis, dilated pupils, or a brief tonic grand mal seizure.

WHEN TO STOP

Survival from out-of-hospital cardiac arrest is greatest when:

- Event is witnessed.
- Bystander starts resuscitation, even if only chest compressions (doubles or triples survival rate).
- Heart arrests in VF or VT (22% survival).
- Defibrillation is carried out at an early stage, with successful cardioversion achieved within 3–5 min (49–75% survival), and not more than 8 min.
  - each minute of delay before defibrillation reduces survival to discharge by 10–12%
  - survival after more than 12 min of VF in adults is less than 5%.

ANAPHYLAXIS

See anaphylaxis algorithm inside front cover.

Anaphylaxis: is an allergic/immunological, IgE-mediated, multi-system reaction that may rapidly follow drug ingestion, particularly parenteral penicillin, a bee or wasp sting, or food such as nuts and seafood.

Non-IgE-mediated, non-allergic anaphylaxis: (previously termed an anaphylactoid reaction) is a clinically identical reaction most commonly following radio-contrast media, or aspirin/NSAID exposure, but which is not triggered by IgE antibodies.

These are both treated the *same* way, with first line drugs including adrenaline, oxygen, and fluids (if shock).

ACUTE CORONARY SYNDROME (ACS)

ACS encompasses the following:

1   **STEMI:** ST elevation myocardial infarction (see p. 230).
2   **NSTEMI:** Non-ST elevation MI; troponin (T or I) +ve.
3   **UA(P):** Unstable angina (pectoris); troponin (T or I) −ve. Angina at rest, increasing in frequency or duration, or abnormality found on provocation testing such as EST.

Clues: Hx of IHD or angina, N&V, sweating, LVF (see p. 234), arrhythmia. Remember atypical pain/silent infarct in DM, elderly or if ↓GCS.

Differential diagnosis of chest pain: see table 4.1 for other causes of chest pain. Suspect and rule out ACS if no alternate diagnosis is made.

ALL ACS

- **O₂:** Do *not* administer routinely, but give supplemental oxygen only if oxygen saturation <93%, or evidence of shock.
- **Aspirin:** 300 mg po stat (chew/dispersible form) unless CI. Check has not already been given by paramedics or GP.
- **Clopidogrel:** 300 mg po (some give 600 mg, esp if immediate PCI planned). Prasugrel (60 mg po loading dose) and ticagrelor (reversible) are alternative ADP-receptor blocking antiplatelet agents used in combination with aspirin – check local guidelines for which to use.
- **Opiate:** most UK centres give diamorphine 2.5–5 mg iv + antiemetic (e.g. metoclopramide 10 mg iv), repeated according to response. Use morphine as an alternative, initially 3–5 mg iv, repeated every few minutes until pain free.
- **GTN:** 1–2 sprays or sl tablets (max 1.2 mg). If pain resistant or if LVF develops, set up ivi titrated to BP and pain. NB: As can

Table 4.1 Causes of chest pain in the ED

Diagnosis	Classic history	Physical examination	Diagnostic testing
Acute coronary syndrome (see p. 226)	Band-like, tight, or pressure pain with radiation to neck and arms, sweating, dyspnoea, cardiac risk factors	May be normal, or may have evidence of heart failure, hypotension	Cardiac biomarkers, ECG, possibly stress testing
Pulmonary embolus (see p. 248)	Sudden onset, pleuritic pain, dyspnoea, risks for venous thrombo-embolism	Tachycardia, tachypnoea, pleural rub, low-grade fever	CXR, V/Q scan, CTPA
Aortic dissection	Sudden, sharp, tearing pain radiating to back, neurologic symptoms	Unequal pulses or BP, new murmur, bruits	CXR, echocardiogram, CT angiogram
Pericarditis	Pleuritic, positional ache, worse lying down	Fever, pericardial rub, tachycardia	ECG, CXR, echocardiogram
Pneumonia (see p. 244)	Cough, fever, dyspnoea, pleuritic pain, malaise	Fever, hypoxia, tachypnoea, tachycardia, abnormal breath sounds	CXR, WCC
Pneumothorax	Pleuritic pain, dyspnoea	Reduced breath sounds over hemithorax	CXR

(Continued)

Table 4.1 (Continued) Causes of chest pain in the ED

Diagnosis	Classic history	Physical examination	Diagnostic testing
Oesophageal rupture (Boerhaave's syndrome)	Constant, severe retrosternal pain, dysphagia	Subcutaneous emphysema	CXR, CT chest
Gastrointestinal causes	Burning, nocturnal pain, gastrointestinal symptoms	Abdominal tenderness, rebound or guarding	Lipase, AXR, ultrasound
Musculoskeletal causes	Pain increased with movement or muscular activity	Chest-wall tenderness to palpation (may occur in ACS!)	Normal

ACS, acute coronary syndrome; AXR, abdominal X-ray; BP, blood pressure; CT, computerized tomography; CTPA, computerized tomography pulmonary angiogram; CXR, chest X-ray; ECG, electrocardiograph; V/Q, ventilation perfusion; WCC, white cell count.

↓BP, do not give if systolic ≤100 mmHg (esp if combined with an antihypertensive), or inferior infarct is suspected (i.e. RV involvement).

Date/ Time	Infusion Fluid	Volume	Additives If Any Drug and Dose	Rate of Admin	Dura-tion	Dr's Signature	Time Start-ed	Time Com-pleted	Set Up by Sig-nature	Batch No.
25/12	N. Saline	50 ml	50 mg GTN	0–10 ml/hr*		TN				
*TITRATE TO PAIN: Stop if systolic BP < 100 mmHg										

Figure 4.1 Drug chart showing how to write up GTN ivi.

Consider:

- β-*blocker*: unless CI (see propranolol p. 139), esp beware ☠ asthma, acute LVF ☠, ↓BP (systolic <100 mmHg), ↓HR (<60/min), 2nd-/3rd-degree HB; get senior help if in doubt.
  - *Can be given po or iv*: often recommended to give iv for STEMI, and po for NSTEMI and UAP. In acute settings, metoprolol is a drug of choice as short $t_{1/2}$ means it wears off quickly if acute LVF develops (in chronic LVF use bisoprolol). Consult local protocol or get senior advice if unsure.
  - *iv*: metoprolol 1–5 mg iv, giving 1–2 mg aliquots at a time while monitoring BP and HR. Repeat to max 15 mg, stopping when BP ≤100 mmHg or HR ≤60. Then decide on starting metoprolol po.
  - *po*: metoprolol 25–50 mg bd. If haemodynamically stable 24 h later, change to long-acting β-blocker, e.g. bisoprolol 5–10 mg od.
  - If already on β-blocker, ensure dose is adequate to control HR.
  - If β-blocker CI and ↑HR consider Ca^{2+} blocker (e.g. diltiazem SR 60–120 mg bd) and get senior ± cardiology advice.
- *iv fluid*: cautious bolus if RV infarct. *Clues*: ↓BP with no pulmonary oedema, ↑JVP, and inferior or posterior ECG Δs (esp ST elevation ≥1 mm in aVF). If suspect, do right-sided ECG and look for ↑ST in V4 i.e. –V4R lead. Then avoid vasodilating drugs (esp nitrates and ACE-i), and care with β-blockers (can ⇒HB).

- *Insulin*: for type I DM and type II DM, or non-diabetics with CBG >11 on admission. Aim to keep CBG in normal range using conventional sliding scale, although this and GIK ivi remain contentious. Contact CCU for advice.

STEMI

- *Reperfusion therapy*: *primary PCI is the preferred option, but if unavailable within 90 min or CI consider thrombolysis.* NB: starting either ASAP is paramount ('time is muscle'!) ∴ if appropriate, initiate/organise during above steps. See below for thrombolysis indications, CIs and choice of agent.
- *Heparin*: iv heparin is given with *recombinant* thrombolytics for 24–48 h to avoid the rebound hypercoagulable states they can cause, but is *not* needed with *streptokinase.*
- If ongoing chest pain or unresolving ECG Δs, get senior advice on further anticoagulation and arrange rescue PCI.
- Consider (consult cardiology on-call/local protocol when unsure):
  - *Glycoprotein IIb/IIIa inhibitor*: esp if not thrombolysed (CI or presentation too late), or PCI planned and still unstable. Use with caution (esp <48 h post-thrombolysis).
  - Rescue PCI: esp if thrombolysis given and doesn't ↓pain (e.g. within 90 min) or non-resolving (e.g ≤50% reduction in) ST elevation on ECG.

Thrombolysis:

Indications (from Resuscitation Council (UK) guidelines 2010):

- Onset of (cardiac) chest pain <12 h + Hx compatible with MI + one of:
  - ST elevation ≥2 mV (= 2 small squares) in ≥2 adjacent chest leads
  - ST elevation >1 mV (= 1 small square) in >2 limb leads
  - new LBBB: must assume it is new if cannot prove is old
- Onset of chest pain 12–24 h ago, but evidence of an evolving infarct, e.g. ongoing chest pain or worsening ECG changes. Get cardiology advice first.

Note:

- Primary PCI is still 1st line treatment for all patients presenting with acute MI if available.
- Posterior infarct is also widely considered to be an indication for primary PCI or thrombolysis. Diagnosis can be hard (look for ST depression + dominant R wave in V1–3); get cardiology advice if suspicious.
- Treatment needs to be started ASAP as 'door to needle time' should be <30 min.

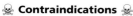 Contraindications

From ESC guidelines 2012 (with permission from *European Heart Journal* 2012; **33**: 2569–2619). As local guidelines/checklists often exist use these if available: consult cardiology ± haematology on-call if in any doubt.

Absolute

- Intracranial haemorrhage or stroke of unknown origin at any time
- Ischaemic stroke in preceding 6 months
- CNS damage, atrioventricular malformation or neoplasm
- Major trauma/surgery/head injury in preceding 3 weeks
- GI bleeding within the last month
- Known bleeding disorder (excluding menses)
- Aortic dissection
- Non-compressible punctures in last 24 h (e.g. liver biopsy, lumbar puncture).

Relative

- TIA in past 6 months
- Refractory hypertension (systolic >180 mmHg and/or diastolic >110 mmHg)
- Oral anticoagulant therapy
- Pregnancy or within 1-wk post partum
- Prolonged or traumatic resuscitation
- Advanced liver disease
- Infective endocarditis
- Active peptic ulcer.

Choice of agent

Use your hospital's protocol when one exists – contact CCU or look on your hospital intranet for details.

Choose between a recombinant thrombolytic such as alteplase, reteplase or tenecteplase and streptokinase. Each hospital tends to stock one in particular; see individual drug entries in common drugs section for dosing regimen.

NICE guidance recommends that, in hospitals, the choice of agent should take account of:

- 'The likely balance of benefit and harm (e.g. stroke) to which each of the thrombolytic agents would expose the individual patient.' Recombinant forms (compared with streptokinase) are probably more efficacious and have ↓incidence of allergic reactions, CCF and bleeding other than stroke. However they have ↑incidence of haemorrhagic stroke.
- 'Current UK clinical practice, in which it is accepted that patients who have previously received streptokinase should not be treated with it again.' Streptokinase is less effective and more likely to cause allergic reaction after first administration (due to Ab production). Do not give if patient has been given it in the past.
- 'The hospital's arrangements for reducing delays in the administration of thrombolysis.' Some agents are quicker to set up and administer and this can reduce 'door to needle' time.

Heparin co-therapy
Recombinant forms always need concurrent iv heparin for 24–48 h (this does not apply for *streptokinase*). Use your hospital's CCU protocol if one exists.

Otherwise use *ESC guideline*: 60 units/kg (max 4000 units) iv bolus, then ivi at 12 units/kg/h for 24–48 h (max 1000 units/h). Monitor APTT at 3, 6, 12, 24 and 48 h, with target APTT (≠APTT ↑ratio!) of 50–70 sec. NB: this is different from 'standard' iv heparin regimens (see p. 210).

NSTEMI or UAP

- *Heparin*: LMWH, e.g. enoxaparin 1 mg/kg bd sc or fondaparinux 2.5 mg od sc esp if PCI planned in 1st 24–36 h after symptom onset.
- Consider (consult local protocol/cardiology on-call if unsure):
  - *Glycoprotein IIb/IIIa inhibitor*: if high risk* (defined by ACC/ESC as: haemodynamic or rhythm instability, persistent pain, acute or dynamic ECG Δs, TIMI risk score >3 (see below), ↓left ventricular function, ↑troponin) and/or ongoing chest pain/ECG Δs.

TIMI risk score for NSTEMI/UA. (Source: Antman E, et al. JAMA 2000; 284: 835–842).

1 point for presence of each of the following:

- Age ≥65 yrs
- ≥3 of following risk factors for IHD: FHx of IHD, ↑BP, ↑cholesterol, DM, current smoker
- Prior coronary stenosis (≥50% occlusion)
- Aspirin use in past 7 days
- Severe angina (≥2 episodes w/in 24 h)
- ST segment deviations (↑ or ↓) at presentation
- +ve serum cardiac markers (troponin).

Score >3 indicates ↑risk (20% or more) of developing cardiac events and death.

SECONDARY PREVENTION

In all ACS unless CI or already started – will be commenced on CCU / medical ward:

- *Next day*: aspirin 75 mg od, 'statin' (e.g. simvastatin 40 mg od) and clopidogrel 75 mg od (for 1 yr[NICE]). If prasugrel used (instead of clopidogrel) 10 mg od unless >75 yrs or <60 kg in which case use 5 mg od.
- *When stable*: β-blocker (e.g. bisoprolol 1.25 mg od once any LVF clears; see above for CI) and ACE-i (e.g. ramipril 2.5 mg

bd po started 2–10 days after MI, then 5 mg bd after 2 days
if tolerated). Consider addition of aldosterone antagonist
eplerenone in established LVF (EF <40 %) and signs of HF after
3 days (closely monitor U&Es).
- Diet/lifestyle Δs (↓Wt, diet Δs, ↑exercise, ↓smoking, etc).

ACUTE LVF

Clues: SOB, S_3 or S_4 gallop, pulmonary oedema with widespread
rales (can ⇒ pink frothy sputum if severe), ↓BP, Hx of IHD, ↑JVP
and peripheral oedema (if also RVF, i.e. CCF).

- O_2: 60–100% to maintain SaO_2 >95% (care if COPD) and keep
  patient upright.
- *Furosemide*: 20–40 mg iv initially (max 100 mg in 1st 6 h);
  consider repeat doses or ivi (5–40 mg/h) later. If not 'in extremis',
  ↓doses (40 or 60 mg) od and monitor urine output.
- *GTN ivi*: see p. 229.
- *Diamorphine* : 0.5–1 mg iv (at 0.5 mg/min) or morphine 1–2.5
  mg iv (1 mg/min) + metoclopramide 10 mg iv. Beware resp
  depression, esp if need to use NIV.

Not responding/worsens. Get senior help and consider:

- *Non-invasive ventilation* (NIV) as continuous positive airways
  pressure (CPAP). Staff must be familiar with its use.
- *Inotropes*: e.g. dobutamine (2–20 microgram/kg/min) if ↓BP, via
  central line. If patient is this sick, will also be needed for CVP
  measurement and CCU care (± intra-aortic balloon pump). Get
  cardiology involved.
- *Underlying cause*: AMI, arrhythmia (esp AF), valve rupture (try
  to listen for new murmur), ↑↑BP; or non-cardiogenic i.e. sepsis,
  ARDS, ICH, AKI with volume overload, hypoalbuminaemia,
  smoke inhalation, and poisons/OD (e.g. aspirin).

ACE-i: once stable and if no CI, e.g. enalapril 2.5 mg od (↑later).

HYPERTENSION AND ACCELERATED HYPERTENSION

HYPERTENSION

Adapted with permission from NICE www.nice.org.uk/guidance/
CG127 (2011 revision).

When to treat

Most hypertensive patients in the ED do *not* require treatment, as
they are usually asymptomatic. *Never* treat a single high BP unless
there are assoc symptoms or signs.

A decision to treat is thus best made by the GP, in the medical
clinic or on the ward, and will depend on severity and other factors:

Severity	Clinic BP[a]		ABPM[b] or HBPM[c]	Drug therapy[d]
Normotensive	<140/90	OR	<135/85	No
Stage 1	≥140/90	AND	≥135/85	Consider[e]
Stage 2	≥160/100	AND	≥150/95	Yes
Severe	SBP≥180 OR DBP≥110			Yes, immediate

[a] All measurements are in mmHg. If 1st clinic BP ≥140/90, repeat. If 2nd measurement
much lower that 1st take 3rd reading; lowest of 2nd & 3rd is taken as clinic BP. Clinic BP
persistently ≥140/90 should be confirmed by ABPM/HBPM unless ≥180 OR 110.

[b] Ambulatory BP monitoring (ABPM); average of ≥14 daytime readings.

[c] Home BP monitoring (HBPM); average of ≥4 days a.m. & evening readings, excluding 1st
days readings.

[d] Encourage lifestyle modifications for all ↑BP: ↓salt, ↓Wt, ↓alcohol, stop smoking, ↑exercise,
↑fresh fruit/vegetables, ↓intake of total and unsaturated fat. For Stage 1 without CVD or
target organ damage*, these measures can be tried before drug therapy.

[e] Indicated in those <80 years old if established CVD or DM, or evidence of target organ
damage*, or 10-yr CVD risk ≥20% (see risk charts at back of BNF or at http://www.bhsoc.org/
Cardiovascular_Risk_Charts_and_Calculators.stm).

*HF, established IHD, CVA/TIA, chronic kidney disease (CKD, ↓GFR, ↑creatinine or proteinuria/
microalbuminuria), hypertensive/diabetic retinopathy or LVH.

Aim for: Clinic BP ≤140/90 mmHg if <80 y.o.; <150/90 if ≥80 y.o. If CKD ≤140/90mmHg. If DM or CKD and >1g/24h proteinuria (urinary albumin:creatinine ratio >70 mg/mmol or protein:creatinine ratio >100 mg/mmol) ≤130/80 mmHg. Consider ABPM/HBPM in those with white coat effect. If target not achieved with Step 1, progress to Step 2 etc.

Primary causes: look for and exclude (esp if treatable), e.g. RAS, Conn's (1° hyperaldosteronism), ↑Ca^{2+}, Cushing's, phaeo (esp if variable BP, headaches, sweats, palpitations), oestrogen-containing contraceptive pills and recreational drugs (e.g. alcohol, cocaine, amphetamines).

NB: stress (inc 'white-coat HTN'), recreational drug use and withdrawal (esp alcohol) are common temporary causes seen in the ED.

Practice points

• It is *rare* to ever need to start new antihypertensive treatment in the ED. Leave this to the medical clinic/ward.

• If you do start treatment make a *written* Rx plan for (other) doctors, nurses and patient. Include target BP and how Rx should change if it is not achieved.

• Age/ethnic origin influence response to drugs (see table below).

• A single agent is rarely successful at achieving target BP. Rather than ↑ing doses, add 2nd and 3rd agents, which often work in an additive or complementary fashion, esp if table below used.

• Exclude/minimise dietary salt and NSAID (inc unrecognised 'over-the-counter') use, as reason for poor treatment response.

Choice of drug: rational combination therapy[NICE/2011]

Step	Younger (<55 yrs) *and* non-black	Older (≥55 yrs) *or* black[a]
1	A[b]	C[c]
2	A[b] + C[c]	
3	A[b] + C + D	
4	Resistant hypertension[d]	

[a] Black = African (not Asian) origin.

[b] β-Blockers are an alternative to ACE-i/ARBS but see notes below.

[c] If C not suitable (e.g. presence or risk of LVF, intolerance, oedema) offer D [thiazide-like diuretic].

[d] Ensure on optimal/best tolerated doses of A+C+D. Check adherence to lifestyle advice. If K+ ≤4.5 mmol/L add spironolactone (e.g. 25 mg od). 💀 CKD, due to risk of ↑K+. If K+ >4.5 mmol/L consider higher dose thiazide diuretic (e.g. chlortalidone 50–200 mg od), α-blocker or β-blocker. Consider missed 1° cause ± specialist referral.

☺ good for, ☹ avoid/caution, 💀 *beware!*

- *A = ACE-i*, e.g. ramipril initially 2.5 mg od (1.25 mg if elderly or CKD). ☺ CKD (but *with caution!*), HF, DM, IHD. ☹ PVD (as assoc with RAS*) 💀. Pregnancy, bilateral RAS*. (*Must monitor U&Es 2 wks after starting, then regularly, esp if vasculopathy or CKD*).

  Angiotensin II receptor blockers (ARBs) preferred to ACE-I in black person of African or Caribbean origin, or if ACE-i not tolerated (esp dt dry cough). Use low cost ARBs. Monitor as for ACE-i. Do not combine ACE-i + ARB.

- *B = β-blocker*, e.g. atenolol 50 mg od. ☺ younger patients with ↑sympathetic drive or childbearing potential, IHD (post-MI/angina), chronic stable LVF, intolerance to ACE-i or ARB. If used for Step 1, add C for Step 2 (in preference to D) to ↓ risk of DM. ☹ dyslipidaemia, PVD, DM (unless also IHD), if on diltiazem. 💀 asthma/COPD, HB, acute LVF, if on verapamil.

- C = *Ca²⁺ -channel blocker*: dihydropyridines such as amlodipine 5 mg or nifedipine LA (e.g. Adalat LA 20–30 mg od) usually 1st-line. ☹oedema, polyuria. ☠ aortic stenosis, recent ACS.

  If IHD 'rate-limiting' types (verapamil, diltiazem) often preferred. ☠ HF, HB, if on other rate-limiting drugs (esp β-blockers).

- D = *thiazide-like diuretic*, e.g. indapamide SR 1.5 mg od or chlorthalidone 25 mg od. ☺ oedema/HF. ☹dyslipidaemia. ☠ gout. If patient on conventional thiazide diuretic (e.g. bendroflumethiazide) and BP controlled, continue this.

NB: starting doses only are given; see main drugs section or SPCs/BNF for doses thereafter.

ACCELERATED HYPERTENSION

Various terms are used sometimes interchangeably such as severe hypertension, hypertensive urgency, hypertensive emergency, hypertensive crisis and malignant hypertension.

The key is whether there is acute end-organ damage or dysfunction. Get senior help before embarking on any treatment – it may be unnecessary!

Practice points

- Accelerated hypertension Dx: diastolic >120 mmHg (or systolic >220 mmHg) *plus* grade III (haemorrhages/exudates) or IV (papilloedema) hypertensive retinopathy.

- ☠ Do not drop BP too quickly as can ⇒ MI, CVA or AKI ☠.

- Patients are often salt and water depleted (look for postural drop of >20 mmHg) *so may require fluid replacement as well as antihypertensives.*

Life-threatening target organ damage

- Encephalopathy, intracranial haemorrhage, aortic dissection, unstable angina, acute MI, acute LVF/pulmonary oedema or pre-eclampsia/eclampsia.

- Get senior help immediately and aim to ↓diastolic to 110–115 mmHg over 1–2 h (systolic to <110 mmHg in aortic dissection) and then more slowly thereafter (e.g. ↓diastolic to 100 mmHg after 48 h).

- This should always be done in the ITU/HDU/CCU setting and generally (but not always) involves an iv antihypertensive and intra-arterial invasive BP monitoring.
- Choose from nitroprusside (most commonly used but can ⇒ cyanide poisoning, esp if used in ↓GFR + may not ↓cerebral vascular resistance as well as labetalol), hydralazine (commonly used in pregnancy), labetalol (in pregnancy but can ⇒ severe ↓BP), phentolamine (esp if phaeo known/suspected), or GTN/ISDN (if pulmonary oedema).

No life-threatening target organ damage

- Uncomplicated acute kidney injury, mild LVF, etc: aim to ↓diastolic BP to 110–115 mmHg over 24–48 h using *oral* medication.
- Choose from nifedipine (e.g. Adalat Retard) 10 mg po. Monitor and reassess; consider repeat doses (e.g. after 2 h) and if required/tolerated aim to get patient on to higher doses (e.g. 20 mg tds). Tablets to be swallowed (not chewed) and avoid quick release or sl preparations. Convert to amlodipine once stable.
- If IHD consider adding β-blocker* later (e.g. atenolol 25–50 mg od).
- When nifedipine CI, consider diltiazem (e.g. 60 mg SR bd initially) or β-blocker instead*: metoprolol (e.g. 12.5–25 mg initially then tds regimen) or labetalol (e.g. 50–800 mg bd/tds) are good choices as short acting and needs no dose adjustment with ↓GFR. When BP controlled withdraw β-blocker except in IHD (risk of new-onset DM). In IHD consider converting to atenolol (e.g. 50 mg po) once stable.
- Other possibilities include ACE-i** (can ⇒ severe ↓BP; if so give iv saline) and diuretics (if patient fluid overloaded).

*If underlying cause is a phaeo (suspect when BP very variable, headaches, sweats or palpitations; get senior help): will need α-blocker (phenoxybenzamine) and may need salt supplements. If tachycardia a problem, must not give β-blocker until several days after α-blocker started.

**If cause is renal artery stenosis (suspect when other clinical vascular disease/multiple CVD risk factors/ ↓GFR): try to avoid renin system blockade (i.e. ACE-i/ARB/direct renin inhibitor) as ☠ risk of severe ↓BP) and monitor U&Es (risk of RF including delayed onset after 3–4 weeks) ☠; if used, starting dose must be low (e.g. enalapril 2.5 mg od).

ATRIAL FIBRILLATION

See ALS tachycardia algorithm on inside back cover.

Clues: Irregularly irregular ↑HR ± SOB, angina or heart failure. Confirm diagnosis with 12 lead ECGs; narrow QRS, absent P waves (esp V1), (irregularly) irregular R-R interval.

Practice point

Treatment (rate or rhythm control) depends on: presence of haemodynamic instability (systolic BP <90 mmHg), acuteness of onset (<48 h) and presence of structural heart disease (e.g. LVH: clinically/ECG/echo) or heart failure (clinically/CXR/echo).

Haemodynamically unstable patient:

- DC cardioversion; ideally after initiating anticoagulation* but this should not delay emergency intervention[NICE]. Procedural sedation will be required (see p. 182).

Haemodynamically stable patient

Acute onset (<48 h)

+ **No evidence of structural heart disease:** flecainide 100 mg bd po or 2 mg/kg iv over 30 min (max 150 mg) with appropriate antithrombotic cover (e.g. enoxaparin 1.5 mg/kg daily); seek cardiology advice if unsuccessful and consider DC cardioversion.

+ **Evidence of structural heart disease (or any doubt):** amiodarone 300 mg ivi over 20–60 min followed by 900 mg ivi over next 24 h and then 1.2–1.8 g/day (po or iv) until 10 g total. Then minimum maintenance dose (100–400 mg/day) to control sinus rhythm. If unsuccessful consider DC cardioversion.

Onset >48 h (or unknown)

+ No evidence of heart failure: β-blocker po (e.g. metoprolol 25–50 mg bd). If β-blocker CI (e.g. COPD/ asthma) use Ca^{2+} channel blocker (e.g. diltiazem MR 120 mg bd).

  + Evidence of heart failure: digoxin 250–500 microgram iv/po loading dose and two repeat half doses at 6–12 h intervals followed by appropriate maintenance dose (62.5–250 microgram). Use half the dose if elderly or RF. Monitor levels and e'lytes on the ward to avoid toxicity.

- All inpatients initially need anticoagulation (e.g. LMWH); for paroxysmal, persistent and permanent AF[NICE] use risk stratification for benefit vs haemorrhagic risk to guide thromboprophylaxis:
  - High stroke risk[NICE]: use warfarin (post stroke/TIA/TE; age ≥75 with HTN, diabetes or vascular disease; structural heart disease or LVF; $CHADS_2$* >3).
  - Moderate risk[NICE]: use warfarin or aspirin (age ≥65 + no risk factors; age <75 and HTN, diabetes or vascular disease).
  - Low risk[NICE]: use aspirin.
- When non-acute (planned) cardioversion anticoagulate ≥3 wks before (and after) cardioversion[NICE].

***CHADS_2 score for risk of stroke in (non-rheumatic) AF*:** JAMA 2001; 285: 2864–2870.

- **C**ongestive heart failure Hx = 1 point
- **H**ypertension Hx = 1 point
- **A**ge ≥ 75 = 1 point
- **D**M Hx = 1 point
- **S**troke symptoms or TIA = 2 points

ACUTE SEVERE ASTHMA

ACUTE SEVERE ASTHMA

Clues: SOB with wheeze and cannot complete sentences in 1 breath, HR ≥110/min, RR ≥25/min, SaO_2 ≥92%, PEF <50% of best*:

- Attach sats monitor.
- 40–60% O_2 through high-flow mask, e.g. Hudson mask.
- Salbutamol 5 mg neb in O_2: repeat up to every 15 min if persisting.
- Ipratropium 0.5 mg neb in O_2: repeat up to every 4–6 h if persisting or fails to respond to salbutamol.
- Prednisolone 40–50 mg po od for at least 5 days. Hydrocortisone 100 mg qds iv can be given if unable to swallow or retain tablets. Both hydrocortisone and prednisolone can be given if seriously ill.

> *Life-threatening features (critical asthma)*
>
> - PEF <33% of best*
> - O_2 sats <92%
> - PaO_2 <8.0kPa, $PaCO_2$ >4.6kPa or pH <7.35
> - Silent chest, cyanosis or ↓respiratory effort
> - ↓HR, ↓BP or dysrhythmia
> - Exhaustion, confusion or coma
>
> *or predicted best (see Figure 4.2).

LIFE-THREATENING/CRITICAL ASTHMA

🕱 NB: patient may not always *appear* that distressed, esp if silent chest 🕱), get senior help and consider the following.

- *$MgSO_4$ ivi*: 1.2–2 g over 20 min (8 mmol=2 g=4 ml of 50% solution) unlicensed indication.
- *Salbutamol ivi*: 5 microgram/kg over 10 min initially (then up to 20 microgram/min ivi according to response): back-to-back or continuous nebs now often preferred.

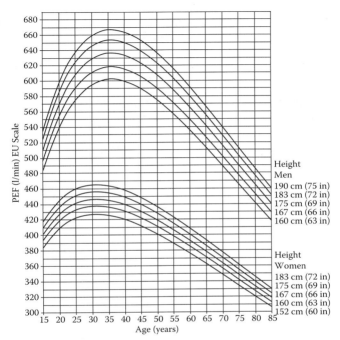

Figure 4.2 Peak expiratory flow (PEF) predictor for normal adults using European standard 'EU' (EN 13826) scale. (Adapted with permission of BMJ group from Gregg I, Nunn AJ. *BMJ* 1989; 298: 1098, corrected to the EN 13826: 2003 scale values by Clement Clarke International Ltd.)

- Call anaesthetist for consideration of ITU admission and/or intubation. Initiate these during the above steps if deteriorating.
- *Aminophylline iv*: give loading dose providing are *not* on maintenance po aminophylline/theophylline (omit if they are) 5 mg/kg iv over 20 min, then ivi at 0.5–0.7 mg/kg/h (0.3 mg/kg/h if

elderly). Risk of serious arrhythmias, hypotension, vomiting and seizures.

PNEUMONIA

COMMUNITY-ACQUIRED PNEUMONIA (CAP)

> *Severity assessment of community acquired pneumonia in hospital*[1]
> 'CURB 65' score – *1 point each for*:
>
> - **C**onfusion; MTS[2] ≤8/10 **or** *new* disorientation in time, place or person
> - **U**rea >7 mmol/l
> - **R**espiratory rate ≥30/min
> - **B**P↓: systolic <90 mmHg **or** diastolic ≤60 mmHg
> - **65**: age ≥65 yrs
>
> <2: **Non-severe***: likely to be suitable for home treatment.
> 2: **Moderate**** with *increased* risk of death: consider admission (or hospital supervised outpatient care) using clinical judgement.
> >2: **Severe**** with *high* risk of death: admit and consider HDU/ITU (esp if ≥4).
> [1]Use 'CRB 65' for assessment in the community, as does not need blood test: 0 = likely to be suitable for home treatment; 1–2 = consider hospital referral; 3–4 = urgent hospital admission.
> [2]MTS = (Abbreviated) Mental Test Score; see p. 293 for details.
> Adapted with permission of BMJ Publishing Group from BTS guidelines. *Thorax* 2001; **56** (suppl IV) and 2004 update.

Treatment
Non-severe*: amoxicillin 500 mg–1 g tds po ± clarithromycin*** 500 mg bd po (if admitted for clinical reasons).

 Severe**: co-amoxiclav 1.2 g tds iv + clarithromycin*** 500 mg bd iv. ± flucloxacillin 1 g qds iv if *S. aureus* (Hx or epidemic of 'flu). ± rifampicin 600 mg bd po/iv if *Legionella* (do urinary Ag test).

- No improvement, consider changing co-amoxiclav to tazocin (piperacillin + tazobactam).
- If risk factors, consider Rx for aspiration (see below) or TB (see p. 267).
- Use clarithromycin*** only if penicillin hypersensitivity.
- ***Clarithromycin is better tolerated than erythromycin (⇒ ↓GI upset); consult local protocol to check preference.

Causes of community-acquired pneumonia (UK adults)
- **48%** *Streptococcus pneumoniae*: esp in winter or shelters/ prison.
- **23%** **viruses**: influenza (A >> B), RSV, rhinoviruses, adenoviruses.
- **15%** *Chlamydia psittaci*: esp from animals, and only 20% from birds (less commonly *Chlamydia pneumoniae*, esp if long-term Hx and headache).
- **7%** *Haemophilus influenzae*.
- **3%** *Mycoplasma pneumoniae*: ↑s during 4-yrly epidemics.
- **3%** *Legionella pneumophila*: ↑d if recent travel (esp Turkey, Spain).
- **2%** *Moraxella catarrhalis*: ↑d in elderly.
- **1.5%** *Staphylococcus aureus*: mostly post-influenza ∴↑s in winter.
- **1.4%** **Gram-negative infection:** *Escherichia coli, Pseudomonas, Klebsiella, Proteus, Serratia.*
- **1.1%** **Anaerobes:** e.g. *Bacteroides, Fusobacterium.*
- **0.7%** *Coxiella burnetii*: ↑s in April–June and in sheep farmers.

NB: As 25% are mixed aetiology this accounts for total >100%. However, in ≥20% of cases, a causative pathogen is *not* identified. Adapted with permission of BMJ Publishing Group from Lim WS, *et al. Thorax* 2001; **56**: 296–301.

The term 'atypical pathogen' or 'atypical pneumonia' is no longer considered useful by the BTS (referring to *Mycoplasma*, *Legionella*,

Chlamydia, *Coxiella*), as there is no clinical presentation characteristic of the pneumonias they cause.

HOSPITAL-ACQUIRED PNEUMONIA

See below for typical causes.

Non-severe: co-amoxiclav 625 mg tds po.

Severe: co-amoxiclav 1.2 g tds iv; or tazocin (piperacillin + tazobactam) 4.5 g tds iv if *Pseudomonas* suspected; or meropenem 1 g tds if penicillin allergy.

DO NOT prescribe meropenem if history of anaphylactic or accelerated allergic reaction – discuss alternatives with microbiologist.

+ gentamicin if septic shock or failure to improve.

+ metronidazole 500 mg tds ivi if aspiration suspected (controversial).

MRSA: teicoplanin/vancomycin if confirmed colonisation/infection.

> *Causes of hospital-acquired pneumonia*
> - *Simple*: (w/in 7 days of admission): *H. influenzae*, *S. pneumoniae*, *S. aureus*, Gram-negative organisms.
> - *Complicated**: Gram-negative organisms (esp *P. aeruginosa*), *Acinetobacter*, MRSA.
> - *Anaerobic***: *Bacteroides*, *Fusobacterium*.
> - *Special situations*:
>   1 Head trauma, coma, DM, RF: consider *S. aureus*.
>   2 Mini-epidemics in hospitals: consider *Legionella*.
> * > 7 days after admission, recent multiple antibiotics or complex medical Hx (e.g. recent ITU/recurrent admissions or severe comorbidity).
> **esp if risk of aspiration, recent abdominal surgery, bronchial obstruction/poor dentition.
> Reproduced with permission from Hammersmith Hospitals NHS Trust Clinical Management Guidelines & Formulary 2001.

Aspiration pneumonia

Treat as for community- or hospital-acquired pneumonia, + metronidazole 500 mg tds ivi or 400 mg tds po.

Cavitating pneumonia

Co-amoxiclav 1.2 g tds iv (or flucloxacillin 1 g qds iv).

- Exclude TB with sputum microscopy and Ziehl–Neelsen staining, culture and PCR/Heaf test ± pleural Bx.
- Consider septic emboli as a cause, e.g. from right-sided endocarditis.
- If MRSA suspected/confirmed use vancomycin iv plus rifampicin po.

> *'TANKS'* Causes of cavitation: **TB**, *Aspergillus, Nocardia, Klebsiella, S. aureus* (and *Pseudomonas*).

COPD EXACERBATION

Clues: Sudden worsening of SOB, productive cough, wheeze, RR >25/min, HR >110 in a patient with emphysema, chronic bronchitis ± asthma.

Treatment

- Attach sats monitor and do baseline ABGs.
- **28% O_2 *via Venturi mask***, which should be *prescribed on drug chart*. ↑dose cautiously if hypoxia continues, but repeat ABGs to ensure CO_2 not ↑ing and (more importantly) pH not ↓ing.
- *Salbutamol 5 mg neb* in O_2: repeat up to every 15 min if ill (seldom necessary to give >hourly).
- *Ipratropium 0.5 mg neb* in O_2: repeat up to every 4–6 h if ill.
- *Prednisolone 30 mg po* then od for ⩽2 wks (usually 7–10 days). Can give 1st dose as hydrocortisone 200 mg iv – rarely used now unless unable to swallow.

- *Doxycycline 200 mg od po* (1st-line), or *amoxicillin/co-amoxiclav* (2nd-line), if 2 out of 3 of Hx of ↑ing SOB, ↑ing volume or ↑ing purulence of sputum.

Not improving, consider

- *Aminophylline ivi*: see Mx of asthma (p. 243) for details.
- *Assisted non-invasive ventilation*: CPAP if just ↓PaO_2 or NIV (BIPAP) if also ↑$PaCO_2$
- *Doxapram* if NIV not available. Get senior advice and or ITU involved.
- *Intubation*: discuss with ITU/anaesthetist.

PULMONARY EMBOLISM

Practice points

- Important symptoms are dyspnoea (73%), chest pain (66% – *not* always pleuritic), cough (37%), apprehension, sweating, haemoptysis and syncope.
- Important signs are tachypnoea > 20/min (70%), crepitations (51%), tachycardia (30%), low grade fever.
- Important laboratory findings are atelectasis or parenchymal abnormality on CXR, PaO_2 under 80 mmHg in absence of lung disease.
- ECG: sinus tachycardia common; AF, RAD, RBBB. Note $S_1Q_3T_3$ is neither sensitive nor specific.
- Hospital mortality is 5% or less.

NB: Absence of dyspnoea plus tachypnoea > 20 / min has a negative predictive value (NPV) for PE of 90%; absence of these and pleuritic pain has NPV of 97%; with absence of CXR changes or a low PaO_2 as well virtually excluding a PE.

Treatment

- *60–100% O_2* if hypoxic. Care if COPD (difficult to know when to suspect PE).

- *Anticoagulation*: LMWH, e.g. enoxaparin or dalteparin. Once PE confirmed, load with warfarin, usually on medical ward (see p. 212). Consider iv heparin if surgery being contemplated, or rapid reversal may be required*.
- *Analgesia*: if xs pain or distress, try paracetamol/ibuprofen 1st; consider opiates if severe or no response (💀 can ⇒ respiratory depression💀).

Massive PE: with worsening hypoxia or cardiovascular instability (↓BP, RV strain/failure) has mortality 30–50%. Seek senior help and consider:

- *Fluids ± inotropes*: if systolic BP <90 mmHg
- *Thrombolysis (e.g. alteplase)*: if ↓BP ± collapse
- *Vena cava filter*: introduced at bedside under ultrasound guidance
- *Embolectomy**: seek urgent cardiothoracic opinion.

ACUTE UPPER GI HAEMORRHAGE

Clues: Haematemesis (fresh red or coffee grounds), and/or melaena/ haematochezia; also consider as differential in unexplained sudden collapse/hypovolaemic shock – at least do a PR.

ASSESS SEVERITY OF BLEEDING
- Pulse >100 or ↑ of >20 bpm
- Systolic BP <100 mmHg (or postural drop >10 mmHg)
- Urine output <0.5 ml/kg/h (30 ml/h)
- Cold, clammy peripheries
- Age over 65 yrs
- Suspected varices – previous variceal bleed, cirrhosis with portal hypertension e.g. alcoholic/hepatitis C, B and D/autoimmune (primary biliary or chronic active hepatitis).

MANAGEMENT

- **Resuscitate:**
  - Give high-flow O_2
  - Insert 2 wide bore intravenous cannulae (14-/16-gauge), and take blood for FBC, INR, U&E, LFT + group and save or cross match 2–6 units depending on severity of bleed.
  - Fluid iv (crystalloid/colloid then blood) to maintain systolic BP >100, but *avoid* over-transfusion in elderly/heart or renal disease. Consider CVP line.
  - Correct clotting with iv fresh frozen plasma if INR >1.5 (NB: although vit K reverses warfarin, it does not alone improve clotting problems due to liver cell failure).
- **Monitor:**
  - Pulse, BP, urine output (consider catheter)
  - Intra-arterial line (suspected varices).
- **Drugs:**
  - Significant non-variceal bleed, give omeprazole 80 mg iv over 40–60 min, then ivi 8 mg/hr for 72 hrs (unlicensed indication, usually following endoscopic treatment)
  - Give 2 mg terlipressin iv 'stat' if variceal bleed suspected (and continue qds – NB: caution in IHD)
  - Suspected variceal bleeds should also receive a short course of prophylactic antibiotics active against Gram negative bacteria to reduce risk spontaneous bacterial peritonitis e.g ceftriaxone 1 g iv, or ciprofloxacin/norfloxacin
  - Stop antihypertensives, diuretics, NSAIDs, anticoagulants.
- **Endoscopy** – Arrange urgently if:
  - Variceal bleed suspected
  - Continued bleeding requiring >4 units blood to maintain systolic BP >100 mmHg
  - Re-bleed after resuscitation
  - Pre-OGD Rockall score $\geq$2 (see *below*).

Rockall score (*Gut* 1996; **38**: 316–321).

		Score			
	Variable	**0**	**1**	**2**	**3**
Pre-OGD Score	Age	<60	60–79	>80	
	Shock	sBP>100; HR<100	sBP>100; HR<100	sBP<100;	
	Comorbidity	nil major		HF, IHD, or any major comorbidity	RF, LF, disseminated malignancy
Post-OGD Score	Diagnosis	Mallory-Weisstear, no lesion, no SRH	All other Dx	Malignancy of upper GI tract	
	Major SRH	None or dark spot only		Blood in upper GI tract, adherent clot, visible or spurting vessel	

OGD = Oesophago gastro duodenoscopy; sBP = systolic blood pressure; SRH = stigmata of recent haemorrhage.
Pre-OGD score 0 or 1 assoc with <2.5% mortality. Can usually be safely endoscoped on the next available list (but w/in 24 hours).
Pre-OGD score >2 assoc with >5% mortality. May require urgent endoscopy.

HYPOGLYCAEMIA

Treat if <3 mmol/l or symptoms: ↑sympathetic drive (↑HR, sweating, aggression/behavioural Δs), seizures or confusion/↓GCS.

- *Glucose orally*: esp sugary drink, mouth gel (e.g. hypostop/ glucogel) or dextrose tablets. Omit this step if confusion/↓GCS, but useful if given at first sign symptoms.
- *Glucose 20–50 ml of 50%* iv stat via large iv cannula. Then flush with saline as 50% glucose is viscous and hypertonic. Repeat if necessary. Can give 5–10% glucose ivi if only mild symptoms or until 50% glucose found, but beware of fluid overload in HF.
- *Glucagon 1 mg* im/iv stat: if symptomatic low glucose or no iv access. Give oral carbohydrate within 10–30 min to prevent recurrence.

NB: look for and correct underlying causes, esp DM Rx (missed meal/undue exertion/excessive insulin), alcohol withdrawal, liver failure, aspirin/sulphonylurea poisoning, and rarely Addison's disease or pituitary insufficiency. If dt sulphonylureas, relapse is common and will need admission.

DKA

Practice points

- *Diagnostic criteria*: include triad of hyperglycaemia, acidaemia and ketonaemia: BG >11.1 mmol/l; pH <7.3 and/or HCO_3 <15 mmol/l; +ve ketones with serum ⩾3 mmol/l or urine dipstick ⩾2+. (NB: urinalysis may miss 3-β hydroxybutyrate early).
- *Precipitating causes*: new diagnosis of diabetes (10–27%), infection (35%), inadequate insulin (30%), surgery, trauma, alcohol, cocaine, other drugs such as steroids/thiazides/ pentamidine. NB: no cause in 19–38%, but poor compliance/ economic reasons frequent.

Clues: Kussmaul's (deep/rapid) breathing, ketotic breath; thirst, polydipsia/polyuria then nausea, vomiting and abdominal pain; dehydration with tachycardia ± hypotension; confusion/↓GCS.

'Joint British Diabetes Societies Inpatient Care Group' published UK guidelines for the Mx of DKA in adults in March 2010 (http://www.diabetes.org.uk/Documents/) or (http://eng.mapofmedicine.com/evidence/map/diabetes4.html). These recommend a fixed rate insulin ivi rather than sliding scale; blood ketone measurement to guide treatment; bedside glucose and ketone meters when available; and use of venous rather than arterial blood gases.

These are increasingly being incorporated into local guidelines, and the treatment below reflects this. However *follow your local diabetes team protocol(s) where applicable*.

Management

- *Initial measures*: O_2 if hypoxic, weigh patient (if possible), 2 wide bore iv cannulae. Consider NGT (if coma), and central line (esp if ↓↓pH or Hx of HF), but urinary catheter usually sufficient.
- *Initial Ix*: CBG then venous BG, U&Es, venous blood gases (ABG if hypoxic), blood ketones, FBC, blood cultures (infection suspected), ECG, CXR, urinalysis and culture.
- *Ongoing biochemical monitoring*: hourly CBG and ketones (bedside if available), venous blood gas (for pH, bicarbonate and K^+) hourly for 1st 2 h, then 2-hourly.
- *Iv fluids and K^+*: initially 0.9% saline guided by pulse, BP, urine output ± CVP. Typical deficits include 100 ml/kg H_2O, 7–10 mmol/kg Na^+ and 3–5 mmol/kg K^+. Thus the following is a guide:
  - *Systolic BP <90 mmHg*: 500 ml 0.9% saline over 15 min. If BP remains <90 mmHg repeat this but call for senior help.
  - *Otherwise* give 0.9% saline more slowly, e.g. 1 litre over 1 h, then 2 litres over 4 h, then 2 litres over 8 h.
  - Add KCl once K^+ <5.5 mmol/l, as will ↓ rapidly dt insulin (but do not give KCl in 1st litre unless K^+ <3.5 mmol/l).
  - About 40 mmol/l K^+ is needed during rehydration: adjust K^+ to individual response with regular checks – best done with

blood gas machine that gives K^+ levels. Use venous samples as long as put in ABG or other heparinised syringe.

- *Insulin*: as soluble insulin ivi (e.g. Actrapid). Use a fixed rate ivi 0.1 units/kg/h (estimate Wt if necessary). Aim for:
  - ↓BG (by 3 mmol/l/h), ↓ketogenesis (↓blood ketones 0.5 mmol/l/h; if no ketone measurement: ↑bicarbonate 3 mmol/l/h), ↓K^+ (keep between 4 and 5 mmol/l).
  - If delay in ivi availability, give 0.1 units/kg im stat (↓dose if BG <20 mmol/l).
  - If patient takes long-acting insulin sc (Lantus or Levemir) continue this at usual dose/time.
  - If blood ketones not ↓ing to target, ↑insulin ivi rate by 1 unit/h.
  - Once BG <14 add 10% glucose 125 ml/h *alongside* 0.9% saline. If BG <7 do *not* stop insulin but ↑rate of glucose ivi.
  - Continue insulin ivi until blood ketones are cleared, pH normal and eating/drinking; then switch to sc regimen (see p. 205).
- *Heparin*: give LMWH until mobile (follow local guidelines – essential with HHS. See below).

Consider also

- *Antibiotics*: search for and treat infection, but note vomiting and acidosis will ↑WCC in absence of infection.
- *Pregnancy test*: for presentation of gestational diabetes.
- *HDU/ITU*: for one-to-one nursing ± ventilation (if coma–think cerebral oedema esp child/or for pulmonary oedema–rare).
- *Diabetes specialist team*: involve ASAP.
- *Bicarbonate*: very rarely needed and potentially dangerous. Get senior help if concerned about pH <7.
- *Complications*: Watch for e'lyte Δs (esp ↓K^+, ↓Na^+, ↓Mg^{2+}, ↓PO_4), TE (esp DVT/PE), *cerebral oedema* (↓GCS, papilloedema, false-localising cranial nerve palsies), *ARDS*, *infection* (esp aspiration pneumonia if ↓GCS).

HHS (HONK)

Hyperosmolar, hyperlycaemic state (HHS) – was formerly known as HONK. Usually seen in older age group than DKA, and is managed similarly but with lower rate of insulin ivi + a slower rate of rehydration.

Practice points

- Key features are severe hyperglycaemia and hyperosmolality (usually >340 mOsmol/l; calculate using $2(K^+ + Na^+)$ + urea + BG, all in mmol/l).
- Generally ↑age of patient and ↑length of Hx of decline/insidious onset (NB: may be 1st presentation and no past Hx).
- Or may be precipitated by intercurrent illness or drugs (e.g. steroids, thiazides).

Clues: as for DKA, but no ketones, normal pH, ↑glucose, ↑dehydration and ↑confusion.

Management

- *Initial measures:* as for DKA; see above.
- *iv fluids:* as for DKA, but correct dehydration *more slowly* over 2–3 days, as will have occurred more gradually, and also ↓s risk of e'lyte abnormalities.
  - A *rough* guide is 1 litre of 0.9% saline over 1 h, then 1 litre over 2 h, then 1 litre over 4 h, then over 6–8 hrs.
  - Less KCl will be needed, as less insulin will be used.
  - Can remain in circulatory collapse despite clinically adequate fluid replacement; if so, give 500 ml colloid and monitor CVP.
  - Consider 0.45% saline if Na^+ >155 mmol/l but get senior (ideally specialist) help first as rapid ↓osmolality can ⇒ cerebral oedema
- *Insulin:* commence insulin ivi but start at lower dose than DKA, e.g. 2 or 3 units/h.
  - Aim to ↓BG by 3–6 mmol/l/h and continue ivi for >24 h (adding glucose if necessary to keep BG normal).

- Seek early senior help and follow local protocols. Sliding scale insulin may be required. Discuss with diabetes team, including need for subsequent sc insulin.
- *Heparin*: usually LMWH (see p. 209). Always give, as ↑↑osmolality ⇒ ↑risk of TE (and consider TEDS).

Consider also
- *Antibiotics*: search for and treat infection, as above.
- *Complications*: watch esp for TE (CVA, IHD), AKI, cerebral oedema.

ADDISONIAN CRISIS

Clues: ↓BP, ↑HR, ↓glucose, ↓Na$^+$/↑K$^+$, ↑urea/↑ CA^{2+}, Hx of chronic high-dose steroid Rx with missed doses or intercurrent illness*.

- O_2 if hypoxic.
- *Fluids iv*: 0.9% saline ± central line if ↓↓BP.
- *Glucose iv*: if hypoglycaemic; see p. 251.
- *Steroids*: usually hydrocortisone 100 mg iv stat then qds (ensure to take a blood sample for cortisol and ACTH *before* first dose if Dx is not certain).
  - Otherwise give 1st dose as dexamethasone 8 mg iv if a Synacthen test is planned (hydrocortisone will affect test result).
  - Consider fludrocortisone once stable and on the medical ward.
- *Antibiotics*: look for and treat infection*: dipstick urine, MSU, CXR and blood cultures. If in doubt, start empiric Rx.

NB: Other pituitary hormones will need to be checked in case of other pituitary dysfunction.

MYXOEDEMA COMA/CRISIS

Clues: 'myxoedema facies' (periorbital puffiness/scanty eyebrows/facial pallor/large tongue/lemon-yellow skin tint–carotenaemia), goitre, thyroidectomy scar, ↓temperature, ↓HR, ↓reflexes, ↓glucose, slow mentation, delirium/seizures, coma. NB: Ψ features common.

- *O₂*: if hypoxic; protect airway.
- *Monitor*: pulse, BP to watch for ↓HR, ↓BP, HF.
- *Glucose iv*: if hypoglycaemic (often coexists); see p. 251.
- *0.9% saline ivi*: slowly as per individual needs (care if HF).
- *Liothyronine* (T_3 / tri-iodothyronine): 5–20 microgram ivi bd for >2 days, then gradually ↑dose with endocrinologist's advice before converting to thyroxine po.
  - Liothyronine can precipitate angina; ↓ rate ivi if occurs.
  - Thyroxine can be given 1st line instead
- *Hydrocortisone*: 100 mg iv tds, until hypopituitarism excluded (↑likelihood when no goitre or past Hx of Rx for ↑T_4).

Consider also

- *Rewarming measures*: e.g. Bair-Hugger (forced-air warming blanket), warm iv fluids / warmed humidified O_2.
- *Antibiotics*: infections are common and may have precipitated decline, so have low threshold for empirical Rx.
- *ITU/Ventilation*: condition has high mortality (25–50%).

THYROTOXIC CRISIS/THYROID STORM

Clues: ↑HR/AF, tremor, agitation, fever, abdominal pain, D&V, confusion, coma. Look for Graves' eye disease, goitre, Hx of ↓compliance with antithyroid Rx. May be precipitated in a thyrotoxic patient by intercurrent illness/trauma/surgery.

- *O₂*: if hypoxic.
- *0.9% saline ivi*: slowly as per individual needs (care if HF).

- *Hydrocortisone*: 100 mg qds iv (or dexamethasone 4 mg qds po). $\downarrow$s $T_4 \Rightarrow T_3$ conversion.
- *Propranolol 40 mg tds po*: aim for HR <100 and titrate up dose as necessary. If $\uparrow\uparrow$HR, give propranolol iv 1 mg over 1 min, repeating if necessary every 2 min to max total of 10 mg. When β-blocker CI, give diltiazem 60–120 mg qds po.
- *Carbimazole*: 15–30 mg qds po ($\downarrow$later on ward under specialist advice).
- *Lugol's solution (iodine)*: 0.1–0.3 ml tds po (normally for 1 wk). Start 4 h after carbimazole. Blocks T_4 release from gland.

Consider also
- *Treat heart failure* (common if fast AF), e.g. furosemide.
- *Digoxin /LMWH* (if AF): DC shock rarely works until euthyroid.
- *Antibiotics*: if evidence/suspicion of infection.
- *Cooling measures*: paracetamol, sponging. NB: avoid aspirin as may displace thyroxine from TBG.

If vomiting, insert NGT for drug administration and to avoid aspiration.

MENINGITIS

TREATMENT
Empirical: (until results of LP known – esp Gram stain).

- *Cefotaxime* 2 g qds ivi: Rx of choice for *N. meningitidis* (meningococcus; commonest cause in UK adults).
  - If Hx of severe hypersensitivity (e.g. anaphylaxis) to cephalosporins (or penicillin, as up to 10% also sensitive to cephalosporins) consider chloramphenicol 1 g tds/qds iv (can $\uparrow$ to 100 mg/kg/day[SPC/BNF]).
  - If allergy (but not anaphylaxis) use meropenem 2 g tds iv.

Consider also

- *Ampicillin* 2 g 4-hrly ivi + gentamicin iv if *Listeria* suspected, e.g. immunosuppression/elderly or indicative CSF with Gram-positive rods.
- *Aciclovir* 10 mg/kg over 1 h tds ivi if HSV encephalitis suspected, e.g. more prominent confusion, behavioural Δs and seizures.
- *TB Rx* (as for pneumonia): if risk factors (HIV/immunocompromise, born or lived in high prevalence country, recent pulm TB contact); or suggestive CSF findings (↑ LØ, ↑protein, ↓glucose).
    - NB: negative CSF stains for acid-fast bacilli do NOT exclude the diagnosis of TB; if clinical suspicion is high, do *not* delay Rx while awaiting microbiological confirmation. Discuss with Infectious Diseases/Microbiology early.

Causes of meningitis in the UK
Common:

- **N. meningitidis**, serotype B: majority (70–80%) of cases.
- **N. meningitidis**, serotype C: ↓ing secondary to vaccine.
- **N. meningitidis**, serotype A: ↓ing again (had been ↓ing).
- **S. pneumoniae**: stable incidence.

Rarer:

- **Listeria monocytogenes**: esp age >60 yr, ↓immunity, neonates.
- **H. influenzae**, type b: ↓ing secondary to Hib vaccine.
- **Gram-negative** bacilli (esp in neonates).

Don't forget:

- **Viral**: HSV/HZV, EBV, HIV, mumps: esp if encephalitic (↓ GCS). Less commonly entero/echo/Coxsackie/polio viruses.
- **TB**, other bacteria, e.g. *Borrelia*: esp if ↓immunity/HIV.
- **Fungi**: *Cryptococcus*, *Candida*: esp if ↓immunity/HIV.
- **Group B Streptococcus**: predominantly in neonates.
- **S. aureus**: if neurosurgery, trauma or ventricular shunt.

SEIZURES

Practice points

- *Status epilepticus* = grand mal seizure lasting >30 min **or** multiple seizures lasting >30 min without full recovery between episodes. However, > 5 min is suggested as a more practical definition to initiate treatment.
  - Mortality: 4% if last < 30 min; 35% if seizures last > 1 hr.
- *Non-convulsive status epilepticus*: consists of two categories (with vastly different aetiology according to age, and prognosis):
  - Absence seizures (petit mal): brief, sudden lapses of consciousness–'staring', that can become multiple and lead to lethargy and confusion. Are easily missed.
  - Complex partial status: prolonged or repetitive complex partial seizures (with a presumed focal onset, often temporal) that produce an 'epileptic twilight state', with fluctuating lack of responsiveness, automatisms, and confusion.
  - NB: complex partial status may also occur in post-ictal phase of multiple grand mal seizures, causing a prolonged confusional state.
  - Differentiate this from subtle status epilepticus, that occurs in the late stages of multiple grand mal seizures, as they 'burn out' and diminish (but continue).

Treatment:

- *Monitor*: attach O_2 sats, ECG and BP monitors and place in recovery position.
- *O_2*: give high-flow O_2 via Hudson mask.
- *Exclude/treat*: reversible causes esp ↓glucose (give thiamine if treating ↓glucose in alcoholic or malnourished patient), ↓O_2.
- *Terminate seizure*: lorazepam 4 mg iv over 2 min (terminates 60–90% of status epilepticus). If not available use diazepam 10 mg iv over 2 min. If no iv access consider midazolam 5–10 mg im, or buccal.
- *0.9% saline ivi*: maintain or ↑mean arterial BP to provide appropriate cerebral perfusion pressure.

- *Protect airway*: with tracheal intubation if seizures continue: call anaesthetist early if concerned.

Seizures continue

- Get senior help
- Repeat lorazepam 4 mg iv over 2 min (or alternatives as above). If no response after 5 min, call anaesthetist and give:
- Phenytoin ivi to total dose 18 mg/kg in normal saline (not compatible with glucose) at 25–50 mg/min then adjust (see p. 132).
  - Fosphenytoin iv is an alternative: see p. 77 for dose, as is different to phenytoin.
  - Monitor BP and HR (both can drop) and ECG (esp QRS, as arrhythmias may occur). Phenytoin will abort 60% of status epilepticus not terminated by lorazepam.
  - Make sure have looked for underlying cause such as head injury or ICH (need CT brain); infection (esp meningitis); alcohol toxicity or withdrawal; other drug poisoning (theophylline, isoniazid). Remember eclampsia.
- If seizures persist, consider phenobarbital ivi 15 mg/kg at 100 mg/min. Can consider giving phenobarbital before phenytoin ivi, if already taking phenytoin po (and plasma levels assumed adequate).
- Seizures still continue = refractory status epilepticus. Requires general anaesthesia with thiopental, or propofol (unlicensed indication) in ICU ideally with EEG monitoring.

TIA AND STROKE

See algorithms for TIA and for stroke on inside back cover.

Practice points

- TIA with stroke symptoms and signs (numbness, weakness or paralysis, slurred speech, blurred vision, confusion) that resolve within 24 hours (usually within 10 min) has forward risk of stroke of 3.9% at 2 days, 5.5% at 7 days and 9.2% at 90 days.

- Risk stratify using ABCD^2 score (see TIA algorithm inside back cover): admit those with score > 4 points.
  - Arrange specialist investigation within one week for those with score ≤4 points and start aspirin po.

STROKE: 80–85% infarction (thrombotic or embolic). May be eligible for time-critical thrombolysis (see below).
  - Rest 15–20% are haemorrhagic (inc SAH), with overall > 50% one month mortality. Treatment is supportive.

Management

- Determine exact time of onset of 1st symptoms. If not clear, the last time patient was known to be normal should be used.
- Ensure glucose normal (e.g. check CBG).
- Perform CT brain imaging immediately if any of the following apply^{NICE}:
  - Indications for thrombolysis (see below) or early anticoagulation treatment.
  - On anticoagulant treatment.
  - Known bleeding tendency.
  - ↓GCS (<13).
  - Unexplained progressive or fluctuating symptoms.
  - Papilloedema, neck stiffness or fever.
  - Severe headache at onset of stroke symptoms.
- Consider thrombolysis for an acute ischaemic stroke: Must be a senior doctor decision with experience in its use, ideally within a specialist stroke centre.
  - Currently only alteplase is licensed for this indication and only if given ≤3 h from symptom onset (although ECASS-III trial shows evidence of benefit ≤4.5 h).
  - Act quickly: 5% ↓ in efficacy per 5 min delay. Aim for 'door to needle' time of 30 min.
  - Indications and contraindications vary according to centre (see below). Research into risk/benefit is ongoing; always ensure you check your local protocol.

   – Consent (where possible) using latest evidence: e.g. 1:8 chance of ↑improvement and 1:30 chance of symptomatic bleed.

   – Give alteplase iv: total dose = 0.9 mg/kg (maximum 90 mg). 10% given as iv bolus over 2 min, remaining 90% given over 60 min via iv pump. Dissolve in water for injection to a concentration of 1 mg/ml or 2 mg/ml.

Indications stroke lysis	Contraindications
Clinical signs of acute stroke	Rapidly improving or minor symptoms
Clear time of onset	Stroke or serious head injury in last 3 months
Treatment within 4.5 h of onset	Past history of intracranial haemorrhage
Haemorrhage excluded on brain imaging	Recent major surgery, GI bleed, etc. BP > 185/110mmHg[a]
Age 18–80 yrs[b]	INR > 1.6 or other clotting disorder
Some centres use NIHSS to define suitable severity (e.g. score of 5–25, but can vary)	Infarction of >1/3 MCA territory seen on CT
	Seizure at onset

[a] If ↑BP is a contraindication can ↓BP with labetalol or GTN; get senior advice.
[b] Often given to older patients. MCA = middle cerebral artery

Post-thrombolysis management

- Observations: every 15 min for 2 h, every 30 min for 6 h, then hrly
- Treat ↓O$_2$/↓glucose if present
- Treat hyperglycaemia BG if >8 mmol/l
- Bed rest for 24 h (flat bed recommended initially)
- No antiplatelet therapy for 24 h. Avoid cannulas, NGTs and ivis
- If BP >180/105 mmHg, consider labetalol 10 mg iv over 1–2 min, then infusion at 2–8 mg/min. Get senior advice.
- If intracranial haemorrhage occurs (CT diagnosis), arrange 5–10 units cryoprecipitate (± platelets ± FFP) and seek neurosurgical opinion.

SEVERE SEPSIS OR SEPTIC SHOCK

Practice points
- *Severe sepsis* = known or suspected infection plus either organ dysfunction, or with features of hypotension or hypoperfusion (e.g. confusion/oliguria/raised lactate).
- *Septic shock* = a subset of severe sepsis with sepsis-induced hypotension (SBP < 90 mmHg), or hypoperfusion abnormality such as lactate ≥ 4 mmol/L persisting despite adequate fluid resuscitation (20–30 mL/kg)

Clues: evidence of infection + ↓BP (MAP <65 mmHg); serum lactate >4 mmol/l; or ↓urine output.

Management
- Get senior help urgently!
- *Oxygen*: 100% via non-rebreather mask (caution if COPD).
- *Fluids*: 1 litre of crystalloid or 300–500ml of colloid (albumin) bolus over 30 min; if still ↓BP measure CVP and consider further iv fluids (20 ml/kg) to achieve CVP ≥8 mmHg and urine output >0.5 ml/kg/h (caution if LVF).
- *Inotropes*: if systolic BP <90 mmHg after fluid resuscitation start noradrenaline (1–10 microgram/min) to maintain MAP >65 mmHg.
  - Measure mixed venous O_2 saturation and if <65–70% need further fluid/packed RBCs to achieve haematocrit >30% (check your local recommended 'sepsis bundle' management).
- *Antibiotics*: Give empiric targeted antibiotics ASAP (w/in 1 h), ensuring all cultures taken 1st (unless significantly delays antibiotics). Note mortality ↑7% per hr delay.
- *Steroids*: consider iv hydrocortisone (200–300 mg/day) when ↓BP responds poorly to adequate fluid resuscitation and vasopressors, especially if begun within 8 hours shock onset.
- *Blood glucose*: aim for <8.3 mmol/l using insulin sliding scale, but *avoid* hypoglycaemia.

- *Deep vein thrombosis prophylaxis*: low-dose LMWH (e.g enoxaparin 40 mg sc od) unless CI.
- *Stress ulcer prophylaxis*: PPI or H_2 antagonist.
- (*Blood products*: the aim is now for a *lower* target such as transfuse to Hb 7–9 g/dl, compared to previously i.e. Hb >10 g/dl).
- (*Activated protein C*: *No* longer recommended and may increase risk of bleeding).

Adapted from Surviving Sepsis Campaign: International guidelines for management of severe sepsis and septic shock: 2008. *Intensive Care Medicine* 2008; **34**(1).

FEBRILE NEUTROPENIA

Clues: If temperature 38°C for $\geq$2 h (or $\geq$38.5°C for $\geq$1 h) and no clues as to the fever's aetiology, give:

- *1st/2nd episodes*: gentamicin 5 mg/kg od iv + Tazocin 4.5 g tds iv (use ceftazidime 2 g tds iv if penicillin allergy).
- *Persistent or recurrent fever at any later stage*: call haematologist/oncologist $\pm$ microbiologist on call for advice.

> NB: Always do full septic screen *before* giving antibiotics inc blood, urine and any other appropriate cultures (e.g. sputum, stool, central/other lines) $\pm$ CXR, providing this does not delay them.

URINARY TRACT INFECTIONS

Clues: dysuria, frequency, suprapubic discomfort, haematuria, nocturia ('lower urinary tract' / simple); systemic malaise, fever/rigors, vomiting, loin/back/abdo pain, occ septic shock ('upper urinary tract' / pyelonephritis). NB: note if recent instrumentation/catheterisation.

Management

- Dipstick urine and obtain microscopy to confirm presence of infection. Request urine culture on clean-catch MSU.
- *Simple UTI*: trimethoprim 200 mg bd po. Another option is nitrofurantoin 50–100 mg qds po (not suitable if RF).
- *Pyelonephritis*: cefotaxime 1 g tds iv. If no response within 24 h (and still no culture results), try co-amoxiclav 1.2 g tds iv + gentamicin.

Causes of UTIs

- Most are caused by *E. coli* (70–80%).
- Remainder caused by Enterococci, or other Gram-negatives – e.g. *Proteus* (assoc. with stones), *Klebsiella*, *Serratia* or *Pseudomonas*.
- *Staph saprophyticus* seen in young women.
- Multi-resistant organisms more likely in catheterised or hospitalised patients.

GI INFECTIONS

Gastroenteritis

- *Simple infections*: Many causes inc traveller's diarrhoea (enterotoxigenic *E. coli*), toxin related (*Staphylococcus/ Bacillus cereus*), viral (rota/Norwalk-like), *Salmonella/Shigella, Campylobacter, Giardia*. These rarely need Rx; take a travel history, focus on rehydration, and contact microbiology department if in doubt.
- *AAC (Clostridium difficile)*: Ask about any antibiotic use in previous 8 weeks, and send stool for *C. difficile* toxin. Give metronidazole 400 mg tds po and *stop other antibiotics if possible*. If no response after 4 days, change to vancomycin 125 mg qds po for 10–14 days.

TB PNEUMONIA

This may well be suspected in the ED, but it is rare to *ever* commence therapy. Should normally be managed by a respiratory or infectious disease physician with expertise in this area.

NB: isolate a potentially infectious patient, and send multiple sputum samples for Ziehl–Neelsen staining / PCR, followed by culture.

NB: notify proven case to public health authorities (usually once on the medical ward).

Treatment

- *Initial phase*: 1st 2 months: ↓s bacterial load and covers all strains: Rifater* (Rifampicin + Isoniazid + Pyrazinamide) + Ethambutol** = 'RIPE'.
- *Continuation phase*: next 4 months (or longer if CNS involvement): Rifinah* (rifampicin + isoniazid) = 'RI'. If resistance to rifampicin/ isoniazid known (or suspected), continue pyrazinamide = 'RIP'.
  - Consider pyridoxine 10 mg od po: ↓s isoniazid neuropathy[BNF].
  - Combined tablets* ⇒ ↑compliance and ease of prescribing.
  - Doses are by weight; see BNF for details.
  - All drugs are hepatotoxic: check LFTs before and during Rx.
- Ethambutol**: is nephrotoxic and can ⇒ optic neuritis: check U&Es and visual acuity before and during Rx. Alternative is streptomycin (also nephrotoxic), or both can be omitted if ↓risk of isoniazid resistance.
- Corticosteroids: usually added to this regimen from the start, if meningeal or pericardial TB.

MALARIA

Practice points

- *Falciparum malaria 'malignant tertian'*: severe cases present with altered conscious level ± convulsions ('cerebral malaria'), jaundice, oliguria or haemoglobinuria ('blackwater fever'), anaemia (Hb < 5 g/dl), hypoglycaemia, metabolic acidosis (HCO_3 <15 mmol/l), ↓BP or resp distress; or have > 5–10% red cells parasitised. Admit to ITU.

- Consider in any returning traveller with fever, rigors, headache, N&V, diarrhoea ± hepatosplenomegaly. Always consult infectious diseases ± microbiology team if malaria suspected/ confirmed.

Clues: travel (even >1 year previously–not with falciparum) + fevers (±3-day cycles ± rigors), jaundice, ↑spleen/liver, ↓Pt, ↓Hb.

Treatment

Confirmed non-falciparum ('benign')

- *Chloroquine* (as base; see below) dose 620 mg po, then 310 mg 6–8 h later, then 310 mg od 24 h later for 2 days (all doses of chloroquine as *base*).
- *Primaquine*: follow, unless pregnant, with 14 days primaquine if *P. ovale* (15 mg od) or *P. vivax* (30 mg od) to kill parasites in the liver and prevent relapses ('radical cure').

Falciparum ('malignant'); or species mixed/unknown. Seriously ill:

- **Quinine** (as salt; see below): load with 20 mg/kg ivi (max 1.4 g) over 4 h (NB: omit loading dose if quinine, quinidine or mefloquine given in past 12 h.) Then, 8 h after the start of the loading dose, give 10 mg/kg (max 700 mg) ivi over 4 h every 8 h for up to 7 days (↓doses to 5–7 mg/kg if RF or >48 h if iv Rx needed), changing to oral quinine (600 mg tds of salt) once able to swallow and retain tablets to complete a 7-day course.
  - Always consult infectious diseases + microbiology team.
- **Doxycycline** 200 mg od po (clindamycin 450 mg tds po if pregnant) with or following quinine course for 7 days.
- **Artesunate or artemether**: consider if patient has been to quinine-resistant areas of SE Asia: get specialist advice.

Stable, normal GCS, able to swallow and retain tablets:

- *Quinine*: 600 mg tds po for 7 days followed by *doxycycline* or *clindamycin*.
- *Proguanil + atovaquone* (Malarone), *artemether + lumefantrine* (Riamet) are alternatives (Rx for 3 days only) to quinine, which only need to be taken for 3 days and do not need any subsequent drugs.

> Quinine doses here are as 'salt' (quinine hydrochloride, dihydrochloride or sulphate). Choloroquine doses are as 'base' (i.e. the chloroquine component of the total drug compound). Specify salt or base on the prescription–don't confuse salt or base doses as they are not equivalent.

ELECTROLYTE DISTURBANCES

HYPERKALAEMIA ($\uparrow K^+$)

Practice points
- *Haemolysis*: if this is possible (poor venesection technique – usually 'difficult vein'), ring lab $\pm$ repeat the sample.
- K^+ >6 mmol/l considered dangerous, with risk of cardiac arrhythmia $\pm$ arrest.
- K^+ >6.5 mmol/l or ECG Δs (tall 'tented' T waves, QRS >0.12 sec (>3 small squares), loss of P waves or sinusoidal pattern) needs immediate treatment plus cardiac monitoring:

Treatment
- *10% Ca^{2+} gluconate*: 10–20 ml iv over 3 min as 'cardioprotection'; or 10 ml of *10% CaCl* iv at $\leq$1ml/min. NB: does *not* alter serum K^+ level.
- *Insulin*: (soluble e.g. Actrapid) 10 units iv + 50 ml 50% glucose ivi over 5–15 min. Stimulates cellular uptake of K^+: aim for drop of 1–2 mmol/l over 30–60 min.
- *Salbutamol*: 5–20 mg nebs. Utilises K^+-lowering fx (unlicensed indication).

- *8.4% **Sodium bicarbonate***: 25–50 ml only if acidotic *and* not volume overloaded (beware dialysis pt).

Consider also

- *Look for and treat cause*: esp AKI (may need urgent dialysis) and drugs; e.g. iv KCl, oral K^+ supplements, ACE-i, ARBs, K^+-sparing diuretics, NSAIDs. Also ciclosporin (do not adjust without specialist advice).

NB: Contrary to popular opinion Calcium Resonium is not useful in the ED.

HYPOKALAEMIA ($\downarrow K^+$)

K^+ <2.5 mmol/l $\Rightarrow$ risk of arrhythmias: attach cardiac monitor.

Treatment

- *Normal saline (0.9%) 1 litre + 40 mmol KCl*: over 4 h via infusion device.
  - If unstable or arrhythmias develop, seek senior help as KCl can be given quicker. Consider possibility of assoc Mg^{2+} deficiency and replace Mg^{2+} as well.
  - Patient may not tolerate faster peripheral ivi due to pain (consider central line).
- *Oral K^+ replacement*: should also be commenced (e.g. Sando-K, Slow-K 2 tablets tds, or as much as can be tolerated – unpleasant taste!).
  - Oral therapy is often sufficient if K^+ >2.5 mmol/l and no clinical features (fatigue, weakness, leg cramps) or ECG Δs (small T waves or large U waves).

HYPERCALCAEMIA ($\uparrow Ca^{2+}$)

Ca^{2+} >2.65 mmol/l is abnormal. Symptoms usually start once Ca^{2+} >2.9 mmol/l.

Clues: 'stones, bones, groans and psychic moans'! Coming from renal colic $\pm$ AKI; bone pain (consider metastases); abdominal pain, constipation $\pm$ vomiting, polyuria and thirst; confusion, psychosis.

Treatment

- Ca^{2+} >3.5 mmol/l or severe symptoms:
- *Normal saline (0.9%) ivi*: average requirements 4–6 litres over 24 h ($\downarrow$ if elderly/HF). Monitor fluid balance carefully and correct electrolytes.

No improvement in Ca²⁺ levels yet rehydrated

- *Loop diuretic*: (e.g. furosemide). *Never* use a thiazide (worsens Ca^{2+}).
- *Bisphosphonate*: (e.g. pamidronate) esp if $\uparrow$PTH or malignancy.
- *Calcitonin*: if no response to bisphosphonate.
- *Steroids*: if sarcoid, lymphoma, myeloma or vitamin D toxicity.
- *Dialysis*: if AKI or life-threatening symptoms (coma).

ALCOHOL WITHDRAWAL

Practice point

Patients dependent on alcohol are common in the ED. Use a simple screening questionnaire CAGE to help identify those at risk (see Table 4.2).

Table 4.2 CAGE screening questionnaire for alcohol abuse.

C	Have you ever felt you should **C**ut down on your drinking?
A	Have people **A**nnoyed you by criticising your drinking?
G	Have you ever felt bad or **G**uilty about your drinking?
E	Have you ever had a drink as an **E**ye-opener first thing in the morning to steady your nerves or help get rid of a hangover?

'Yes' to two or more indicates probable chronic alcohol abuse or dependence

PREVENTION OF AGITATION, SEIZURES AND DELIRIUM TREMENS

Start a long-acting benzodiazepine in a tapered regimen as follows (will need medical admission):

Alcohol withdrawal regimen. Courtesy of Professor H. Ghodse, St George's Hospital.

Day	Chlordiazepoxide	*OR*	Diazepam
1	30 mg qds		15 mg qds
2	30 mg tds		10 mg qds
3	20 mg tds		10 mg tds
4	20 mg bd		5 mg qds
5	10 mg bd		5 mg tds
6	10 mg od		5 mg bd
7	10 mg prn		5 mg od

> *This is only a suggested initial average regimen*
> Ideal regimens involve an initial 24-h assessment of prn doses, but require adequate training and staff time to monitor closely and ensure no under- (or over-) treatment occurs. Start with dose of 20–40 mg chlordiazepoxide or 10–20 mg diazepam and add up doses used in 1st 24 h, then reduce by 1/5th (–1/7th) per day for 5(–7) days.

- Chlordiazepoxide usually 1st line, but diazepam preferred if Hx of seizures (esp if occurred in context of alcohol withdrawal).
- Significant liver failure (e.g. ↑AST or ALT): consider shorter-acting benzodiazepines such as oxazepam or lorazepam at equivalent doses; avoids xs metabolite build up and sedation (but marginal ↑seizure risk).
- Only start once acute alcohol intoxication has resolved.

THIAMINE (VIT B₁) AND OTHER SUPPLEMENTS

Give thiamine (vit B_1) for Px or Rx of suspected Wernicke's encephalopathy (WE) with one or more of: ophthalmoplegia, ataxia, acute confusion, memory disturbance, unexplained hypotension, hypothermia or coma.

Thiamine must be given *before* patient receives any carbohydrate load po or iv (which can precipitate WE).

☠ ∴ Take particular care if hypoglycaemic and iv glucose needed! ☠

- ***Parenteral thiamine (iv or im)***: e.g. Pabrinex (contains other B and C vits); prescribe as '1 pair Pabrinex vials' or 'Pabrinex 1 and 2'. British Association for Psychopharmacology substance abuse guidelines 2004/2012 update (Journal of Psychopharmacology 2012) recommends:
  — *WE* suspected (see below) or established: 2 pairs tds iv (or im) for 3–5 days, then 1 pair od for a further 3–5 days.
  — *High risk* of WE (malnourished/chronic severe abuse):1 pair od iv or im for 3–5 days.
  — *Low risk* of WE: no parenteral treatment needed, but give oral thiamine.

☠ Pabrinex can ⇒ *anaphylaxis*
∴ have resus facilities at hand. NB: ↑risk if given iv too quickly; ensure mixture of both vials either given as injection over ⩾10 min or as infusion (with 50–100 ml saline) over ⩾30min ☠.

- Oral vitamins and supplements:
  — Thiamine 100 mg bd/tds po; should be given for 1 month if no parenteral treatment required.
  — Multivitamins 1 tablet/day long-term; cheap and potentially important if future diet likely to be poor.

Wernicke's encephalopathy
Caused by thiamine deficiency and often missed; only 10% have classical triad of confusion, ataxia and eye signs (ophthalmoplegia or nystagmus; seen in only 30% of cases). Suspect diagnosis if any evidence of chronic alcohol misuse and any one of: acute confusion, ataxia, ophthalmoplegia, ↓BP + ↓temp, ↓GCS or ↓memory.

> If unsure whether intoxication or WE is causing any of these, always assume it is WE and give treatment. Rarely WE is caused by other malnutrition, e.g. malabsorption, eating disorders, protracted vomiting, CRF, AIDS and other drug misuse.
> NB: $\downarrow Mg^{2+}$ can $\Rightarrow$ Rx refractory WE $\therefore$ check $\pm$ correct Mg^{2+} too.

MAINTENANCE OF ABSTINENCE

It is essential to:

- Encourage abstinence and refer to local alcohol liaison practitioner (if available) $\pm$ addiction services.
- Arrange adequate social support, and look for and treat assoc depression.
- The following are used as aids:
  - *Acamprosate*: modulates alcohol withdrawal fx & limits –ve reinforcement of drinking cessation $\Rightarrow \downarrow$ cravings and $\downarrow$ relapse rate.
  - *Disulfiram*: $\Rightarrow$ unpleasant symptoms if alcohol consumed.
  - *Naltrexone*: $\downarrow$s pleasurable fx of alcohol and $\downarrow$s craving and relapse rate. Specialist use only (unlicensed in UK for this indication).

ACUTE POISONING

Deliberate self-harm is a common problem seen in the ED. Methods inc cutting or self-mutilation, or more commonly ingestion of drugs (inc over-the-counter/herbal remedies), chemicals (industrial or household), plants and biologicals.

The following sources should always be consulted:

- **TOXBASE** *(www.toxbase.org)*: authoritative and updated regularly. Should be used in the 1st instance to check clinical features and Mx of the poison(s) in question.

- You need to sign in under your departmental account username and password.
- *UK National Poisons Information Service (NPIS)*: if in UK phone 0844 892 0111 (if in Ireland 01 809 2566) for specialist advice if unsure of TOXBASE instructions, and for rarer/complex poisonings.

GENERAL MEASURES

- *Activated charcoal*: if w/in 1 h of significant ingestion, but CI if ↓GCS (unless ET tube *in situ*), if bowel sounds absent or if corrosive substance/petroleum ingested.
  - Repeated doses and administration later than 1 h suggested for certain drugs (e.g. quinine, carbamazepine, theophylline, or sustained release preparations).
  - Charcoal *not* effective for lithium, iron, organophosphates, ethylene glycol, ethanol, methanol.
  - See TOXBASE for dosing guide for activated charcoal. NB: 'routine' GI decontamination is no longer recommended.
- *Gastric lavage*: Rarely ever used now. Only consider if w/in 1 h of life-threatening ingestion that cannot be removed effectively (e.g. iron). *Must* protect the airway, esp if ↓GCS. CI if corrosive/petroleum distillate ingested.
- Check a paracetamol level in any patient who is unable/unwilling to give an accurate Hx of the exact poisons ingested, and perform an ECG. Send a salicylate level if pt symptomatic 'salicylism', or comatose / unexplained metabolic acidosis.
- Other drug levels will depend on suspected ingestion, but note the majority of poisonings are managed supportively, and only a few have a specific antidote.

SIDE EFFECT PROFILES

Knowledge of side effect profiles (SEs) together with a drug's mechanism(s), allow anticipation of that drug's SEs or toxic effect (toxidrome).

CHOLINOCEPTORS

ACh stimulates muscarinic and nicotinic receptors.

Anticholinesterases ⇒ ↑ACh and ∴ stimulate both receptor types and have 'cholinergic fx'.

↓**cholinoreceptor** action drugs do this mostly via muscarinic receptors (antinicotinics used only in anaesthesia) and are ∴ more accurately referred to as 'antimuscarinics' rather than 'anticholinergics'.

Cholinergic fx	Antimuscarinic fx
Generally ↑*secretions*	*Generally* ↓*secretions*
Diarrhoea	**C**onstipation
Urination	**U**rinary retention
Miosis (constriction)	**M**ydriasis↓accommodation[a]
Bronchospasm/bradycardia[b]	**B**ronchodilation/tachycardia
Excitation of CNS (and muscle)	**D**rowsiness, **D**ry eyes, **D**ry skin
Lacrimation↑	
Saliva/sweat↑	
Commonly caused by:	
Anticholinesterases:	Atropine, ipratropium (Atrovent)
MG Rx, e.g. pyridostigmine	Antihistamines (inc cyclizine)
Dementia Rx, e.g. rivastigmine, donepezil	Antidepressants (esp TCAs)
	Antipsychotics (esp 'typicals')
	Hyoscine, Ia antiarrhythmics

[a] ↑blurred vision and ↑IOP. [b] Together with vasodilation ⇒ ↓BP.

ADRENOCEPTORS

α generally excites sympathetic system (except*):

- **α1** ⇒ GI smooth-muscle relaxation*, otherwise contracts smooth muscle: vasoconstriction, GI/bladder sphincter constriction (uterus, seminal tract, iris (radial muscle)). Also ↑salivary secretion, ↓glycogenolysis (in liver).

- $\alpha 2 \Rightarrow$ inhibition of neurotransmitters (esp NA and ACh for feedback control), Pt aggregation, contraction of vascular smooth muscle, inhibition of insulin release. Also prominent adrenoceptor of CNS (inhibits sympathetic outflow).

β **generally inhibits sympathetic system** (except*):

- $\beta 1 \Rightarrow \uparrow$ HR*, $\uparrow$ contractility* (and $\uparrow$ s salivary amylase secretion).
- $\beta 2 \Rightarrow$ vasodilation, bronchodilation, muscle tremor, glycogenolysis (in hepatic and skeletal muscle). Inhibits further mediator release from mast cells via $\uparrow$ intracellular cAMP (important in anaphylaxis). Also $\uparrow$ s renin secretion, relaxes ciliary muscle and visceral smooth muscles (GI sphincter, bladder detrusor, uterus if not pregnant).
- $\beta 3 \Rightarrow$ lipolysis, thermogenesis (of little pharmacological relevance).

SEROTONIN (5HT)

'Serotonin syndrome' $\Rightarrow$ *relative excess*: occurs with antidepressants at $\uparrow$ doses, or if swapped without an adequate 'tapering' or 'washout period'. Causes restlessness, sweating and tremor, progressing to shivering, myoclonus and confusion, and, if severe enough, convulsions/death.

'Antidepressant withdrawal/discontinuation syndrome' $\Rightarrow$ *relative deficit*: occurs when antidepressants stopped too quickly; likelihood depends on $t_{1/2}$ of drug. Causes 'flu-like symptoms (chills/sweating, myalgia, headache and nausea), and dizziness, tinnitus, anxiety, irritability, insomnia, vivid dreams. Rarely $\Rightarrow$ movement disorders and $\downarrow$ memory/concentration.

DOPAMINE (DA)

Relative excess: causes behaviour Δ, confusion and psychosis (esp if predisposed, e.g. schizophrenia). Seen with L-dopa and DA agonists used in Parkinson's (and some endocrine disorders, e.g. bromocriptine).

Relative deficit: causes extrapyramidal fx (see below), $\uparrow$ prolactin (sexual dysfunction, female infertility, gynaecomastia), neuroleptic malignant syndrome. Occurs with DA antagonists, esp antipsychotics and certain antiemetics such as metoclopramide, prochlorperazine and levomepromazine.

EXTRAPYRAMIDAL EFFECTS

Abnormalities of movement control arising from dysfunction of basal ganglia.

- *Parkinsonism*: rigidity and bradykinesia ± tremor.
- *Dyskinesias* (= abnormal involuntary movements):
  - *Dystonia* (= abnormal posture): dynamic (e.g. oculogyric crisis) or static (e.g. torticollis).
  - *Tardive (delayed onset) dyskinesia*: esp orofacial movements.
  - *Others*: tremor, chorea, athetosis, hemiballismus, myoclonus, tics.
- *Akathisia* (= intolerable sense of inner restlessness): seen with antipsychotic or neuroleptic drugs, but also with antiemetics (e.g. metoclopramide, prochlorperazine).

All the above are more commonly caused by antipsychotics (esp older 'typical' drugs) but are a rare complication of antiemetics (e.g. metoclopramide, prochlorperazine – esp in young women). Dyskinesias and dystonias are common with antiparkinsonian drugs (esp peaks of L-dopa doses).

Most respond to stopping (or ↓dose of) the drug – if not possible, fails or immediate Rx needed add an antimuscarinic drug (e.g. procyclidine) – this does not work for akathisia (try β-blocker, or benzodiazepine) + can worsen tardive dyskinesia: seek neurology ± psychiatry opinion if in doubt.

CEREBELLAR EFFECTS

Esp antiepileptics (e.g. phenytoin) and alcohol.

- **D**ysdiadokokinesis, dysmetria (= past-pointing) and rebound
- **A**taxia of gait (wide-based, irregular step length) ± trunk
- **N**ystagmus: towards side of lesion; mostly coarse and horizontal
- **I**ntention tremor (also titubation = nodding-head tremor)

- Speech: scanning dysarthria – slow, slurred or jerky
- Hypotonia (less commonly hyporeflexia or pendular reflexes).

CYTOCHROME P450 (CYP)

Substrates of P450 that often result in significant interactions (these drugs can ↑ severe problems if rendered ineffective or toxic by interactions ∴ always check for interactions when prescribing):

- **Inhibitors** and **inducers** can affect warfarin, phenytoin, carbamazepine, ciclosporin and theophyllines. Interactions can ∴ ⇒ toxicity or treatment failure.
- **Inducers** also affect OCP so can ↑ failure as contraceptive ∴ recommend alternate barrier method.

> *NB*
> CYP system is complex and mediated by many isoenzymes (> 60 key forms with hundreds of genetic variations); predicting significant interactions requires understanding which drugs are metabolised by which isoenzymes as well as which, and to what degree, other drugs affect these isoenzymes.
> Look for P450 symbols in this book as a rough guide; check SPCs if concerned (available online at www.medicines.org. uk/emc/), and for a full overview of the CYP system see www. edhayes.com/startp450.html.

PARACETAMOL

Significant poisoning is >75 mg/kg in any 24 h period (serious toxicity may occur if >150 mg/kg, toxicity uncommon if 75–150 mg/kg).

Initial management

Dependent on time since ingestion.

0–8 h post-ingestion:

- *Activated charcoal*: if w/in 1 h of significant poisoning.
- *Acetylcysteine*: wait until 4 h post-ingestion then take urgent sample for paracetamol level (result is meaningless before 4 h post). If presents at 4–8 h post-ingestion, take immediate sample.

- Level above the treatment line (see nomogram): use the following acetylcysteine regimen:
  - 150 mg/kg in 200 ml 5% glucose ivi over 1 hr.
  - 50 mg/kg in 500 ml 5% glucose ivi over 4 h.
  - 100 mg/kg in 1000 ml 5% glucose ivi over 16 h.

NB: if patient weighs >110 kg, use 110 kg (rather than their actual weight) for these calculations.

> Do not delay acetylcysteine beyond 8 h post-ingestion if waiting for a paracetamol level after a significant ingestion (beyond 8 h, efficacy ↓s substantially) – ivi can always be stopped if the level comes back below treatment line and timing of ingestion is certain, and INR, ALT and creatinine normal.

8–15 h post-ingestion:

- *Acetylcysteine*: give above regimen ASAP if significant ingestion. Do not wait for urgent paracetamol level result. Acetylcysteine can be stopped later (see note).

15–24 h post-ingestion:

- *Acetylcysteine*: give above regimen ASAP unless certain that significant ingestion has not taken place–do not wait for paracetamol level result. Presenting this late ⇒ severe risk, and treatment lines are unreliable: always finish the course of acetylcysteine.

- Be aware that paracetamol level might be over treatment line but reported as undetectable (e.g. a level of 16 mg/L may be reported as <20 mg/L); if in doubt, TREAT.

>24 h post-ingestion:

- Acetylcysteine is controversial when presenting this late. Check creatinine, LFTs, INR, glucose, and paracetamol concentration, and consult TOXBASE or NPIS.

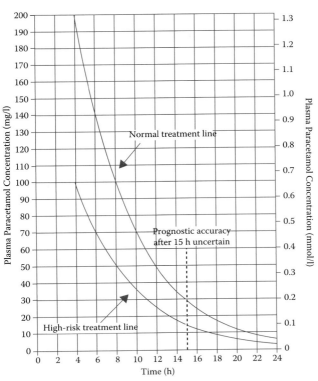

Figure 4.3 Treatment lines for acetylcysteine treatment of paracetamol overdose. (Reproduced courtesy of Medicines and Healthcare products Regulatory Agency (UK).)

> **Important points regarding acetylcysteine**
>
> - Have lower threshold for initiating Rx if doubts over timing of ingestion, if it was staggered, if present 24–36 h post-ingestion, or if evidence of LF/severe toxicity regardless of time since ingestion. Contact NPIS if unsure.
> - Anaphylactoid reactions common esp at initial faster rates. Reduce infusion rate or stop temporarily until reaction settles. Give antihistamine (e.g. chlorphenamine 10–20 mg iv over 1 min) if required. Give salbutamol nebs if significant bronchospasm. Once reaction settles restart acetylcysteine, and consider giving the second bag at half normal rate (i.e. 50 mg/kg over 8 h). A past Hx of such a reaction is not an absolute CI to future treatment. Pretreatment with chlorphenamine 10 mg iv **or** administration of 1st ivi at slower rate may reduce risk of reaction.
> - Acetylcysteine $\Rightarrow$ mildly $\uparrow$INR itself; so if after treatment ALT is normal but INR is $\leqslant$1.3 no further monitoring or treatment is needed. But if ALT is $\uparrow$ continue acetylcysteine ivi at rate of 150 mg/kg given over 24 h (unless substantial pause in ivi further loading dose not needed), and seek immediate TOXBASE/liver unit advice.

Subsequent management

Patients may be *medically* fit for discharge once acetylcysteine ivi is completed, and INR, ALT, creatinine and HCO_3^- ($\pm$pH) are normal (or recovering in two successive checks if additional acetylcysteine has been administered).

Psychiatric evaluation must still be undertaken for all patients who have taken tablets deliberately.

A patient with laboratory abnormalities despite acetylcysteine, seek immediate TOXBASE/liver unit advice.

SALICYLATE/ASPIRIN

Much less commonly seen now. A complex poisoning to manage.

Initial management:

- *Activated charcoal* and consider *gastric lavage* (if airway protected): if w/in 1 h of ingestion of >125 mg/kg. As aspirin delays gastric emptying (esp if enteric-coated tablets), both may be considered >1 h after ingestion. Can repeat activated charcoal every 4 h, if salicylate level continues to rise despite measures below. Consult TOXBASE.

- *Measure/monitor* U&Es, glucose, clotting, ABGs (or venous pH and HCO_3^-) and fluid balance (often need large volumes of iv fluid). Send a salicylate level if ingested >120 mg/kg; take sample at least 2 h post-ingestion if symptomatic or 4 h post-ingestion if not. Repeat in both cases 2 h later if severe toxicity suspected (hyperthermia, dehydration, agitation, confusion, seizures, ↓GCS, metabolic acidosis) in case absorption was delayed (repeating until levels↓). Note that peak concentrations are often delayed after large ingestions.
  - If significant biochemical abnormalities, get senior help and contact ITU for advice, then consider the following.

- *Sodium bicarbonate ivi*: give 1.5 litres 1.26% over 2 h (or 225 ml of 8.4%) if metabolic acidosis and salicylate levels >500 mg/l (3.6 mmol/l) – will minimise movement of salicylate into tissues, and enhance renal elimination. Beware risk of tissue necrosis if extravasation. Bicarbonate administration may cause hypokalaemia: watch K^+ closely, and hypoglycaemia. Monitor arterial blood gases to ensure correction of acid–base disturbance.

- *Haemodialysis*: salicylate levels >700 mg/l (5.1 mmol/l) or unresponsive to the above measures. Also consider if AKI, CCF, non-cardiac pulmonary oedema, severe metabolic acidosis, convulsions or any CNS fx that are not resolved by correction of pH, and in patients aged >70 yrs due to increased risk of toxicity.

OPIATES

Clues: pinpoint pupils, ↓respiratory rate, ↓GCS, drug chart and Hx/signs of opiate abuse (e.g. collapsed vein 'track marks').

- O_2 + maintain airway ± ventilatory support.
- *Naloxone 0.4–2 mg iv* (or im) stat initially, repeating after 2 min if no response (check pupils). Note that large doses (>2 mg) may be required in some patients.
  - Start with a smaller dose naloxone 0.1 mg if chronic user and build up, to avoid precipitating acute withdrawal.

BENZODIAZEPINES

- O_2 + maintain airway with positioning ± ventilatory support.

> ☠ Flumazenil is *not* to be used as a diagnostic test, and must *not* be given routinely ☠. Risk of inducing seizures (esp if epileptic or habituated to benzodiazepines) and arrhythmias (esp if co-ingested TCA or amphetamine-like drug).

Surgical emergencies

Acute abdomen   286
Orthopaedic infections   287
ENT infections   288
Eye infections   288

ACUTE ABDOMEN

The aims are to resuscitate critically ill patients; differentiate those requiring referral to a surgical, gynaecological, urological or medical team; and to determine who can be allowed home.

MANAGEMENT IF SERIOUSLY ILL

- Resuscitate:
  - Give high-flow O$_2$.
  - Insert 1 or 2 large bore intravenous cannulae (14-/16-gauge), and take blood for FBC, U&E, BG, LFT, amylase/lipase, lactate + group and save or cross match blood, if haemorrhage suspected (ruptured AAA, ectopic pregnancy–check pregnancy test).
  - *Fluid iv*: crystalloid/colloid (blood if haemorrhage) to maintain systolic BP >100 mmHg, but avoid over-transfusion in elderly/heart or renal disease + if ongoing bleeding (need operation!). Consider CVP line.
- Investigate:
  - Bloods as above, urinalysis, preg test, ECG (abdo pain in the elderly); CXR (perforation, basal pneumonia).
  - *USS* to look for ruptured AAA, free fluid from ectopic.
  - *CT* scan once resuscitated and stabilised.
- Treat:
  - *Analgesia*: morphine titrated to effect ± antiemetic. Morphine does *not* mask intra-peritoneal signs, and it is inappropriate and inhumane to withhold it.
  - *Antibiotics*: cefuroxime 1.5 g iv or gentamicin 5 mg/kg, and metronidazole 500 mg iv for generalized peritonitis.
  - *NGT*: bowel obstruction, ileus or peritonitis.
- Refer:
  - Involve the surgical team early.

ORTHOPAEDIC INFECTIONS

BONE AND JOINT INFECTIONS
Septic arthritis
Suspect if severe pain, redness and swelling, with decreased movement (active and passive). Perform joint aspiration and refer to orthopaedic team for admission.

- Treat as for osteomyelitis (see below), but consider changing after urgent Gram stain, e.g. to iv 3rd-generation cephalosporin (cefotaxime, ceftriaxone) if *H. influenzae* suspected (Gram-negative bacilli, esp in non-immunised child).
- Suspect Salmonella in sickle cell disease; or TB/fungi if immunocompromised.

Osteomyelitis
Suspect in any deep DM ulcer, or postoperative joint pain/redness. *Staph aureus* is usual cause, but in spinal infection consider also Gram-negatives (discuss with Microbiology).

- *Flucloxacillin* 1–2 g qds iv + *fusidic acid* 500 mg tds po (can give iv in severe cases, but is poorly tolerated and often not required).
- MRSA suspected: consult local guidelines ± microbiologist.
- *Co-amoxiclav* 1.2 g tds iv instead of flucloxacillin, if associated with chronic ulceration.
- *Clindamycin* 600 mg qds iv, if penicillin allergy.

Cellulitis

- *Mild*: co-amoxiclav 625 mg tds po or flucloxacillin 500 mg qds po.
- *Severe* (systemically unwell): benzylpenicillin 1.2 g iv 4–6-hrly + flucloxacillin 1 g qds iv.
  - Add metronidazole 500 mg tds ivi if suspect anaerobes, e.g. abdominal wound (admit surgical).
  - Consider vancomycin 1 g bd ivi if confirmed MRSA colonisation/infection.

ENT INFECTIONS

Acute epiglottitis

- Becoming uncommon since Hib vaccination. Call senior help immediately before doing anything else!
- *Cefotaxime* 1 g tds iv + *metronidazole* 500 mg tds ivi (or Tazocin (piperacillin + tazobactam) 4.5 g tds iv).

Pharyngitis/tonsillitis

- *Penicillin V* (phenoxymethylpenicillin) 500 mg qds po for 'Strep' throat *only* when recent Hx of otitis media, confirmed group A Strep infection, or 3 of the following 4 clues that infection is bacterial (rather than viral)—tender cervical lymphadenopathy, purulent tonsils, Hx of fever or absence of cough.

Sinusitis/otitis media

- *Amoxicillin* 500 mg tds po if systemically unwell with fever and vomiting, or when does not resolve in 2–3 days (as would be expected if viral). Also regular analgesia such as paracetamol.

Otitis externa

- *Topical steroid + antibiotic combination*: Sofradex or Otomize.
- Less commonly fungal (look for black spores); give topical Otosporin or Neo-cortef.
- If does not resolve or evidence of perichondritis (inflamed pinna), cellulitis, boil/local abscess, refer to ENT for advice and systemic Rx (e.g. amoxicillin, co-amoxiclav, flucloxacillin) with local aural toilet (esp if fungal).

EYE INFECTIONS

Orbital cellulitis

- *Co-amoxiclav* po if preseptal 'periorbital' (lids only, related to local infection) ⇒ can be managed as outpatient with close observation.

- *Ceftriaxone* 2 g iv + *flucloxacillin* 2 g iv if postseptal (true 'orbital', usually arising from paranasal sinuses or occ orbital trauma) ⇒ admit.

Corneal ulcer

- *Ofloxacin* 0.3% 1 drop hrly (day and night) for 48 h, then hrly daytime. Urgent ophthalmology referral.
  - Suspect in contact lens wearer with painful red eye
  - Give antibiotic drops once scrape taken for Gram stain/ culture.
  - Do not allow patient to self-administer topical anaesthetic for analgesia as ⇒ epithelium to slough ☠.

Conjunctivitis

- *Chloramphenicol* 0.5% 1 drop qds. Only if mucopurulent/ prolonged.

Blepharitis

- Lid margin/eyelash: scrubs/hygiene only.
- If severe or lid hygiene alone insufficient ⇒ Maxitrol ointment (dexamethasone 0.1% & neomycin 0.35%) to eyelashes bd for 1 month + lid hygiene. Hypromellose artificial tears help reduce symptoms.

Stye (external hordeolum)

- Regular warm compresses to release cyst (antibiotics usually not required).
- If concern early cellulitis ⇒ co-amoxiclav po may be given.

Meibomian abscess (internal hordeolum)

- Infected Meibomian gland within tarsal plate, which does not discharge as readily as an external stye. May leave a residual Meibomian lipogranulomatous cyst (chalazion).
- Give co-amoxiclav po. Warm compresses do not help.

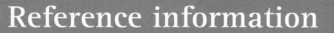

Reference information

Glasgow coma scale	292
Mental state examination	293
Acid-base nomogram	294
Useful formulae	295
Common laboratory reference values	297

GLASGOW COMA SCALE

A standardised assessment tool to describe the level of consciousness originally introduced in 1974 for head injured patients, now used universally. GCS score 8 or less usually means 'unconscious'. See Table 6.1

NB: 'Medical' causes of a low GCS score may be rapidly reversible such as dt hypoglycaemia, whereas in head trauma the GCS can be used as a guide to severity:

- GCS 13–15 = minor
- GCS 9–12 = moderate
- GCS <9 = severe injury

Table 6.1 The Glasgow Coma Scale (GCS) score

Score		Score
Eye opening	Spontaneously	4
	To speech	3
	To pain	2
	None	1
Verbal response	Oriented	5
	Confused	4
	Inappropriate	3
	Incomprehensible	2
	None	1
Motor response	Obeys commands	6
	Localizes pain	5
	Withdraws (pain)	4
	Flexion (pain)	3
	Extension (pain)	2
	None	1

The maximum score is 15. Any reduction in score indicates deterioration in the level of consciousness.

MENTAL STATE EXAMINATION

Abbreviated Mental Test Score (AMTS)

Most basic assessment of cognitive impairment; popular due to its brevity (esp for use in the elderly).

Score: **<8/10** is abnormal and suggests delirium / dementia (look for these).

W World War II: what year did it end?[1]
H Hospital (what is name of building you are in?).
A Address: 42 West St (ask to remember and repeat at end of test*).
T Time: to the nearest hour.
Y Year.
E Elizabeth II (who is current monarch/prime minister etc ?)[1].
A Age (of patient).
R Recognition of 2 persons: e.g. Dr and other[2].
B Birthday (patient's date of birth).
C Count backwards from 20 to 1.
? ? Can you repeat that address?*.

[1]If culturally inappropriate change to relevant question or omit.
[2]If alone with patient omit.

When a question is omitted, record why and reduce denominator of score.

Mini Mental State Examination (MMSE)

Best validated 30-point, basic cognitive assessment that includes orientation, attention and calculation, immediate and short-term recall, language and ability to follow simple verbal and written commands.

Score: **≥25** is effectively normal; **21–24** is mild cognitive impairment; and **≤20** indicates moderate to severe cognitive impairment suggesting delirium/dementia (look for these).

(Questions to ask are in bold):

Orientation:

Time – (1–3) **Date?** 1 point each for day, month and year.
(4) **Season?** (5) **Day of week?**   5

Place – (1) **Country?** (2) **County/state (or l arge city)?**   5
(3) **Town (or city area)?** (4) **Building?** (5) **Floor?**

Registration: Say[1] **ball, flag, tree.** Repeat until success or 5 attempts. 3

Attention/concentration: **Spell 'WORLD' backwards**[2].   5

Recall: **Can you remember those 3 items?** (ball, flag, tree). 3

3-stage command: **Take paper in R hand, fold in half and put on floor.**   3

Language: **What is this?** Point to pen and then wristwatch. 2

Repeat exactly after me: 'No ifs, ands or buts.'   1

Reading/comprehension: **Do what the sentence below instructs**[3]. 1

Praxis: **Write a sentence of your choice.** Provide dotted line. 1

Copy this shape as best you can alongside it[4].   1

1 Precede with 'I will mention 3 objects to you. Please repeat them to me once I have finished all 3.' Allow 1 s between objects. At end say 'I will ask you to remember these later' which is tested in Recall in next, but one section – should be done after 1 min.

2 'Serial 7s' can also be used which obviously tests calculation too so remember to take into account premorbid numeracy skills.

3 Write out in large, clear capital letters 'CLOSE YOUR EYES'.

4   Only correct if makes 4-sided shape formed by 2 intersecting pentagons.

- Allow 1 min for tasks, except 30 s for 3-stage command and writing of sentence.
- Frontal lobe tests are not covered; useful to add these e.g. abstract thinking, verbal fluency etc.

ACID-BASE NOMOGRAM

Plot the arterial blood gas results on the acid-base nomogram (Flenley) below and read off the interpretation. See Figure 6.1.

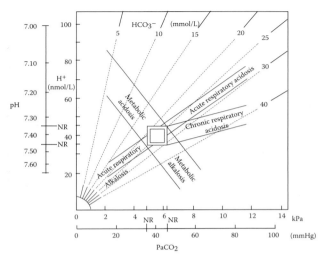

Figure 6.1 Acid-base nomogram for plotting interpretation of the arterial blood gas result (NR = normal range).

Alternatively, to determine the likely acid-base disorder from the pH, $PaCO_2$ and HCO_3 see Table 6.2.

USEFUL FORMULAE

A-a gradient= $P_AO_2 - P_aO_2$, where $P_AO_2 = (F_iO_2 \times (760 - 47)) - (P_aCO_2 / 0.8)$.
Normal is <10 torr (mmHg), or roughly < (Age/4) + 4 in yrs.

Serum osmolality=1.86 $(K^+ + Na^+)$+urea+glucose
NB: all units are in *mmol/l* and this calculation is an *estimate* (actual osmolality usually differs by ±13 mosm/kg).

Table 6.2 Determining the likely acid-base disorder from the pH, PaCO$_2$ and HCO$_3$

pH	PaCO$_2$	HCO$_3$	Acid-base disorder
↓	N	↓	**Primary metabolic acidosis**
↓	↓	↓	Metabolic acidosis with respiratory compensation
↓	↑	N	**Primary respiratory acidosis**
↓	↑	↑	Respiratory acidosis with renal compensation
↓	↑	↓	**Mixed metabolic and respiratory acidosis**
↑	↓	N	**Primary respiratory alkalosis**
↑	↓	↓	Respiratory alkalosis with renal compensation
↑	N	↑	**Primary metabolic alkalosis**
↑	↑	↑	Metabolic alkalosis with respiratory compensation
↑	↓	↑	**Mixed metabolic and respiratory alkalosis**

Note: respiratory compensation occurs rapidly by changes in PaCO$_2$. Renal compensation occurs more slowly by changes in HCO$_3$. N, normal.

Anion gap $= (Na^+ + K^+) - (Cl^- + HCO_3^-)$
Normal range 8–16 mEq/l
>16 = loss of HCO_3^- w/o concurrent increase in Cl^-.

Creatinine clearance = [Urine creatinine] $\times$ urine flow rate/[Plasma creatinine]

Body mass index = Weight (kg)/height (m)^2
'Normal' (target) = 18.5–25

Ideal body weight (kg) Men = [(height (cm) − 154) $\times$ 0.9] + 50
Women = [(height (cm) − 154) $\times$ 0.9] + 45.5

Metric conversions:

Weight   1 kg = 1000 g; 1 g = 1000 mg; 1 mg = 1000 micrograms;
1 microgram = 1000 nanograms
1 stone = 6.35 kg; 1 kg = 2.2 lb

Temp.	Fahrenheit to Celsius: (°F − 32) × 5/9 = °C
	Celsius to Fahrenheit: °C × 9/5 + 32 = °F
Pressure	1 kPa = 7.5 mmHg
Length	1 foot = 0.3048 metres; 1 inch = 25.4 mm
	1 metre = 3 feet 3.4 in; 1 cm = 0.394 in
Volume	1 tablespoon = 15 ml (approx.); 1 teaspoon = 5 ml (approx)
	1 litre = 1.76 pints (UK imperial) = 2.11 pints (USA liquid)

COMMON LABORATORY REFERENCE VALUES

NB: normal ranges often vary between laboratories. The ranges given here are deliberately narrow to minimise missing an abnormal result, but this means that your result may be normal for your laboratory's range, which should always be checked if possible.

Biochemistry

Na^+	135–145 mmol/l
K^+	3.5–5.0 mmol/l
Urea	2.5–6.5 mmol/l
Creatinine	70–110 µmol/l
Ca^{2+}	2.15–2.65 mmol/l
PO_4	0.8–1.4 mmol/l
Albumin	35–50 g/l
Protein	60–80 g/l
Mg^{2+}	0.75–1.0 mmol/l
Cl^-	95–105 mmol/l
Glucose (fasting)	3.5–5.5 mmol/l
LDH	70–250 iu/l
CK	25–195[a] u/l (↑in blacks)

(Continued)

Biochemistry (Continued)

Trop I	<0.4 ng/ml (=microgram/l)
Trop T	<0.1 ng/ml (=microgram/l)
D-dimers	<0.5[b] mg/l
Bilirubin	3–17 μmol/l
ALP	30–130 iu/l
AST	3–31 iu/l
ALT	3–35 iu/l
GGT	7–50[a] iu/l
Amylase	0–180 u/dl
Cholesterol	3.9–5.2 mmol/l
Triglycerides	0.5–1.9 mmol/l
LDL	<2.0 mmol/l
HDL	0.9–1.9 mmol/l
Urate	0.2–0.45 mmol/l
CRP	0–10 mg/l

[a] Sex differences exist: females occupy the lower end of the range.

[b] D-dimer normal range can vary with different test protocols: check with your lab.

Haematology

Hb male	13.5–17.5 g/dl
Hb female	11.5–15.5 g/dl
Pt	150–400 $\times$ 10^9/l
WCC	4–11 $\times$ 10^9/l
NØ	2.0–7.5 $\times$ 10^9/l (40–75%)
LØ	1.3–3.5 $\times$ 10^9/l (20–45%)
EØ	0.04–0.44 $\times$ 10^9/l (1–6%)
PCV (Hct)	0.37–0.54[a] l/l
MCV	76–96 fl

Haematology (Continued)

ESR	<age in years *(+10 in women)*/2
HbA$_{1C}$	2.3–6.5%

[a] Sex differences exist: females occupy the lower end of the range.

Clotting

APTT	35–45 s
APTT ratio	0.8–1.2
INR	0.8–1.2

Haematinics

Iron	11–30 µmol/l
Transferrin	2–4 g/l
TIBC	45–72 µmol/l
Serum folate	1.8–11 microgram/l
B$_{12}$	200–760 pg/ml (5 ng/l)

Arterial blood gases

PaO$_2$	>10.6 kPa
PaCO$_2$	4.7–6.0 kPa
pH	7.35–7.45
HCO$_3^-$	24–30 mmol/l
Lactate	0.5–2.2 mmol/l
Base xs	$\pm$2 mmol/l

Thyroid function

Thyroxine (total T$_4$)	70–140 nmol/l
Thyroxine (free T$_4$)	9–22 pmol/l
TSH	0.5–5 mU/l

INDEX

A-a gradient 295
Abbreviated Mental Test Score (AMTS) 293
Abbreviations xvii–xxvi
Abciximab (ReoPro) 2
Acamprosate (Campral EC) 2, 274
Acarbose 2–3
Accelerated hypertension 238–240
  life-threatening target organ damage 238–239
  non-life-threatening target organ damage 239–240
  practice points 238
ACE inhibitors 237
Acetazolamide (Diamox) 3
Acetylcysteine (Parvolex) 3–4, 279–282
Aciclovir (acyclovir) 4, 259
Acid-base disorders 296
Acid-base nomogram 294–295
Acidex 3
ACS, see Acute coronary syndrome (ACS)
Activated charcoal, see Charcoal
Activated protein C 265
Acute abdomen 286
Acute confusional state 219–220

Acute coronary syndrome (ACS) 226–234
  NSTEMI 226, 233
  secondary prevention 233–234
  STEMI 226, 230
  thrombolysis 230–232
  unstable angina (pectoris) 226, 233
Acute epiglottitis 288
Acute LVF (left ventricular failure) 234
Acute poisoning, see Poisoning, acute
Acute sedation 219–221
Acute severe asthma 242–244
Acute thrombosis 214–215
Acute upper GI haemorrhage 249–251
  assessment of severity of bleeding 249
  clues 249
  management 250–251
Acute use insulin 204
Addisonian crisis 256
Adenosine 4–5
Adrenaline 5–6, 187
Adrenoceptors 276–277
Advil, see Ibuprofen
Aggrastat, see Tirofiban
Agomelatine (Valdoxan) 6–7
Akathisia 278
Albumin 199, 201

Alcohol, warfarin and 215
Alcohol withdrawal 271–274
  maintenance of abstinence 274
  practice point 271
  prevention of agitation, seizures and delirium tremens 271–272
  regimen 272
  supplements for 272–274
Alendronate (Fosamax) 7
Alendronic acid 7
Alfacalcidol 7
Aliskiren 7–8
Allopurinol 8–9
Alphagan, *see* Brimonidine
Alteplase 9, 192, 232, 263
Aluminum hydroxide 9
Amantadine 10
Amfebutamone, *see* Bupropion
Amiloride 10
Aminophylline 11, 187, 243–244, 248
Amiodarone 11–12, 187
Amitriptyline 12–13
Amlodipine (Istin) 13
Amoxicillin 13–14, 248, 288
Ampicillin 14, 259
Anaerobes 245
Anaesthesia, local 181–182
Analgesia 178–179
  general rules 178–179
  ladder 178

procedural sedation and 182–184
  for pulmonary embolism 249
Anaphylaxis 225–226
Angina 226
Angiotensin II receptor blockers (ARBs) 237
Anion gap 296
Antabuse, *see* Disulfiram
Antacids, *see* Alginates; Co-magaldox
Antibiotic-associated colitis (AAC) 266
Antibiotics 254, 256, 258, 264
Anticholinesterases 276
Anticoagulants
  dabigatran 216–217
  fondaparinux 212
  heparin 209–212
  how to prescribe 209–217
  for pulmonary embolism 249
  warfarin 212–216
Antidepressant withdrawal/ discontinuation syndrome 277
Antiemetics 179–181
  general rules 180
  ladder 180
Antihistamines 181
Antipsychotics 220–221
Aortic dissection 227
Aqueous cream 14

Aripiprazole (Abilify) 14–15
Artemether 268
Arterial blood gases 299
Artesunate 268
Arthritis, septic 287
Arthrotec 15
Asacol 15; see also Mesalazine
Aspart (NoboRapid) 204
Aspiration pneumonia 247
Aspirin 15–16, 226, 233, 283
Assisted non-invasive
    ventilation 248
Asthma
    acute severe 242–244
    life-threatening/critical
        242–244
Atenolol 16
Atorvastatin (Lipitor) 16–17
Atracurium 17, 186
Atrial fibrillation 240–241
Atropine (sulphate) 17–18,
    185
Atrovent, see Ipratropium
Augmentin, see Co-amoxiclav
Azathioprine 18–19
Azithromycin 19
Azopt, see Brinzolamide
AZT, see Zidovudine

Baclofen 19–20
Bactroban, see Mupirocin
Beclometasone 20
Becotide, see Beclometasone
Bendroflumethiazide 20–21
Benzamine 180, 181

Benzodiazepines 220,
    271–272, 284
Benzylpenicillin 21
Beta-blockers 229, 233, 237
Betahistine (Serc) 22
Betamethasone cream 22
Betnovate, see Betamethasone
    cream
Bezafibrate 22–23
Bicarbonate, see Sodium
    bicarbonate
Bimatoprost eye drops
    (Lumigan) 23
Biochemistry 297–298
Biphasic insulins 205
Bisphosphonate 271
Bisoprolol 23
Blepharitis 289
Blood products 265
BMI, see Body mass index
    (BMI)
Body mass index (BMI) 296
Boerhaave's syndrome 228
Bone and joint infections 287
Bosentan (Tracleer) 23–24
Bowel preparations 24
Bricanyl, see Terbutaline
Brimonidine eye drops
    (Alphagan) 24
Brinzolamide (Azopt) 24–25
Bromocriptine 25
Buccastem 25
Budesonide 25–26
Bumetanide 26
Bupropion (Zyban) 26–27

Burinex 27
Buscopan, *see* Hyoscine
    butylbromide
Butyrophenone 180

Cacit D3, *see* Calcium
    carbonate
CAGE screening for alcohol
    abuse 271
Calcichew, *see* Calcium
    carbonate
Calcichew D3 27
Calciferol 65
Calcipotriol ointment and
    cream 27
Calcitonin 27–28, 271
Calcium + ergocalciferol
    28–29
Calcium carbonate 28
Calcium channel blockers 238
Calcium chloride 28
Calcium gluconate 29
Calcium resonium 29
Calcium sandoz 29
Calpol 29–30
Candesartan (Amias) 30
Canesten 30
CAP, *see* Community-acquired
    pneumonia (CAP)
Captopril 30–31
Carbamazepine (Tegretol)
    31–32
Carbimazole 32, 258
Cardiopulmonary resuscitation
    (CPR) 225

Carvedilol 32–33
Cavitating pneumonia 247
Cefaclor 33
Cefalexin 33
Cefotaxime 33–34, 258–259,
    288
Cefradine 34
Ceftazidime 34
Ceftriaxone 34, 289
Cefuroxime 34–35
Celecoxib (Celebrex) 35
Cellulitis 287
Cetirizine (Zirtek) 36
CHADS$_2$ score 241
Charcoal 36, 275, 279, 283
Chest pain
    causes of 227–228
    differential diagnosis
        of 226
Chlamydia psittaci 245
Chloramphenicol 289
    eye drops 37
    iv (and po) 36–37
Chlordiazepoxide 37, 272
Chlorhexidine 37
Chloroquine 37–38, 268
Chlorphen(ir)amine
    (Piriton) 38
Chlorpromazine 38–39
Cholinoceptors 276
Chronic obstructive pulmonary
    disease (COPD) 247–248
Ciclesonide (Alvesco) 39
Ciclosporin 40
Cimetidine 40

Ciprofloxacin 41

Citalopram (Cipramil) 41–42

Citramag, *see* Bowel preparations

Clarithromycin 42, 245

Clexane, *see* Enoxaparin

Clindamycin 42–43, 269, 287

Clobetasol propionate cream/ ointment (Dermovate) 43

Clobetasone butyrate cream/ ointment (Eumovate) 43

Clonazepam 43, 188

Clopidogrel (Plavix) 43–44, 226

Clostridium difficile 266

Clotrimazole (Canesten) 44

Clotting 299

Clozapine 44–45

Co-amilofruse 46

Co-amilozide 46

Co-amoxiclav (Augmentin) 46, 248, 287, 288

Co-beneldopa (Madopar) 46–47

Co-careldopa (Sinemet) 47

Co-codamol 47

Co-Danthramer, *see* Dantron

Codeine (phosphate) 47–48

Co-dydramol 48

Colchicine 48

Colestyramine 48–49

Colloids 199–200, 201

Co-magaldrox antacid 49

Combivent 49

Community-acquired pneumonia (CAP) 244–246

Conjunctivitis 289

Controlled drugs 221–222

Cooling measures 258

COPD exacerbation 247–248

Corneal ulcer 289

Corsodyl 49

Corticosteroids 217–219, 267

common 217

interactions 218–219

side effects 217–218

therapeutic effects 217

withdrawal effects 219

Co-triamterzide 49

Co-trimoxazole (Septrin) 50

Coxiella burnetii 245

CPR, *see* Cardiopulmonary resuscitation (CPR)

Creatinine clearance 296

Critical asthma 242–244

Crystalloids 196–199, 201

Cushing's syndrome 217

Cyclizine 50, 181

Cyclopentolate eye drops (Mydrilate) 50–51

Cyclophosphamide 51

Cyclosporin, *see* Ciclosporin

CYP, *see* Cytochrome P450 (CYP)

Cyproterone acetate 51–52

Cytochrome P450 (CYP) 279

Dabigatran (etexilate)
(Pradaxa) 52, 216–217
Dalteparin (Fragmin) 52–53
Dantron 53
Darbepoetin, *see* Erythropoietin
Deep vein thrombosis
prophylaxis 265
Delirium 219–220
Delirium tremens 271–272
Dermovate, *see* Clobetasol
propionate cream/
ointment
Desferrioxamine 53
Detemir 205
Dexamethasone eye drops
(Maxidex) 53
Dexamethasone phosphate
54, 217
Dextran 200
Dextrose 200
5% 197
10% 198
50% 198
DF118 54
Diabetic ketoacidosis
(DKA) 252–254
clues 252
complications 254
diagnostic criteria 252
management 253–254
practice points 252–253
precipitating causes 252
Dialysis 271
Diamorphine (heroin
hydrochloride) 54, 234

Diazemuls 54
Diazepam 55, 183, 185, 220,
272
Diclofenac 55–56
Diet, warfarin and 215
Difflam 56
Digibind 56
Digoxin 56–57, 258
Dihydrocodeine 57
Dilating eye drops 57
Diltiazem 57–58
Diprobase 58
Dipyridamole (Persantin) 58
Disodium etidronate, *see*
Pamidronate
Disodium pamidronate, *see*
Pamidronate
Disturbed patients 220
Disulfiram (Antabuse) 59,
274
Diuretics 238, 271
DKA, *see* Diabetic ketoacidosis
(DKA)
Dobutamine 59, 188
Docusate sodium 59
Domperidone 60, 181
Donepezil (Aricept) 60
Dopamine (DA) 60–61, 188,
277–278
Dorzolamide (Trusopt) 61
Doses xvi
Doxapram 61–62, 248
Doxazosin (Cardura) 62
Doxycycline 62–63, 248,
268, 269

Drug infusion guideline
186–193
critical care area 187–193
safe usage 186
Drug selection 177–193
analgesia 178–179
antiemetics 179–181
drug infusion
guidelines 186–193
local anaesthesia 181–182
procedural sedation and
analgesia 182–184
rapid sequence
induction 184–186
Duloxetine (Cymbalta/
Yentreve) 63
Dyskinesias 278

Ear, nose, and throat (ENT)
infections 288
Edrophonium 63
Efexor XL 172
Eformoterol 77
Electrolytes
daily requirements
201–202
disturbances 269–271
Enalapril (Innovace) 63–64
Endotracheal tube (ETT) 184
Enoxaparin (Clexane) 64
Ensure 64
Epaderm 64
Epilim, see Valproate
Epinephrine, see Adrenaline
Epoetin, see Erythropoietin

Eprosartan (Teveten) 64
Eptifibatide (Integrilin) 64–65
Ergocalciferol 28–29, 65
Erythromycin 65–66
Erythropoietin 66
Escitalopram (Cipralex) 66
Esmolol 66–67
Esomeprazole (Nexium) 67
Etanercept (Enbrel) 67
Ethambutol 67, 267
Etomidate 68, 183
Etoricoxib (Arcoxia) 68–69
Eumovate, see Clobetasone
butyrate cream/ointment
Extrapyramidal effects 278
Eye drops
dilating 57
fusidic acid 78
hypromellose 0.3% 88
ofloxacin 122
phenylephrine 132
travoprost 167
tropicamide 168–169
Eye infections 288–289

Falciparum malaria 267–268
Fansidar 69
Febrile neutropenia 265
Felodipine (Plendil) 69
Fentanyl 69–70, 183, 185,
188
Ferrous fumarate 70
Ferrous gluconate 71
Ferrous sulphate 71
Fibrinolytics 210

50% dextrose 198
50% glucose 201
Finasteride 71
5% dextrose 197
5% glucose 196
5HT$_3$ antagonists 181
Flagyl, *see* Metronidazole
Flecainide 71–72
Fleet (phospho-soda) 72
Flixotide 72, 75
Flomaxtra XL, *see* Tamsulosin
Flucloxacillin 72–73, 287, 289
Fluconazole 73
Fludrocortisone 73, 219
Fluid challenges 203–204
Fluids
  daily requirements, 201–202
  oral 203
Flumazenil 74, 284
Fluoxetine (Prozac) 74–75
Fluticasone (Flixotide) 72, 75
Folate 75–76
Folic acid 75–76
Fomepizole 76
Fondaparinux (Arixtra) 76, 212
Formoterol (Foradil, Oxis) 77
Formulae 295–297
  a-a gradient 295
  anion gap 296
  body mass index (BMI) 296
  creatinine clearance 296

ideal body weight (IBW) 296
metric conversions 296–297
serum osmolality 295
Fosphenytoin 77
Fostair 77
Fragmin, *see* Dalteparin (Fragmin)
Frusemide, *see* Furosemide
Furosemide 77–78, 234
Fusidic acid (Fucidin) 78
Fusidic acid 1% eye drops (Fucithalmic) 78
Fybogel 78

Gabapentin 79
Gastric lavage 275
Gastrocote 79
Gastrointestinal (GI) infections 266
Gastrointestinal causes, of chest pain 228
Gaviscon (advance) 79
Gelofusine 79, 199, 201
Gentamicin 79–80
GI infections 266
Glargine 205
Glasgow Coma Scale (GCS) 292
Glibenclamide 80–81
Gliclazide 81
Glimepiride 81
Glipizide 81–82
Glucagon 82, 252

Glucose 252, 264
  5% 196
  10% 201
  20% 201
  50% 201
Glucose saline 196
Glulisine (Apidra) 204
Glycerin suppositories 82
Glycerol suppositories 82
Glyceryl trinitrate, see GTN
Glycoprotein IIb/IIIa
    inhibitor 230, 233
Gram-negative infection 245
Granisetron 82, 181
GTN (glyceryl trinitrate) 83,
    188, 226, 229, 234

Haemaccel 200, 201
Haematinics 299
Haematology 298–299
Haemodialysis 283
Haemolysis 269
Haemophilus influenzae 245
Haemorrhage, acute upper
    GI 249–251
Half normal saline 197
Haloperidol 83–84, 180, 221
Hartmann's solution 84, 196,
    197
Heart failure 203
Heparin 84, 209–212
  co-therapy 232
  for DKA 254
  for HHS 256
  LMWHs 209–210

monitoring 211–212
  for NSTEMI or UAP 233
  overtreatment/overdose
    212
  for STEMI 230
  unfractionated 210
Heparin-induced
    thrombocytopenia
    (HIT) 209–210
Herbal remedies, warfarin
    and 215
HHS, see Hyperosmolar,
    hyperlycaemic state (HHS)
HONK, see Hyperosmolar,
    hyperlycaemic state (HHS)
Hospital-acquired
    pneumonia 246
Humalog 84, 204
Humulin 85
Humulin I 85
Humulin M 85
Humulin S 85
Hydralazine 85
Hydration, clinical markers
    of 203
Hydrocortisone butyrate
    cream 85
Hydrocortisone cream/
    ointment 85–86
Hydrocortisone iv/po 86, 217,
    242, 257, 258
Hydroxocobalamin 86
Hydroxycarbamide 86
Hydroxychloroquine
    (Plaquenil) 87

Hydroxyurea 86
Hyoscine butylbromide
(Buscopan) 87
Hyoscine hydrobromide
87–88
Hypercalcaemia 270–271
Hyperkalaemia 269–270
Hyperosmolar, hyperlycaemic
state (HHS) 255–256
management 255–256
practice points 255
Hypertension 235–238
accelerated 238–240
practice points 236–238
primary causes 236
when to treat 235–236
Hypertonic (5%) saline 201
Hypoglycaemia 251–252
Hypokalaemia 270
Hypotonic (0.45%) saline
201
Hypromellose 0.3% eye
drops 88

Ibugel 88
Ibuprofen 88–89
IBW (ideal body weight) 296
Ideal body weight (IBW) 296
Indapamide 89
Indometacin 89–90
Inducers 279
Infections
bone and joint 287
ENT 288
eye 288–289

GI 266
orthopaedic 287
urinary tract 265–266
Infliximab (Remicade) 90
Inhibitors 279
Inotropes 234, 264
Insulatard 90
Insulin 90, 189
for acute coronary
syndrome 230
for DKA 254
for HHS 255–256
how to prescribe 204–209
for hyperkalaemia 269
initial dose and
adjustments 207–208
sliding scale 205–209
types 204–205
Integrilin, see Eptifibatide
(Integrilin)
Intermediate-acting
insulins 205
Intravenous fluids
for acute coronary
syndrome 229
colloids 199–200, 201
composition of commonly
used 197–200
crystalloids 196–199, 201
daily fluid and electrolyte
requirements 201–202
hints for 203–204
how to prescribe 196–204
K+ considerations 202
Intubation 248

Iodide, *see* Lugol's solution
Iodine, *see* Lugol's solution
Ipocol, *see* Mesalazine
Ipratropium   106, 242, 247
Irbesartan (Aprovel)   91
Iron tablets, *see* Ferrous
    sulphate/fumarate/
    gluconate
ISMN, *see* Isosorbide
    mononitrate
ISMO, *see* Isosorbide
    mononitrate
Isoniazid   91
Isophane   205
Isoprenaline   189
Isosorbide mononitrate
    (ISMN)   91–92
Isotonic crystalloids   196
ISTIN, *see* Amlodipine (Istin)
Itraconazole (Sporanox)   92
Ivabradine (Procoralan)
    92–93

IV procedural sedation drug
    doses   183

Joint infections   287

K+   202
Kay-cee-L   93
Ketamine (Ketalar)   93–94,
    183, 185, 189
Ketoconazole (Nizoral)
    94–95
Klean-Prep   95; *see also* Bowel
    preparations

Labetalol   95
Laboratory reference
    values   297–299
Lacri-Lube   95
Lactulose   96
Lamisil, *see* Terbinafine
Lamotrigine (Lamictal)   96
Lansoprazole (Zoton)   96
Lariam, *see* Mefloquine
Lasix, *see* Furosemide
Latanoprost (Xalatan)   97
Leflunomide (Arava)   97
Left ventricular failure
    (LVF)   234
Legionella pneumophila   245
Length conversions   297
Levobunolol   98
Levodopa (L-dopa)   98
Levomepromazine   99, 180
Levothyroxine, *see* Thyroxine
Librium, *see* Chlordiazepoxide
Lidocaine   99–100, 185, 189
Lignocaine, *see* Lidocaine
Liothyronine sodium   100,
    257
Lisinopril   100
Lispro (Humalog)   204
Lithium   100–101
Liver failure   203
Local anaesthesia   181–182
    features of systemic
        toxicity   183
    safe usage   181–182
Locoid, *see* Hydrocortisone
    butyrate cream

Lofepramine 102
Long-acting insulins 205
Loop diuretics 271
Loperamide (Imodium) 102
Loratadine 102
Lorazepam 102–103, 220
Losartan (Cozaar) 103
Losec, *see* Omeprazole
L-tri-iodothyronine
    sodium 100
Lugol's solution 103, 258
LVF, *see* Acute LVF (left
    ventricular failure)
Lymecycline 104

Madopar, *see* Co-beneldopa
Magnesium sulphate (iv) 104,
    190
Maintenance use insulin
    204–205
Malaria 267–269
    practice points 267–268
    treatment 268–269
Mannitol 104
Maxolon, *see* Metoclopramide
Mebeverine 105
Medical emergencies 223–284
    accelerated
        hypertension 238–240
    acute coronary
        syndrome 226–234
    acute LVF 234
    acute poisoning 274–284
    acute severe asthma
        242–244

acute upper GI
    haemorrhage 249–251
Addisonian crisis 256
alcohol withdrawal
    271–274
anaphylaxis 225–226
atrial fibrillation 240–241
cardiopulmonary
    resuscitation 225
COPD exacerbation
    247–248
diabetic ketoacidosis
    (DKA) 252–254
electrolyte
    disturbances 269–271
febrile neutropenia 265
GI infections 266
hyperosmolar, hyperlycaemic
    state (HHS) 255–256
hypertension 235–238
hypoglycaemia 251–252
malaria 267–269
meningitis 258–259
myxoedema coma/crisis
    257
pneumonia 244–247
pulmonary embolism
    248–249
seizures 260–261
severe sepsis or septic
    shock 264–265
TB pneumonia 267
thyrotoxic crisis/thyroid
    storm 257–258
TIA and stroke 261–263

urinary tract infections
265–266
Mefenamic acid (Ponstan)
105
Mefloquine (Lariam) 105–106
Meibomian abscess (internal
hordeolum) 289
Meningitis 258–259
causes of 259
treatment 258–259
Mental state
examination 293–294
Meropenem 106
Mesalazine 106, 242, 247
Mesna 107
Metformin 107
Methadone 107–108
Methionine 108
Methotrexate 108–109
Methotrimeprazine 99; see also
Levomepromazine
Methyldopa 109–110
Methylprednisolone 110, 190,
217
Metoclopramide
(Maxolon) 110, 180
Metolazone 110–111
Metoprolol 111
Metric conversions 296–297
Metronidazole (Flagyl) 111,
288
MgSO₄ ivi 242
Miconazole 112
Midazolam 112, 183, 185,
190, 220

Mineralocorticoids 219
Mini Mental State Examination
(MMSE) 293–294
Minocycline 112–113
Minoxidil 113
Mirtazapine (Zispin) 113
Misoprostol 114
MMF, see Mycophenolate
mofetil
Modified Hartmann's 197
Mometasone (furoate) cream/
ointment (Elocon) 114
Montelukast (Singulair)
114–115
Moraxella catarrhalis 245
Morphgesic SR 115
Morphine (sulphate) 115–116,
183, 185, 190
MST Continus 116
Mupirocin (Bactroban) 116
Musculoskeletal causes, of chest
pain 228
MXL Capsules 116
Mycophenolate mofetil
(MMF) 116–117
Mycoplasma pneumoniae 245
Myocardial infarction 226
Myxoedema coma/crisis 257

N-acetylcysteine, see
Acetylcysteine
Naloxone 117, 284
Naltrexone 117–118, 274
Naproxen 118
Naratriptan (Naramig) 118

Narcan, see Naloxone
Nausea, causes of 179
Nicorandil 118–119
Nicotinic acid (Niaspan) 119
Nifedipine 119–120
Nimodipine 191
Nitrofurantoin 120
Non-convulsive status epilepticus 260
Non-IgE-mediated, non-allergic anaphylaxis 225–226
Non-invasive ventilation (NIV) 234
Non-isotonic crystalloids 201
Non-prescription drugs, warfarin and 215
Noradrenaline 121, 191
Norepinephrine 121, 191
Norethisterone 121
Normal saline 196, 197, 270, 271
NSTEMI (non-ST elevation myocardial infarction) 226, 233
Nurofen, see Ibuprofen
Nystatin 122

O₂ 226, 234, 247, 248
Octreotide 191
Oesophageal rupture 228
Ofloxacin 0.3% eye drops (Exocin) 122, 289
Olanzapine (Zyprexa) 122–123
Olmesartan (Olmetec) 123

Omega-3-acid ethyl esters 90 (Omacor) 123
Omeprazole (Losec) 124
Ondansetron 124, 181
Opiates 226, 284
Oral fluids 203
Oramorph 125
Orbital cellulitis 288–289
Orthopaedic infections 287
Osteomyelitis 287
Otitis externa 288
Otitis media 288
Otosporin 125
Oxybutynin 125
Oxycodone (hydrochloride) (Oxynorm) 125–126
Oxytetracycline 126

Pabrinex 126, 273
(Disodium) Pamidronate 126–127
Pancuronium 127, 186
Pantoprazole 128
Paracetamol 128, 279–282
Parkinsonism 278
Paroxetine (Seroxat) 128–129
Parvolex, see Acetylcysteine
Peak expiratory flow (PEF) 243
Penicillamine 129
Penicillin G, see Benzylpenicillin
Penicillin V, see Phenoxymethylpenicillin
Pentasa, see Mesalazine
Peppermint oil 130

Peptac 130
Pericarditis 227
Perindopril (Coversyl) 130
Pethidine 130–131
Pharyngitis 288
Phenobarbital 131, 191
Phenobarbitone 131, 191
Phenothiazine 180
Phenoxymethylpenicillin
    (penicillin V) 131, 288
Phentolamine 131–132
Phenylephrine eye drops 132
Phenytoin 132–133, 191
Phosphate enema 133
Phyllocontin continus, see
    Aminophylline
Phytomenadione 133
Picolax 134; see also Bowel
    preparations
Pioglitazone (Actos) 134
Piperacillin 134
Piriton, see Chlorphen(ir)amine
Plasma-Lyte 199
Plavix, see Clopidogrel
Pneumonia 227, 244–247
    aspiration 247
    cavitating 247
    community-acquired
        244–246
    hospital-acquired 246
    TB 267
Pneumothorax 227
Poisoning, acute 274–284
    adrenoceptors 276–277
    benzodiazepines 284

cerebellar effects 278–279
cholinoceptors 276
cytochrome P450
    (CYP) 279
dopamine 277–278
extrapyramidal effects 278
general measures 275
opiates 284
paracetamol 279–282
resources 274–275
salicylate/aspirin 283
serotonin (5HT) 277
side effect profiles 275
Post-thrombolysis
    management 263
Potassium tablets 134–135; see
    also Kay-cee-L; Sando-K;
    Slow-K
Pramipexole (Mirapexin) 135
Pravastatin (Lipostat) 135
Prednisolone 135–136, 217,
    242, 247
Pregabalin (Lyrica) 136
Pregnancy
    testing 254
    warfarin and 215–216
Prescribing
    anticoagulants 209–217
    controlled drugs 221–222
    insulin 204–209
    intravenous fluids 196–204
    safety xvii–xxix
    sedation 219–221
    steroids 217–219
Pressure conversions 297

Primaquine   268
Procainamide   192
Procedural sedation and analgesia   182–184
  criteria for discharge following   184
  IV drug doses   183
Prochlorperazine (Stemetil)   136–137
Procyclidine   137
Promethazine   137–138
Propofol   138–139, 183, 185, 192
Propranolol   139–140, 258
Propylthiouracil   140
Proscar, see Finasteride
Protamine (sulphate)   140–141
Proxymethacaine   141
Prozac, see Fluoxetine
Pulmicort, see Budesonide
Pulmonary embolism   248–249
Pulmonary embolus   227
Pyelonephritis   266
Pyrazinamide   141
Pyridostigmine   142

Quetiapine (Seroquel)   142–143
Quinine   143, 268, 269

Rabeprazole (Pariet)   143
Ramipril (Tritace)   143–144
Ranitidine (Zantac)   144

Rapid sequence induction (RSI)   184–186
  drugs for   185–186
  general principles   184–185
Reference information
  acid-base nomogram   294–295
  Glasgow Coma Scale   292
  laboratory reference values   297–299
  mental state examination   293–294
  useful formulae   295–297
Renal failure   203
ReoPro, see Abciximab
Reperfusion therapy   230
Reteplase (r-PA)   144, 232
Rifabutin   144–145
Rifampicin   145
Rifater   145
Ringer's lactate   197
Risedronate   146
Risperidone (Risperdal)   146–147
Rituximab (Mabthera)   147
Rivastigmine (Exelon)   147–148
Rizatriptan (Maxalt)   148
Rockall score   251
Rocuronium   148–149, 185
Ropinirole (Requip, Adartrel)   149
Rosuvastatin (Crestor)   149–150
Routes   xvi

r-PA 193
(R)tPA, *see* Alteplase

Safety, prescription, xvii–xxix
Salbutamol 150, 193, 242, 247, 269
Salicylate 283
Saline
 glucose 196
 half normal 197
 hypertonic (5%) 201
 hypotonic (0.45%) 201
 normal 196, 197, 270, 271
Salmeterol (Serevent) 150–151
Salofalk, *see* Mesalazine
Sandocal 151
Sando-K 151, 270
Scopolamine 87–88
Sedation
 acute 219–221
 how to prescribe 219–221
 procedural 182–184
Seizures 260–261
 practice points 260
 treatment 260–261
Self-harm 274
Senna (Senokot) 151
Sepsis 264–265
Septic arthritis 287
Septic shock 264–265
Septrin, *see* Co-trimoxazole
Serc, *see* Betahistine
Seretide 151
Serotonin (5HT) 277

Serotonin syndrome 277
Seroxat, *see* Paroxetine
Sertraline (Lustral) 152
Serum osmolality 295
Sevelamer hydrochloride 152
Severe sepsis 264–265
Sevredol 152
Short-acting insulins 205
Sildenafil (Viagra, Revatio) 152–153
Simvastatin (Zocor) 153–154
Sinemet, *see* Co-careldopa
Sinusitis 288
Sliding scale insulin 205–209
Slow-K 154, 270
Sodium bicarbonate iv 154, 198, 201, 254, 270, 283
Sodium chloride 197, 198
Sodium nitroprusside 193
Sodium valproate, *see* Valproate
Soluble insulin 204
Sotalol 154–155
Spiriva, *see* Tiotropium
Spironolactone 155
Staphylococcus aureus 245
Status epilepticus 260
Stemetil, *see* Prochlorperazine
STEMI (ST elevation myocardial infarction) 226, 230
Steroids
 for Addisonian crisis 256
 corticosteroids 217–219
 how to prescribe 217–219

for hypercalcaemia   271
mineralocorticoids   219
for sepsis or septic
   shock   264
Streptococcus
   pneumoniae   245
Streptokinase   156, 193, 232
Streptomycin   156
Stress ulcer prophylaxis   265
Stroke   261–263
   CHADS₂ score for risk
      of   241
Strontium ranelate
   (Protelos)   156
Stye (external hordeolum)
   289
Sulfasalazine   156–157
Sumatriptan (Imigran)   157
Surgical emergencies
   acute abdomen   286
   ENT infections   288
   eye infections   288–289
   orthopaedic infections   287
Suxamethonium   157–158,
   185
Symbicort   158
Synacthen   158–159

Tacrolimus (FK 506)   159
Tadalafil (Cialis, Adcirca)
   159
Tamoxifen   160
Tamsulosin (Flomaxtra
   XL)   160
Tazocin   160

TB pneumonia   267
Tegretol, see Carbamazepine
Teicoplanin   160–161
Telmisartan (Micardis)   161
Temazepam   161, 222
Temperature conversions   297
10% dextrose   198
10% glucose   201
Tenecteplase (TNK-tPA)
   (Metalyse)   161, 232
Terazosin (Hytrin)   162
Terbinafine (Lamisil)   162
Terbutaline (Bricanyl)   162
Tetracycline   162–163
Theophylline   163
Thiamine (vitamin B1)   164,
   272–273
Thiazide-like diuretics   238
Thiopentone   185
Thrombolysis   230–232, 262
Thyroid function   299
Thyroid storm   257–258
Thyrotoxic crisis   257–258
Thyroxine (levothyroxine)
   164
TIA, see Transient ischemic
   attack
TIMI risk score   233
Timolol eye drops
   (Timoptol)   164
Tinzaparin (Innohep)   165
Tiotropium (Spiriva)   165
Tirofiban (Aggrastat)
   165–166
Tolbutamide   166

Tolterodine (Detrusitol)   166
Tonsillitis   288
TOXBASE   274–275
Tramadol   166–167
Trandolapril (Gopten)   167
Tranexamic acid   167
Transient ischemic attack
    (TIA)   261–263
Travoprost eye drops
    (Travatan)   167
Triamterene   167–168
Tri-iodothyronine   168
Trimethoprim   168
Tropicamide eye drops
    168–169
Tropisetron   181
Turbohaler   169
20% glucose   201

UAP, see Unstable angina
    (pectoris)
UK National Poisons
    Information Service
    (NPIS)   275
Unfractionated heparin   210
Unstable angina
    (pectoris)   226, 233
Urinary tract infections
    (URIs)   265–266
URIs, see Urinary tract
    infections

(Sodium) Valproate   169
Valsartan (Diovan)   169–170
Vancomycin   170

Vardenafil (Levitra)   170–171
Vecuronium (bromide)   171,
    185
Venlafaxine (Efexor)
    171–172
Ventolin, see Salbutamol
Verapamil   172–173
Viagra, see Sildenafil
Violent patients   220
Vitamin K, see Phytomenadione
Voltarol, see Diclofenac
Volume conversions   297
Vomiting, causes of   179

Warfarin   173, 212–216
    for acute thrombosis
        214–215
    basics   212–213
    interrupting   215
    loading regimen   214–215
    monitoring   213
    overtreatment/overdose
        216
    pregnancy and   215–216
Weight conversions   296
Wernicke's encephalopathy
    (WE)   272, 273–274

Xalatan, see Latanoprost
    (Xalatan)

Zaleplon   173–174; see also
    Zopiclone
Zantac, see Ranitidine
Zestril, see Lisinopril

Zidovudine (AZT) 174
Zirtek, *see* Cetirizine
Zoledronic acid
   (Zometa) 174–175
Zolmitriptan (Zomig) 175

Zolpidem 175
Zomorph 175
Zopiclone 175–176
Zoton, *see* Lansopraxole
Zyban, *see* Bupropion

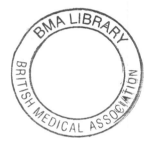
BMA LIBRARY
BRITISH MEDICAL ASSOCIATION

Adult tachycardia (with pulse) algorithm

European Resuscitation Council Guidelines 2010

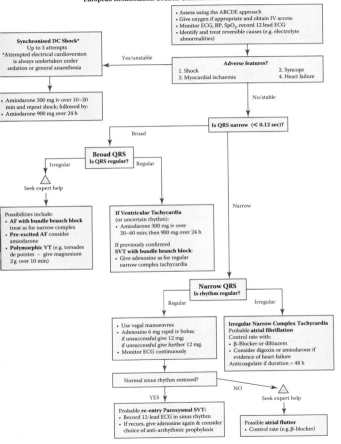

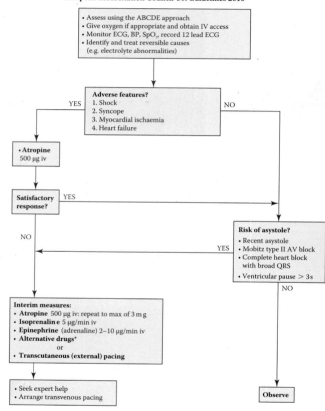

Adult bradycardia algorithm

European Resuscitation Council UK Guidelines 2010

- Assess using the ABCDE approach
- Give oxygen if appropriate and obtain IV access
- Monitor ECG, BP, SpO₂, record 12 lead ECG
- Identify and treat reversible causes (e.g. electrolyte abnormalities)

Adverse features?
1. Shock
2. Syncope
3. Myocardial ischaemia
4. Heart failure

YES   NO

- **Atropine** 500 µg iv

Satisfactory response?   YES

NO

Risk of asystole?
- Recent asystole
- Mobitz type II AV block
- Complete heart block with broad QRS
- Ventricular pause > 3s

YES   NO

Interim measures:
- **Atropine** 500 µg iv: repeat to max of 3 mg
- **Isoprenaline** 5 µg/min iv
- **Epinephrine** (adrenaline) 2–10 µg/min iv
- **Alternative drugs***
  or
- **Transcutaneous (external) pacing**

- Seek expert help
- Arrange transvenous pacing

Observe

*Alternatives include: Aminophylline, Dopamine, Glucagon (if β-blocker or Ca⁺⁺ channel blocker overdose) or Glycopyrrolate (can be used instead of atropine)